FOURTH EDITION

Motor Speech Disorders

DIAGNOSIS AND TREATMENT

FOURTH EDITION

Motor Speech Disorders

DIAGNOSIS AND TREATMENT

Donald B. Freed, PhD

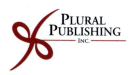

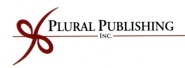

9177 Aero Drive, Suite B
San Diego, CA 92123

email: information@pluralpublishing.com
website: https://www.pluralpublishing.com

Copyright © 2025 by Plural Publishing, Inc.

Typeset in 11/13 ITC Garamond Std by Achorn International Inc.
Printed in the China by Regent Publishing Services, Ltd.

All rights, including that of translation, reserved. No part of this publication may be reproduced, stored in a retrieval system, or transmitted in any form or by any means, electronic, mechanical, recording, or otherwise, including photocopying, recording, taping, web distribution, or information storage and retrieval systems without the prior written consent of the publisher.

For permission to use material from this text, contact us by
Telephone: (866) 758-7251
Fax: (888) 758-7255
email: permissions@pluralpublishing.com

Every attempt has been made to contact the copyright holders for material originally printed in another source. If any have been inadvertently overlooked, the publisher will gladly make the necessary arrangements at the first opportunity.

Library of Congress Cataloging-in-Publication Data

Names: Freed, Donald B., author.
Title: Motor speech disorders : diagnosis and treatment / Donald B. Freed.
Description: Fourth edition. | San Diego, CA : Plural Publishing, [2025] |
  Includes bibliographical references and index.
Identifiers: LCCN 2023029341 (print) | LCCN 2023029342 (ebook) |
  ISBN 9781635506075 (paperback) | ISBN 1635506077 (paperback) |
  ISBN 9781635504460 (ebook)
Subjects: MESH: Dysarthria—diagnosis | Dysarthria—therapy
Classification: LCC RC423 (print) | LCC RC423 (ebook) | NLM WL 340.2 |
  DDC 616.85/5—dc23/eng/20230929
LC record available at https://lccn.loc.gov/2023029341
LC ebook record available at https://lccn.loc.gov/2023029342

Contents

Preface ix
About the Author xiii

CHAPTER 1. A Brief Historical Review of Motor Speech Disorders — 1

Case Reports From Ancient Greece — 3
Case Reports From the Middle Ages and Renaissance — 6
Two Early Theories on the Localization of Reason — 7
From the 19th Century to Today — 9

CHAPTER 2. The Motor System — 15

Components of the Motor System — 16
Structure and Function of the Motor System — 27
Summary of the Motor System — 53
Study Questions — 53

CHAPTER 3. Evaluation of Motor Speech Disorders — 55

Goals of a Motor Speech Evaluation — 57
Speech Production Components and Disorders — 58
Standardized Tests for Dysarthria — 63
Standardized Tests for Apraxia of Speech — 65
Conducting a Motor Speech Evaluation — 68
Instructions for the Motor Speech Evaluation — 70
Auditory-Perceptual Evaluations of the Motor Speech Mechanism — 78

Summary of the Evaluation of Motor Speech Disorders   85
Study Questions   85
Appendix 3–1: Motor Speech Examination   87

CHAPTER 4. Flaccid Dysarthria   99

Definitions of Flaccid Dysarthria   100
Neurologic Basis of Flaccid Dysarthria   101
Causes of Flaccid Dysarthria   114
Speech Characteristics of Flaccid Dysarthria   119
Key Evaluation Tasks for Flaccid Dysarthria   123
Treatment of Motor Speech Disorders   124
Treatment of Flaccid Dysarthria   128
Summary of Flaccid Dysarthria   142
Study Questions   142

CHAPTER 5. Spastic Dysarthria   145

Definitions of Spastic Dysarthria   146
Neurologic Basis of Spastic Dysarthria   146
Causes of Spastic Dysarthria   150
Speech Characteristics of Spastic Dysarthria   152
Spastic Dysarthria Versus Flaccid Dysarthria   157
Key Evaluation Tasks for Spastic Dysarthria   158
Treatment of Spastic Dysarthria   159
Summary of Spastic Dysarthria   167
Study Questions   168

CHAPTER 6. Unilateral Upper Motor Neuron Dysarthria   169

Definitions of Unilateral Upper Motor Neuron Dysarthria   170
Neurologic Basis of Unilateral Upper Motor Neuron Dysarthria   171
Causes of Unilateral Upper Motor Neuron Dysarthria   174
Speech Characteristics of Unilateral Upper Motor Neuron Dysarthria   177
Key Evaluation Tasks for Unilateral Upper Motor Neuron Dysarthria   181

	Treatment of Unilateral Upper Motor Neuron Dysarthria	181
	Summary of Unilateral Upper Motor Neuron Dysarthria	183
	Study Questions	184

CHAPTER 7. Ataxic Dysarthria — 185

Definitions of Ataxic Dysarthria	186
Neurologic Basis of Ataxic Dysarthria	186
The Cerebellum and Speech	191
Causes of Ataxic Dysarthria	192
Speech Characteristics of Ataxic Dysarthria	196
Key Evaluation Tasks for Ataxic Dysarthria	200
Treatment of Ataxic Dysarthria	201
Summary of Ataxic Dysarthria	207
Study Questions	208

CHAPTER 8. Hypokinetic Dysarthria — 209

Definitions of Hypokinetic Dysarthria	210
Neurologic Basis of Hypokinetic Dysarthria	210
Causes of Hypokinetic Dysarthria	215
Speech Characteristics of Hypokinetic Dysarthria	218
Key Evaluation Tasks for Hypokinetic Dysarthria	223
Treatment of Hypokinetic Dysarthria	223
Summary of Hypokinetic Dysarthria	239
Study Questions	240

CHAPTER 9. Hyperkinetic Dysarthria — 241

Definitions of Hyperkinetic Dysarthria	242
Neurologic Basis of Hyperkinetic Dysarthria	243
Causes of Hyperkinetic Dysarthria	246
Key Evaluation Tasks for Hyperkinetic Dysarthria	264
Treatment of Hyperkinetic Dysarthria	265
Summary of Hyperkinetic Dysarthria	270
Study Questions	271

CHAPTER 10. Mixed Dysarthria — 273

- Definitions of Mixed Dysarthria — 274
- Neurologic Basis of Mixed Dysarthria — 274
- Causes of Mixed Dysarthria — 277
- Treatment of Mixed Dysarthria — 288
- Summary of Mixed Dysarthria — 292
- Study Questions — 292

CHAPTER 11. Apraxia of Speech — 295

- Definition of Apraxia of Speech — 296
- Overview of the Apraxias — 298
- Neurologic Basis of Apraxia of Speech — 302
- Causes of Apraxia of Speech — 304
- Speech Characteristics of Apraxia of Speech — 305
- Assessment of Apraxia of Speech — 309
- Differential Diagnosis of Apraxia of Speech — 310
- Additional Diagnostic Considerations — 313
- Treatment of Apraxia of Speech — 318
- Summary of Apraxia of Speech — 333
- Study Questions — 333

References — *335*
Glossary — *353*
Index — *365*

Preface

This is the fourth edition of *Motor Speech Disorders: Diagnosis and Treatment*. In the 24 years since the first edition, knowledge about motor speech disorders has evolved quite a lot, and research into this topic continues to be a dynamic area of study. Information about specific conditions associated with motor speech disorders has grown; a number of assessment instruments have become more accurate in diagnosing disorders; and evaluations of treatment procedures appear frequently in the research literature. Perhaps the most exciting development over the past two and a half decades is the creation of new evidence-based behavioral treatments for apraxia of speech and hypokinetic dysarthria. In addition, older treatments have been refined, adapted, or combined to enhance their ability to address motor speech disorders.

This fourth edition remains dedicated to students and beginning clinicians, both in its uncomplicated presentation of neurological conditions and its accessible writing style. Each chapter was written with the author's own students in mind. Their questions during lectures and their performance on tests and in clinics helped shape the content and tone of the book. To further help all students understand the complexity of these disorders, over two hours of clinical videos and case histories are available on the PluralPlus companion website (see the inside front cover for the URL and your access code), along with eFlashcards with all the of the key terms and definitions from the text. For instructors, PowerPoint slides that highlight important details within each chapter and an image bank containing high-resolution images from the book are also included on the website.

Organization

The overall organization of the book is the same as the prior edition. Chapter 1 is a historical introduction to the study of motor speech disorders. It examines ancient case reports that might involve dysarthria or apraxia of speech. Chapter 2 is an introduction to the motor system, one of the most remarkable parts of the human body. Clinicians must have at least a basic understanding of the motor system if they are to accurately diagnose and treat motor speech disorders. Chapter 3 discusses the assessment of these disorders. It includes a detailed explanation of the complete motor speech examination that is at the end of the chapter (Appendix 3–1). Chapters 4 through 11 examine the six pure dysarthrias, mixed dysarthria, and apraxia of speech. Throughout these chapters, a consistent organization is maintained to facilitate the reader's understanding of the disorders. Each chapter begins with the neurologic basis of the condition, then continues with the etiologies and causes of the disorder, an examination of the relevant speech characteristics, and key evaluation tasks specific to the disorder; and concludes with treatment procedures.

New to This Edition

This fourth edition includes many updated references and citations in nearly every chapter. Other additions to the book include these items:

- Newly published information on conditions that can cause dysarthria.
- New illustrations that provide insight into how certain diseases affect the motor system.
- Recent developments in assessment of dysarthria and apraxia of speech.
- Recent developments in treatment tasks, with particular attention given to evidence-based procedures.

Finally, a few extra words need to be added about the videos on the PluralPlus companion website. As has been said in the preface of each edition of this book, grateful acknowledgment must be given to the individuals who allowed themselves to be videotaped.

It takes a special person to face the world while demonstrating a significant neurologic disorder, yet they were all pleased to do it, especially when told that the video would help students learn about these disorders. So, thanks once again to all the generous individuals in those videos.

About the Author

Donald B. Freed, PhD, is a chair emeritus in the Department of Communicative Sciences and Deaf Studies at California State University, Fresno. He received both his MS and PhD from the University of Oregon. Prior to joining the Fresno faculty, he worked as a speech-language pathologist in acute care and rehabilitation facilities and served as a research speech pathologist at the Portland Veterans Affairs Medical Center. His research has concentrated on aphasia and motor speech disorders. He has published articles in journals such as *Aphasiology, Clinical Aphasiology, American Journal of Speech and Language Pathology,* and *Journal of Speech and Hearing Research.*

In memory of Clyde E. Freed (1927–2019).

Chapter 1

A Brief Historical Review of Motor Speech Disorders

Case Reports From Ancient Greece
Case Reports From the Middle Ages and Renaissance
Two Early Theories on the Localization of Reason
From the 19th Century to Today

The term *motor speech disorders is an apt description of the deficits that are examined in this textbook. For readers who are new to the study of motor speech disorders, it will be beneficial to discuss the meaning of each word in this term. First of all,* motor *refers to the part of the nervous system that controls voluntary movements. Neuroanatomists call this portion of the nervous system the* **motor system**. Speech *is communication through the use of vocal symbols, sometimes also defined as the physical production of language.* Disorders *means an abnormality of function; the plural indicates that there is more than one abnormality in this condition. Motor speech disorders, therefore, are a collection of speech production deficits that are caused by the abnormal functioning of the motor system. Altogether, this collection of motor speech disorders consists of seven types of dysarthria and one type of apraxia.*

Although the following chapters contain detailed discussions of dysarthria and apraxia, these disorders should be briefly defined now. The literal definition of dysarthria is "disordered utterance" ("dys" means disordered or abnormal; "arthria" means to utter distinctly, from the Greek, arthroun). A more comprehensive definition is that dysarthria is the impaired production of speech because of disturbances in the muscular control of the speech mechanism. The layperson's concept of dysarthria is someone with slurred speech, but this disorder certainly includes many more speech production deficits than just poor articulation. It can involve respiration, prosody, resonance, and phonation as well.

Apraxia of speech also is a motor speech disorder. Apraxia means without action ("a" means absence of; "praxia" means performance of action, from the Greek, praxis). Actually, apraxia of speech is a deficit in the ability to smoothly sequence and place the tongue, lips, and jaw during speech. Apraxia of speech primarily affects articulation and prosody. Although apraxia of speech occurs frequently when the left hemisphere of the brain is damaged, the general public seems to be less aware of the characteristics of this disorder than they are of dysarthria.

1. A BRIEF HISTORICAL REVIEW OF MOTOR SPEECH DISORDERS

This chapter reviews a small selection of ancient medical reports that mention speech and language disorders. It is important to examine these early reports because a valuable part of any study is understanding the historical context from which the subject developed. Whether the topic is science or entertainment, a historical perspective adds a sense of depth and continuity that is otherwise difficult to obtain. While reading the following pages, keep in mind that some of the individuals in these case studies experienced their speech and language disorders more than 2,000 years ago.

*One of the most remarkable aspects of preparing this chapter was the discovery of how "modern" many of these ancient medical writers were. From today's perspective, it is easy to view them as quaint at best or frightfully ignorant at worst. But when examined in the context of the time in which they lived, these physicians' conclusions about **anatomy** and **physiology** show that most of them were trying to take an analytical approach to medicine. When reading their descriptions of their medical practice, it is easy to imagine them as today's state-of-the-art practitioners.*

Case Reports From Ancient Greece

Some of the earliest written accounts of speech and language disorders appear in the Greek texts known as the **Hippocratic Corpus**. Originally, these texts were a collection of 70 volumes that described numerous medicines, diseases, and treatments, as observed by ancient Greek physicians. Only about 60 of these volumes survive to the present, and they contain descriptions of anatomy, explanations of symptoms, and case studies of patients. A sampling of the individual titles gives an idea of the wide-ranging topics covered in these works—"On Ancient Medicines," "On Fractures," "The Book of Prognostics," and "Of the Epidemics." There are even volumes devoted to ulcers and hemorrhoids. Some of these works were written for educated physicians and contain surprising amounts of specific information about medical disorders and how to treat them. Other volumes were written for the general public and are, accordingly, more plainspoken in their advice.

The authorship of the Hippocratic Corpus is a bit of a mystery. Although it carries his name, **Hippocrates** (ca. 460–377 BC) was not the sole writer of this collection (Figure 1–1). In fact, it is not certain that he wrote any of the volumes. Most experts believe that numerous writers contributed to the collection over a period of at least 100 years. It is possible that the actual writers were physicians who were part of a school founded by Hippocrates on the Greek island of Kos.

Among the many descriptions of disorders in the Hippocratic Corpus are numerous references to patients being "speechless" or having "loss of speech." A few of these seem to be references to neurologically based speech or language disorders. For example, in Book One in "Of the Epidemics" (ca. 400 BC), there is a description of what could be an instance of **aphasia** and right hemiplegia.

> A woman, who lodged on the Quay, being three months gone with child, was seized with fever, and immediately began to have pains in the loins. On the third day, pain of the head and neck, extending to the clavicle, and right hand; she immediately lost the power of

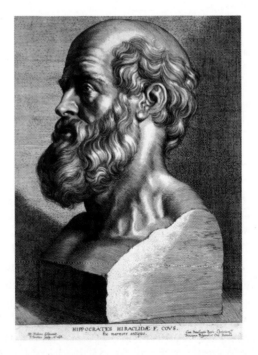

FIGURE 1–1. An artist's representation of Hippocrates (ca. 460–377 BC), who might or might not have contributed to the ancient medical texts that carry his name. *Source*: Image obtained from the History of Medicine database of The National Library of Medicine.

speech; was paralyzed in the right hand, with spasms, after the manner of paraplegia; was quite incoherent; passed an uncomfortable night. ("Of the Epidemics," ca. 400 BC/1995)

Fortunately, the woman's speech or language deficit, whatever it might have been, was only temporary because on the next day, she "recovered the use of her tongue," and on the sixth day, she "recovered her reason."

Another volume in the Hippocratic Corpus contains descriptions that also could be references to neurologically based speech or language disorders. In the "Aphorisms" (ca. 400 BC/1995), the writer makes an intriguing comment about the rapid onset of a condition that is accompanied by speechlessness: "When persons in good health are suddenly seized with pains in the head, and straightway are laid down speechless, and breathe loudly, they die in seven days, unless fever comes on." Although it is impossible to determine with certainty, this could be a description of the sudden onset of a stroke or some other neurologic disorder. Garrison (1925/1969) suggested that this passage describes a subarachnoid hemorrhage, a condition that is nearly always accompanied by a sudden, painful headache and the rapid onset of other neurologic signs.

A second intriguing comment from the "Aphorisms" seems to be a reference to the loss of speech after a head injury: "In cases of concussion of the brain produced by any cause, the patients necessarily lose their speech." As with the prior quote, it is difficult to determine which modern-day condition this might be describing. It could be that the loss of speech is the result of aphasia, severe dysarthria, or merely a temporary loss of consciousness.

One of the more detailed accounts of head injury resulting in a speech or language deficit is found in Book Five of "Of the Epidemics." It describes what happened to a young woman who was playing with a friend.

> The pretty virgin daughter of Nerius was twenty years old. She was struck on the bregma (front of the head) by the flat of the hand of a young woman friend in play. At the time she became blind and breathless, and when she went home fever seized her immediately, her head ached, and there was redness about her face. On the seventh day foul-smelling pus came out around the right ear, reddish, more than a cyathus [one-fifth of a cup]. She seemed better, and was relieved. Again she was prostrated by the fever; she was depressed, speechless; the right side of her face was drawn up; she had difficulty breathing; there was a spasmodic trembling. Her tongue was paralyzed, her eye stricken. On the ninth day she died. (Smith, 1994, p. 191)

This description indicates clearly that the author believed that the cause of the woman's speechlessness was the blow to her head. However, the type of speech or language disorder she had is difficult to determine. A modern-day reader might assume that dysarthria was a part of the problem because of the reference to a paralyzed tongue and facial contractions, but this conclusion would be little more than a guess.

Numerous examples of disordered voice are found in Book Seven of "Of the Epidemics." One of the more interesting reports describes a woman with arthritis whose "voice was checked during the night and up to midday." Although she could not talk, "she could hear, her mind was clear; she indicated with her hand that the pain was around the hip joint" (Smith, 1994, p. 399). That her auditory comprehension was functional and that she could gesture appropriately suggests that her speechlessness was from a laryngeal disorder, although it is difficult to say with certainty. Another case report tells of a man in Olynthus who had a "fever" for 17 days. The writer described him as having a "dreadful disorganization of body" and that his "voice [was] broken, a task to hear it, but intelligible" (Smith, 1994, p. 377). Once again, the author's imprecise description of the man's deficits makes it difficult to know what was wrong with his speech or voice. The man might have been demonstrating the effects of a neurologic speech impairment such as dysarthria or, perhaps, his voice was only soft and breathy from his weakened condition.

All of these case studies from the Hippocratic Corpus show that the ancient Greeks understood that speech difficulties could be the result of physical injury. Most important, these writings indicate that the Greeks knew that injury to the head could cause speechlessness (O'Neill, 1980). It is less certain whether they had a modern-day understanding of how voice, speech, and language differ, as can be seen in their vague medical descriptions of these communicative processes. Nevertheless, the influence of the Hippocratic Corpus on Western medicine was long-lasting; it was part of the standard medical curriculum for nearly 2,000 years. As late as the 18th century, some physicians were still studying and practicing the Hippocratic teachings on medicine.

Case Reports From the Middle Ages and Renaissance

Early descriptions of speech and language disorders did not end with the Greeks. The Byzantine physician, Paulus Aegineta (625–690), included numerous references to conditions that could result in speechlessness in his Medical Compendium in Seven Books. Later medical texts from the Middle Ages and Renaissance also provide various examples of these problems. For instance, in the early 1300s, a physician named Bernard of Gordon described individuals who omitted and added syllables to their speech (O'Neill, 1980). His examples of their spoken words (e.g., saying "Aristoles" for "Aristoteles") are intriguing and have characteristics that are similar to those in apraxia of speech or aphasia. As with the case studies from the Hippocratic Corpus, though, the exact nature of these patients' speech disorders cannot be determined from the writer's descriptions.

Another example of a speech or language disorder from the medieval era comes from an Italian physician, Lanfranc. He wrote about an incident in which a man fell from a horse and injured his head. After regaining consciousness, the man's initial attempts at speech were filled with what Lanfranc described as a child's babble—something that today might be labeled neologistic jargon or perhaps language of confusion. The man did survive the accident, and his speech eventually became intelligible again. Unfortunately, the recovery was not complete, because Lanfranc reported that the man never regained all of his mental abilities.

In the mid-1500s, a physician named Niccolo Massa recorded the details of another head injury that resulted in disordered speech. His case report is of a young man who was hit in the head with a spear, which apparently pierced deeply into his skull.

> Also returned to health by my work is the noble youth, Marcus Goro who was wounded by the sharp point of a spear. . . . There was fracture of not only the cranial bone, but of the **meninges**, and of the brain substance as far as to the basilar bone. . . . Besides all his other difficulties, the young man had been speechless for eight days. . . . Since the physicians declared they had seen no bone, I thought that the reason for the extinction of the voice was that there was a piece of bone fixed in the brain, and taking an instrument from a certain surgeon who was there, I extracted the bone from the wound, and immediately, he began to speak, and said, "Praise God, I am healed." (O'Neill, 1980, p. 185)

Two Early Theories on the Localization of Reason

Early medical writings were not confined to case reports of injuries. Many of them also included the authors' thoughts on how the human body functioned. Some of the most interesting of these are the theories of where human reasoning (and by implication, speech and language) was located in the body. One of the most long-lasting theories stated that reasoning was housed in the four cerebral ventricles. It was thought that the two lateral ventricles were where the body received sensory information from the outside world. This sensory information was believed to then move to the third ventricle, which contained the intellect. It was thought that the intellect analyzed the information and extracted meaning from sensory information. The fourth ventricle was responsible for memory—storing sensory information once it had been analyzed.

Evidence for this theory was described by such writers as Galen (ca. 130–200 BC), who observed that the closer a wound was to the ventricles, the more serious were the consequences for the patient. For instance, a surface wound to the brain usually did not result in deficits that were as significant as a wound that penetrated deeply into cerebral tissue. Because the deeper wound caused more serious damage and was closer to the ventricles, it was hypothesized that the ventricles must play an important role in cognitive abilities. Although this theory of ventricular localization was incorrect, it was nevertheless nearer to the truth than an earlier theory that placed the centers for speech and emotion in the heart. The ventricle hypothesis was an enduring one. It lasted from ancient times to the 16th century. This theory also had many noted followers, such as Leonardo da Vinci (1452–1519), who included the ventricles in many of his anatomical drawings of the nervous system (Figure 1–2). It finally was discredited when Vesalius (1514–1564) reasoned that because the cerebral ventricles in animals' brains were so similar in shape and number to those in human brains, it was unlikely that the ventricles played an especially important part in human reasoning.

A second, contemporaneous theory about the center for human reasoning held that the senses and movement were controlled by the meninges—the membranes that cover the brain and spinal cord. In brief, this theory was based on the observation that whenever the meninges were damaged by an injury, there almost always was some deficit in a patient's reasoning abilities, whether it was memory, movement, sensation, speech, or some other mental faculty. The wide acceptance of this theory is reflected by the fact that many early case studies of head injury frequently mentioned whether there was damage to the meninges, as seen in the prior quote from Massa. Another example of this can be found in a 1514 medical text by Giovanni da Vigo. He described a nobleman who was seriously injured when he fell from a horse and was kicked in the head. The man's subsequent speechlessness was attributed to sharp bone fragments that had pierced his meninges. No mention

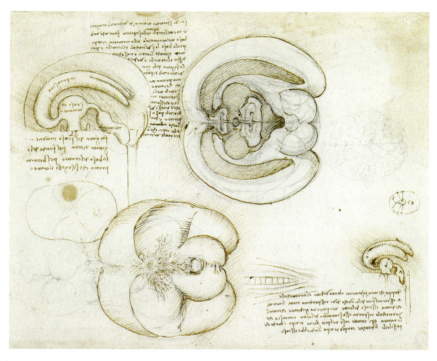

FIGURE 1–2. Leonardo da Vinci (1452–1519) believed that the cerebral ventricles were the containers of human intellect, and he featured them prominently in many of his anatomical drawings. This drawing is almost certainly of an ox's brain. *Source*: Image obtained from the History of Medicine database of The National Library of Medicine.

was made that the fragments might have damaged the underlying brain tissue. The meningeal theory was accepted widely for many centuries. Some physicians were still ascribing to it as late as the 16th century (O'Neill, 1980).

From the 19th Century to Today

Before the 19th century, most descriptions of speech and language disorders were too vague to be identified as definite historical instances of motor speech disorders. Reports that seemed to describe a motor speech disorder had to remain intriguing possibilities because details were lacking. This began to change in the early 1800s, when case reports and medical descriptions became much more specific. Numerous descriptions of modern-day motor speech disorders can be found in medical texts from that period. For instance, in his 1817 account of his patients' "shaking palsy,"

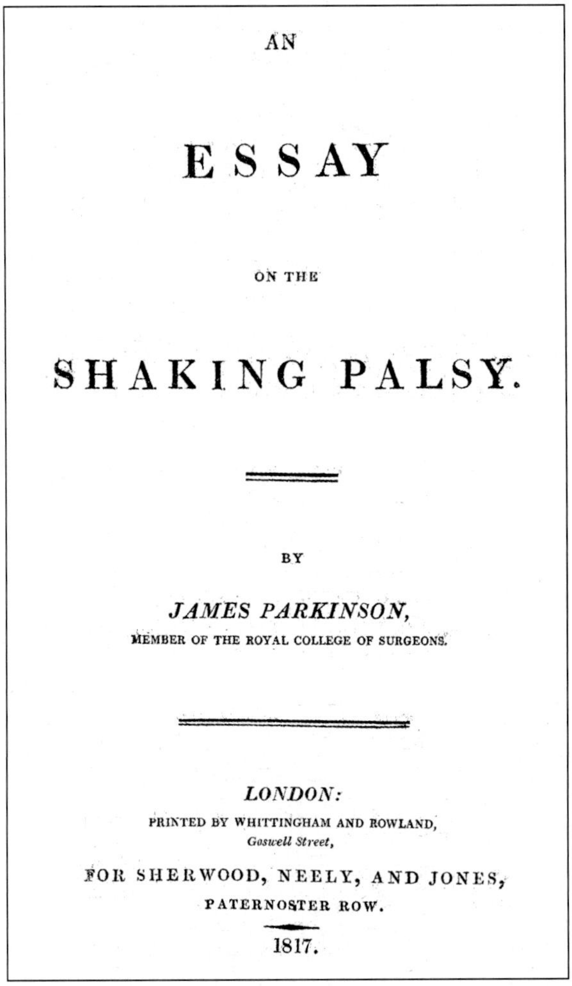

AN

ESSAY

ON THE

SHAKING PALSY.

BY

JAMES PARKINSON,
MEMBER OF THE ROYAL COLLEGE OF SURGEONS.

LONDON:
PRINTED BY WHITTINGHAM AND ROWLAND,
Goswell Street,
FOR SHERWOOD, NEELY, AND JONES,
PATERNOSTER ROW.
1817.

FIGURE 1–3. The title page from James Parkinson's (1825–1824) 1817 essay on the disease that now bears his name. *Source*: Image obtained from the History of Medicine database of The National Library of Medicine.

James Parkinson (1755–1824) described their symptoms, including speech, with stark and surprising clarity (Figure 1–3). Here is an excerpt about a middle-age gardener with the shaking palsy:

> As the debility increases and the influence of the will over the muscles fades away, the tremulous agitation becomes more vehement. It now seldom leaves him for a moment; but even when exhausted nature seizes a small portion of sleep, the motion becomes so violent as not only to shake the bed-hangings, but even the floor and sashes of the room. The chin is now almost immoveably bent down upon the sternum. The slops with which he is attempted to be fed, with

the saliva, are continually trickling from the mouth. The power of articulation is lost. (Parkinson, 1817, p. 9)

Jean-Martin Charcot (1825–1893), often called the father of modern neurology, published influential descriptions of several diseases that have dysarthria as a prominent symptom, such as multiple sclerosis (MS), amyotrophic lateral sclerosis, and Parkinson's disease (Figure 1–4). In 1877, Charcot described the speech of individuals with MS, saying that, "The affected person speaks in a slow drawling manner, and sometimes almost unintelligibly. . . . The words are as if measured or scanned; there is a pause after every syllable, and syllables themselves are pronounced slowly" (Darley, 1983, p. xiv). The speech deficits described so clearly by Charcot most resemble the motor speech disorder called **ataxic dysarthria**. Today, it is known that individuals with MS can have ataxic dysarthria, although it is more typical for them to have another type of dysarthria, known as mixed dysarthria.

In their 1897 paper on the speech and language abilities of individuals with right hemisphere lesions, Marie and Kattwinkel described yet another type of dysarthria. They reported that the

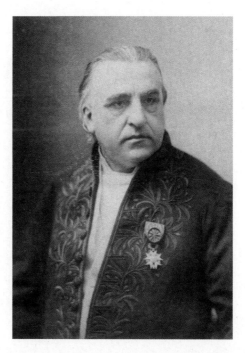

FIGURE 1–4. Jean-Martin Charcot (1825–1893) published a number of early descriptions of diseases that have dysarthria as a prominent symptom. *Source:* Image obtained from the History of Medicine database of The National Library of Medicine.

most obvious speech or language deficit after right hemisphere damage was "the mechanical functioning of speech, the articulation of words; it is really a question of dysarthria and not of aphasia" (Cole & Cole, 1971, p. 24). This type of dysarthria is now called unilateral upper motor neuron dysarthria and, just as described in 1897, it is primarily a disorder of articulation. Liepmann is credited with being the first to clearly describe apraxia of speech, which, as mentioned at the beginning of this chapter, is a deficit in an individual's ability to smoothly produce the voluntary motor movements needed for normal speech (Wertz et al., 1991). Although his 1900 report was mostly a description of his patient's limb apraxia (i.e., difficulties in sequencing the movements of the limbs), Liepmann also included detailed discussions of the patient's speech deficits. At about the same time, Carl Wernicke described another type of apraxia (Figure 1–5). In his last published work (in 1906), Wernicke described the characteristics of nonverbal oral apraxia, a disorder that often co-occurs with apraxia of speech. Although he was not the first to comment on this type of apraxia, his description is remarkable for its clarity and concise detail:

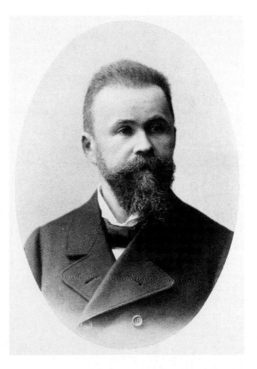

FIGURE 1–5. Carl Wernicke (1848–1905) studied a number of neurologic disorders in his productive career, including those associated with motor speech disorders and aphasia. *Source*: Image obtained from the History of Medicine database of The National Library of Medicine.

For example, many such patients typically cannot protrude the tongue upon command, puff out the cheeks, show their teeth, or even open their mouth without protruding their tongue, etc. The unsuccessful attempts to carry out such actions, which before this were common everyday movements, clearly reveals the loss of ability to organize the execution of such movements. (Eggert, 1977, p. 229)

For today's speech-language pathologist, the work of Darley et al. (1969a, 1969b, 1975) must certainly rank as one of the most important accomplishments in the field of acquired speech and language deficits. These researchers' descriptions and classification of motor speech disorders are still much in use. Prior to their work, the medical terms used to describe the dysarthrias varied from profession to profession. Sometimes, the name of a disorder was used as the name of the associated speech deficit. For example, the term "**bulbar** palsy" would be used as the name for weakness in the facial musculature as well as for the speech deficit caused by the weakness. A dysarthria also could be known by several terms that described the characteristics of the deficit. For instance, the dysarthria associated with damage to the cerebellum might have appeared variously as "scanning speech," "ataxic speech," or "cerebellar speech." Through their research, publications, and presentations, Darley and his colleagues introduced a more standardized method of naming and classifying motor speech disorders. Furthermore, Darley et al. (1969a, 1969b) also compiled an invaluable listing of the speech errors that occur in motor speech disorders.

Dysarthria and apraxia of speech continue to be rich areas of research, with both medical and behavioral studies examining these disorders. Recent contributions to the motor speech disorders literature have been made by many contemporary researchers, and important studies examining dysarthria and apraxia of speech continue to be published. Advances in computers and other instrumentation continue to open new opportunities for research that were impossible just a few years ago. The ultimate beneficiaries of this work will be the patients who have motor speech disorders.

Chapter 2

The Motor System

Components of the Motor System
  Brain
    Cerebrum
    Brainstem
    Cerebellum
  Nervous System Cells
    Types of Neurons
    Other Nervous System Cells
    Tracts and Nerves
    Transmission of Neural Impulses
  Summary of Motor System Components

Structure and Function of the Motor System
  The Desire to Move
  Primary and Association Cortices
  Basal Ganglia and Cerebellum
    Basal Ganglia
    Cerebellum
  Thalamus
  Primary Motor Cortex
  Descending Motor Tracts
    Pyramidal System
    Extrapyramidal System
  Cranial and Spinal Nerves
    Cranial Nerve Nuclei
    Spinal Nerve Nuclei
  Neuromuscular Junction

Summary of the Motor System

Study Questions

The parts of the nervous system that control voluntary movement are known collectively as the motor system. Understanding how this system works is an important part of being an effective diagnostician of motor speech disorders. Familiarity with the workings of upper and lower motor neurons, the basal ganglia, the cerebellum, and the pyramidal and the extrapyramidal systems is essential in making the correct diagnosis of a motor speech disorder and in designing appropriate treatment plans. This chapter provides an overview of the motor system to lay the foundation for the more specific investigations of the motor speech disorders presented in later chapters.

The motor system is what allows thought to be turned into movement, whether it is moving a hand, a leg, or the tongue. By any measure, the motor system is extremely complex. The nerve cells of the motor system are arranged into many different pathways, with each pathway performing different functions. Some parts of the motor system work at a conscious level and others at a subconscious level. The system's scope also is impressive. It ranges from the very highest cognitive centers of the brain down to the body's simplest muscles. A properly functioning motor system allows movements of the fingers, vocal folds, feet, and eyebrows, all at the same time and in a coordinated manner. When a portion of it is damaged, though, the result can be a debilitating movement disorder. The type of disorder is dependent on the location and extent of the damage to the motor system. For example, lesions in the basal ganglia can result in involuntary movements that seriously interfere with an individual's voluntary attempts to speak, walk, or do any number of other things. Because of this relationship between the type of disorder and the site of damage, it is important to understand the basics of the motor system.

Components of the Motor System

The motor system is actually one of several subdivisions of the nervous system. Consequently, any discussion of the motor system is difficult, if not impossible, without a basic understanding of the

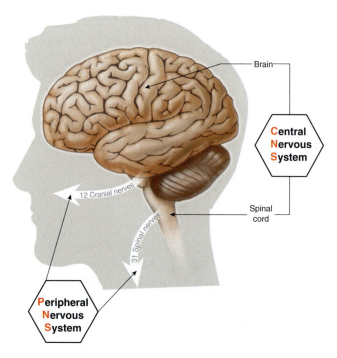

FIGURE 2–1. The central nervous system consists of the brain and spinal cord. The peripheral nervous system contains the 12 cranial nerves and the 31 spinal nerves.

nervous system. Because of the link between these two systems, the first portion of this chapter reviews the fundamental structures of the nervous system before moving on to the specifics of the motor system. The nervous system is organized into the central and peripheral nervous systems (Figure 2–1). The **central nervous system (CNS)** consists of the brain and the spinal cord. The **peripheral nervous system (PNS)** is composed of 12 pairs of cranial nerves and 31 pairs of spinal nerves. The **cranial nerves** are so named because they project from parts of the CNS that are within the cranium (i.e., inside the skull). They innervate many organs and muscles of the head, neck, thorax, and abdomen. In contrast, the **spinal nerves** branch from the spinal cord and innervate most of the other muscles of the body, including the chest, arms, and legs.

Brain

The brain is the key component, and the most complex part, of the nervous system. Almost all activity in the nervous system originates in or is ultimately processed by the brain. Voluntary motor commands to the muscles originate in the brain. The brain also receives sensory information from the body and controls the cognitive functions, including reasoning, memory, language, and problem solving.

Humans have large brains relative to their body size, as compared with most other animals. The normal adult brain weighs about 2.5 to 3.5 lb. It has an amazingly complex number of interconnections among its various parts, as well as connections with the other portions of the nervous system. The following sections review the parts of the brain that are most relevant to understanding the motor system.

Cerebrum

The brain is divided into the **cerebrum**, **brainstem**, and **cerebellum** (Figure 2–2). The largest and most prominent of these is the cerebrum. It is split into two hemispheres by the longitudinal fissure, which runs front to back along the middle of the brain. The cerebrum is organized into four areas called lobes. The **frontal lobe** is located on the **anterior** (front) portion of the cerebrum. The **temporal lobe** lies on the lower sides of the cerebrum. The **parietal lobe** is found on the upper sides of the cerebrum behind the frontal lobe. Finally, the **occipital lobe** is on the rearmost portion of the cerebrum, behind both the parietal and temporal lobes. The most obvious feature of the cerebrum is its deep convolutions. Each convolution is called a **gyrus** (plural, gyri), and the groove between the gyri is called a **sulcus** (plural, sulci).

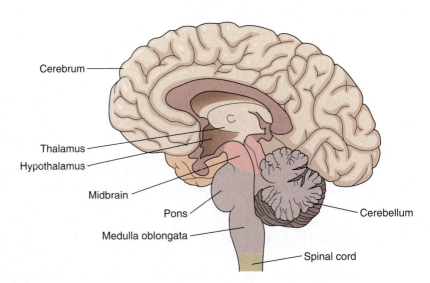

FIGURE 2–2. The brain consists of the cerebrum, brainstem (midbrain, pons, and medulla), and cerebellum.

2. THE MOTOR SYSTEM

The gyri and sulci of the cerebrum create several significant landmarks that will be referred to frequently in this textbook (Figure 2–3). The first of these is the **lateral sulcus**, certainly the most prominent sulcus on the cerebrum. It runs horizontally along the lateral sides of each hemisphere and separates the temporal lobe from the frontal lobe. Another landmark is the **central sulcus**,

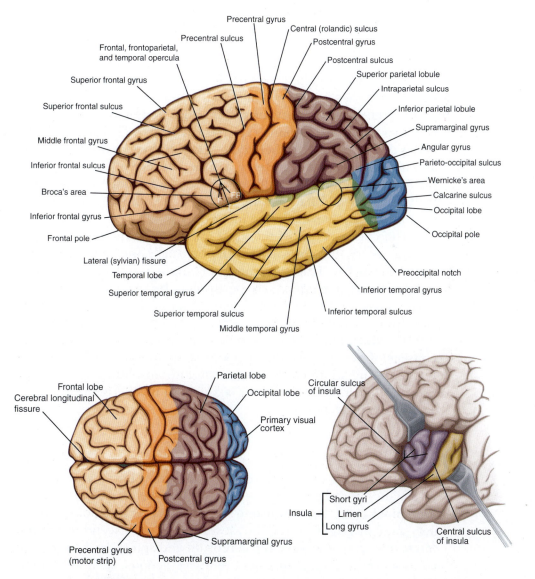

FIGURE 2–3. Four of the most prominent landmarks on the lateral surface of the brain are the lateral and central sulci and the precentral and postcentral gyri.

probably the second most prominent sulcus on the cerebrum. It is located near the center of the lateral sides of each hemisphere (hence its name) and extends vertically from the very top of the hemisphere down to the lateral sulcus. The central sulcus separates the frontal lobe from the parietal lobe.

The gyrus immediately in front of the central sulcus is known variously as the **precentral gyrus**, the **primary motor cortex**, or the **motor strip**. The nerve cells located in this gyrus play a very important role in controlling the voluntary movements of the body. The gyrus just behind the central sulcus is called either the **postcentral gyrus**, the **primary sensory cortex**, or the **sensory strip**. Here, the higher centers of the brain receive sensory information from the body via the PNS and other portions of the CNS.

The surface of the cerebrum is called the **cerebral cortex**. Its thickness varies between 2 mm and 5 mm, and it is composed of six different layers of nervous system cells. In its entirety, the cortex contains about 15 billion nerve cells (neurons). The cortex is gray and is often described as being the "**gray matter**" of the brain. Only about one third of the cortex is visible because of the cerebrum's many convolutions; the other two thirds are hidden between the many sulci. If laid flat, the total surface area of the cortex would be approximately 340 square inches.

The cortex is one of the most important parts of the nervous system. In this thin cortical layer of nerve cells, the higher cognitive activities, such as language, motor planning, problem solving, and much sensory perception, are performed. Because it is so thin, the cortex makes up only a small percentage of the cerebrum's total size. Most of the cerebrum is actually composed of large groupings of **white matter** located below the cortex. This white matter consists of nerve-cell axons that course to and from other parts of the CNS. The white color is from the fatty myelin that covers the axons. More information about axons and myelin is presented in a subsequent section.

Brainstem

The brainstem is divided (from top to bottom) into the **midbrain**, **pons**, and **medulla** (Figure 2–4). It sits between the cerebrum and the spinal cord. The brainstem's importance is threefold. First, it acts as a passageway for the descending and ascending neural tracts that travel between the cerebrum and spinal cord. Second, it controls certain integrative and reflexive actions, such as respiration, consciousness, and some functions of the cardiovascular system. Third, and probably most important with regard to the motor speech system, it contains the places where the cranial nerves

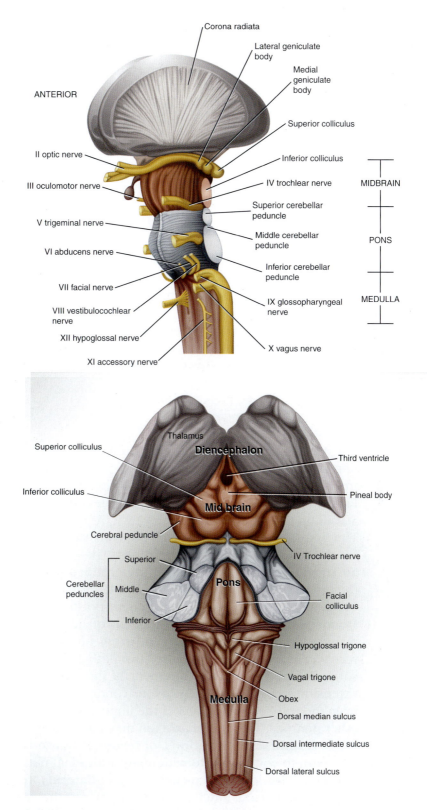

FIGURE 2–4. The brainstem is divided into the midbrain, pons, and medulla. These figures also illustrate the roots of the cranial nerves.

project out from the CNS. It is the cranial nerves that convey motor impulses from the CNS to the muscles of the larynx, face, tongue, pharynx, and velum. The cranial nerves are attached to the brainstem at points called the **cranial nerve nuclei**.

Cerebellum

The cerebellum is shaped somewhat like the cerebrum, but it is much smaller. It is attached to the back of the brainstem, where it makes neural connections with the cerebral cortex and numerous other parts of the CNS. The most important function of the cerebellum is to coordinate voluntary movements, so that muscles will contract with the correct amount of force and at the appropriate times. Cerebellar damage can cause significant deficits in the performance of both gross and skilled motor actions. Movements such as walking, writing, and speech can become uncertain and awkward when the cerebellum is not functioning properly. The cerebellum is examined in more detail later in this chapter and in Chapter 7.

Nervous System Cells

The nervous system contains many different types of cells. The most important are the **neurons** (Figure 2–5), which transmit the electrochemical signals that control nearly every function of the body. Estimates of the number of neurons in the human body range from 50 billion to 100 billion. Neurons have three primary components. The first is the **cell body**, which contains the nucleus responsible for the cell's vital metabolic functions. The cell bodies of neurons are gray. When many cell bodies are grouped together, they cause the distinctive grayish tint that is visible in many structures in the CNS, such as the cortex and the central portion of the spinal cord. **Dendrites** are the second component of neurons. These are the many short processes that extend from the cell body. Dendrites receive electrochemical impulses from other neurons or from sensory organs. The third component is the **axon**, the single long extension from the cell body. Axons conduct neural impulses away from the cell body and transfer the impulses to muscles, glands, or other neurons. The end of an axon may have many small branches called **terminal ramifications**, or **terminal boutons**, which allow one axon to communicate with many additional neurons. An axon also may have longer branches called **collaterals**, further extending the influence of a neuron to other parts of the nervous system.

Most axons are covered by **myelin**, a white, lipid-protein membrane that covers the length of the axon. Myelin insulates a neu-

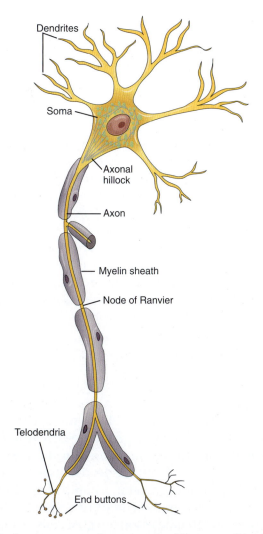

FIGURE 2-5. A neuron contains many dendrites, a cell body, and a single axon.

ron's electrochemical impulses from the surrounding tissues and fluids, which would otherwise degrade the strength of an impulse as it travels the length of the axon. Myelin acts very much like the insulation on household electrical wiring to prevent the leakage of electrical energy.

Types of Neurons

Neurons are categorized by their shape and size. The cell body of some neurons is in the middle of the axon, and in others it is to the side. Some have very large cell bodies; others do not. Some neurons have axons that are only a fraction of a millimeter long; others have axons up to a meter in length. In addition, neurons are classified by the types of information they carry. **Motor neurons** transmit neural impulses that cause contractions in muscles (and thereby cause movement). **Sensory neurons** carry information related to sensory stimuli. **Interneurons** link neurons with other neurons and are the most common type of neuron. Because they form connections with many other neurons, interneurons play an important role in controlling movement.

Yet another distinction between neurons is the direction in which they convey neural impulses. Neurons that transmit their impulses away from the CNS are called **efferent neurons**. Those sending their impulses toward the CNS are called **afferent neurons**. In general, motor neurons are efferent, and sensory neurons are afferent. It is not unusual to use these terms to describe the flow of neural information from one area of the nervous system to another. For instance, the cortex may be said to receive afferent input from sensory neurons.

Other Nervous System Cells

Although neurons are the most important cells of the nervous system, they are certainly not the only ones, nor are they the most numerous. The other cells in the nervous system, called **glial cells** (or the neuroglia), include **Schwann cells**, which provide the myelin sheath around axons in the PNS; **microglia**, which act as scavengers and remove dead cells and other waste; **oligodendroglia**, which form myelin around axons in the CNS; and **astrocytes**, which make up the connective tissue of the CNS. It is believed that there are 10 times as many glial cells as neurons and that they make up more than half the volume of the nervous system. Glial cells play a vital supporting role in the functioning of the nervous system.

Tracts and Nerves

Axons are usually found coursing throughout the nervous system in bundles. The axons in these bundles are often functionally related to each other. For example, a prominent bundle of motor neuron axons travels together from the cortex to the spinal cord, all transmitting motor impulses. Another example is the bundle of sensory neuron axons extending from the retina of the eye to the visual centers of the brain. When bundles of axons such as these are found in the CNS, they are most often called **neural tracts**. When found in the PNS, they are called **nerves**. The bundles of axons in the prior two examples are called the corticospinal tract and the **optic nerve**, respectively. Note that the wording of the term *corticospinal* indicates the direction in which neural impulses travel within this tract. In this example, the flow is from the cortex (cortico) to the spinal cord (spinal).

Transmission of Neural Impulses

Stated simply, the function of a neuron is to transmit neural impulses from one part of the nervous system to another. A neuron accomplishes this by conducting a small electrochemical charge along the length of its axon. When this charge reaches the axon's terminal ramifications, small amounts of a substance called a **neurotransmitter** are released from these end points. The neurotransmitter crosses a microscopic gap (the **synaptic cleft**) between the active neuron and an adjoining neuron (Figure 2–6). Some neurotransmitters have an excitatory function—they increase the probability of an electrochemical impulse being stimulated in the adjoining neuron. Other neurotransmitters are inhibitory—they decrease the probability of an impulse occurring in the adjoining neuron. If enough of an excitatory neurotransmitter is received in specialized receptors in the adjoining neuron, an electrochemical impulse will be initiated in this neuron. In contrast, if too much inhibitory neurotransmitter is present, the impulse will not be transmitted to the adjoining neuron. **Acetylcholine** and **dopamine** are two important neurotransmitters in the motor system.

It is misleading, however, to concentrate too narrowly on the functioning of just a few neurons when describing the transmission of neural impulses. The true picture is really much more complicated. There are two important points to remember when visualizing how neurons communicate. The first is that a single neuron may have synaptic connections with the terminal ramifications or collaterals of many different axons. In fact, a typical neuron has several thousand synaptic connections with other neurons. Consequently, a single neuron may synapse with some axons that are producing excitatory neurotransmitters and with others producing inhibitory neurotransmitters.

This leads to the second important point. A receiving neuron will fire its own electrochemical impulse only when a certain threshold of excitation is reached, and then only if the amounts of excitatory neurotransmitters exceed the influence of inhibitory neurotransmitters. The nervous system depends on this complex interplay of excitatory and inhibitory neurotransmitters to effectively convey neural impulses. When this interplay is not kept in

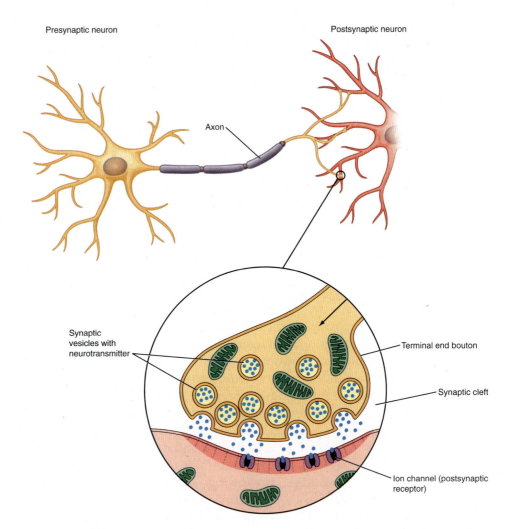

FIGURE 2–6. Neurons communicate with each other across microscopic gaps called synaptic clefts.

balance, the results can be serious. In the motor system, an imbalance between excitatory and inhibitory neurotransmitters could be a cause of spasticity. For example, if a stroke or physical trauma damages a tract of inhibitory motor neurons, those neurons will not be able to contribute their inhibitory neurotransmitters to their synaptic connections with other motor neurons. In this case, there will be a disproportionate amount of excitatory neurotransmitters affecting those other neurons, resulting in excessive contractions of the muscles innervated by the highly excited neurons that did not receive the counterbalancing inhibitory neurotransmitters. The causes of spasticity are explored in more detail in later sections of this book.

Summary of Motor System Components

- The nervous system is divided into the CNS and the PNS. The CNS includes the brain and the spinal cord. The PNS includes the spinal and cranial nerves.
- The brain is organized into the cerebrum, brainstem, and cerebellum. The cerebrum is divided into four lobes: frontal, temporal, parietal, and occipital.
- The most important cells of the nervous system are neurons. They are the means by which neural impulses are transmitted from one part of the nervous system to another.

Structure and Function of the Motor System

The remainder of this chapter concentrates on the structure and function of the motor system. We present a model of how the motor system is organized and how its components interact during movement. Admittedly, it is a simplified model. Some components of the motor system have been combined, others glossed over, and a few omitted. For example, the influence of sensory information on movement is not examined in detail, nor are the **limbic system**'s contributions included. (The limbic system is a subcortical area of the brain that influences emotion, memory, learning, and related behaviors.) Refer to Figure 2–7 frequently while reading the following sections because each box in the diagram is detailed individually. The boxes represent parts of the motor system, and the arrows indicate the flow of neural information from one part to another.

The Desire to Move

The starting place for any voluntary movement is the desire to move. It is the first step in picking up an object, walking, standing, phonating, or any of a hundred other actions that are performed every day. Taking that desire and turning it into a movement is something most individuals can do quite easily. It seems like a simple task; in reality, however, it is exceedingly complex. In fact, it is not clearly understood how the brain transforms the desire to move into a sequence of motor neuron firing. The nature of the neurologic "spark" that begins the whole process of planning a movement is unknown. One textbook jokingly described it as a small person inside the brain pulling the appropriate strings when an individual wants to move.

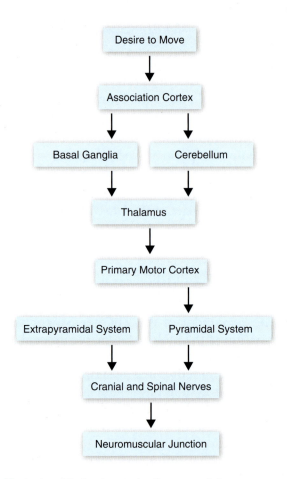

FIGURE 2-7. A simplified schematic diagram of the motor system.

Currently, it can only be assumed that thought somehow triggers the firing of the correct neurons that lead to a desired movement. Although it is not known how the desire to move initiates movement, many of the subsequent steps in the motor system are better understood. It is known, for example, that there is a significant increase in metabolic activity over large **bilateral** areas of the cortex, called the **association cortex**, about 800 ms before a voluntary movement is actually performed. Consequently, it is believed that the association cortex plays an especially important role in the initial planning of voluntary movements.

Primary and Association Cortices

A discussion of the association cortex needs to be preceded by an examination of the four primary cortices because the association cortex receives much of its sensory input from three of these areas. The **primary cortex** comprises the parts of the cerebrum that are dedicated to the analysis of a single type of neural input. Individually, these areas are known as the primary auditory cortex, primary visual cortex, primary sensory cortex, and primary motor cortex (Figure 2–8). The first three are responsible for the initial cortical processing of auditory, visual, and somatosensory (i.e., bodily sensation) information, respectively. The processing performed in these areas is relatively basic as compared with the more complex analysis performed in higher centers of the brain. For example, the **primary auditory cortex**, which is located on the uppermost portion of the temporal lobe, is thought to analyze tone patterns and sound properties. It also might help in the localization of sounds. The more sophisticated analyses of sound are completed in the association cortex.

The **primary visual cortex** is located at the posterior end of the occipital lobe. It performs a preliminary analysis of depth and perhaps integration of visual information from both eyes. Damage to this area can result in the loss of conscious awareness of visual stimulation.

The **primary sensory cortex** is located on the postcentral gyrus. This is where the cortex receives the first neural input about bodily sensation. The analysis includes sensations of pressure, temperature, touch, and proprioception (i.e., the position and movement of joints and limbs).

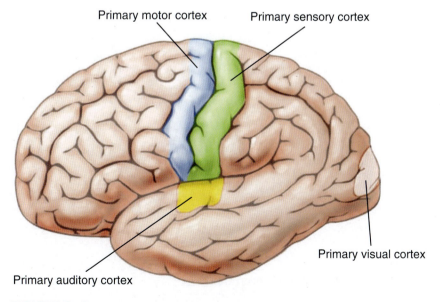

FIGURE 2–8. The four areas of the primary cortex.

These three primary cortex areas are similar in that they are the first cortical areas to analyze sensory information. The **primary motor cortex**, which is located on the precentral gyrus, works in a comparable but reversed manner. It receives planned motor impulses from cortical and subcortical areas of the brain (to be discussed later in this chapter) and sends those impulses down through the brainstem and spinal cord, where they eventually are sent to the muscles. An important point to remember is that most planning for voluntary movement does not originate in the primary motor cortex. The initial planning of a voluntary movement is formulated elsewhere in the brain, primarily in the association cortex.

The association cortex is the area of the cortex that, in conjunction with other parts of the brain, "makes sense" of the sensory impulses that have been initially analyzed by the primary cortices. The association cortex, however, is not a single region of the brain. It actually is divided among four areas of the cortex—the temporal association area, parietal association area, frontal association area, and occipital association area (Figure 2–9). Although each area is covered individually in the following paragraphs, it would be a mistake to think of them as independent centers for specific types of processing. The association areas of the cortex are heavily interconnected with many other parts of the brain, and they function together in various combinations during mental tasks. The parietal association area, for example, has neural connections with at least

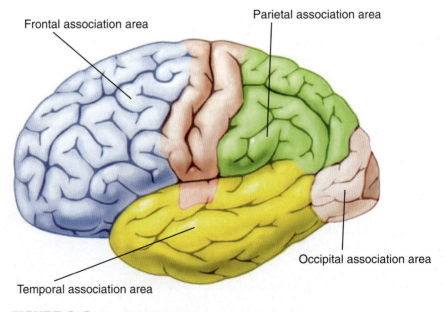

FIGURE 2–9. The four areas of the association cortex.

eight other cortical areas, including the primary sensory cortex, the temporal association area, and the frontal association area. Given these many cortical connections (and their numerous connections with subcortical structures), it is not surprising to find that the association cortex operates in a highly integrated fashion.

The **temporal association area** covers much of the upper and central parts of the temporal lobe. It has neural connections with the frontal association area, the primary auditory cortex, certain visual processing regions along the bottom, rear edge of the temporal lobe, and subcortical areas involved with memory. The workings of the temporal association area are diverse. It is involved with the recognition of complex visual stimuli, integrating auditory stimuli with other centers of the brain, and the formation of memories. Damage to this area can result in visual agnosia, amnesia, and high levels of distractibility.

The **frontal association area** is found on the forwardmost half of the frontal lobe. This area of the brain is sometimes called the prefrontal cortex, to differentiate it from the cortical motor areas that also are located on the frontal lobes (see Figure 2–9). The frontal association area has many neural connections with the other lobes of the cerebrum. Because of these numerous pathways, this area has access to all the sensory centers of the brain. The frontal association area also receives information on emotion and motivation from subcortical structures. Through the integration of this information, the frontal association area undoubtedly plays an important role in initiating and planning volitional movements. Bilateral damage to this area can result in decreased spontaneity and initiative, shortened attention span, and difficulties with abstract problem solving.

The **parietal association area** is located between the primary sensory cortex and the occipital lobe. It has many important neural connections with the prefrontal and motor areas of the frontal lobe, as well as with the occipital lobe. A key responsibility of the parietal association area is integrating bodily sensations with visual information. As part of the motor system, the parietal association area plays an important role in the control of visually guided movements (e.g., hand–eye coordination). Damage here can cause impairments in manipulating objects, sensory neglect of half the body, and certain reading and writing deficits.

The **visual association area** is a band of the cortex that runs between the primary visual cortex and the parietal and temporal lobes. It has many connections with the primary visual cortex, through which it receives visual sensory impulses. Its main function is to perform very complex analyses of visual impulses from the primary visual cortex. The contributions of the visual association cortex to the motor system include its input to the parietal association area regarding visually guided movements. Although selective damage to the visual association area is rare, it can result in several unusual disorders. One is motion blindness. In this rare condition, affected individuals have difficulty perceiving the movement of objects. For instance, running water will appear to be frozen in a fixed position; people walking into a room will seem to suddenly appear and disappear; or an oncoming train will first seem to be far away and then suddenly it will be very close. Other disorders associated with visual association area damage are color blindness and prosopagnosia (the inability to recognize familiar faces).

In a process that is not well understood, these four cortical association areas, along with other parts of the brain, are able to take that nebulous desire to move and turn it into a planned pattern of muscular contractions. At this early stage of creating a movement, however, the planned contractions are believed to be rough and exaggerated approximations of what is really needed to successfully accomplish the desired movement. Further processing of the planned movement is required; this is where the basal ganglia, cerebellum, and thalamus enter the picture. The association cortex sends this rough sequence of motor impulses down to these subcortical structures for further processing and refining.

Basal Ganglia and Cerebellum

The association cortex sends its neural signals of an intended motor movement to both the basal ganglia and the cerebellum. These two structures seem to have different, equally important, effects on planned movements. Each has its own separate looping neural circuit, often called control circuits. Through these circuits, the basal ganglia and cerebellum link the association cortex with the primary motor cortex. That is, they take the rough motor impulses from the association cortex, smooth them out, coordinate them, and then send them (via the thalamus) up to the primary motor cortex.

Basal Ganglia

Basal ganglia is a collective name for three large subcortical structures located near the lateral ventricles (Figure 2–10). Individually, they are the **caudate nucleus**, the **putamen**, and the **globus pallidus** (Andreatta, 2023; Seikel et al., 2020). The three structures are interconnected with assorted neural fibers. The caudate nucleus and putamen are known together as the **striatum**. Because they are dense with gray matter (i.e., the cell bodies of neurons), the

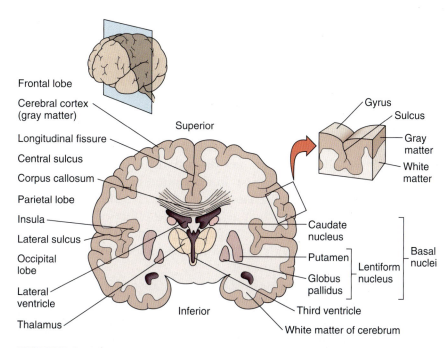

FIGURE 2–10. A **coronal** section of the brain showing the positions of the basal ganglia (caudate nucleus, putamen, globus pallidus), thalamus, and other landmarks of the cerebrum.

basal ganglia are quite distinct visually from the surrounding white matter. The basal ganglia contain an extremely complex network of neural pathways and have connections with many cortical and subcortical areas. Most cortical input to the basal ganglia goes to the striatum. In turn, most of the output from the basal ganglia is sent from the globus pallidus to the thalamus (another subcortical gray matter structure that is discussed later in this chapter).

The workings of the basal ganglia are very intricate. In general, the basal ganglia seem to act as a "filter" that prevents unwanted movements. This filter action is best observed when the basal ganglia are impaired. For example, when the basal ganglia are hyperexcited because of decreased levels of dopamine, voluntary movements are greatly compressed and attenuated (see the example below of Parkinson's disease). On the other hand, when basal ganglia neurons degenerate and lose their inhibitory abilities, movements can be exaggerated and purposeless (see the description below of Huntington's disease). The basal ganglia are believed to be especially important in the planning and refining of slow, continuous movements. They are quite active during those types of actions and, in turn, are mostly inactive during rapid, back-and-forth movements.

Several other subcortical gray matter structures influence the basal ganglia. One of them is the **substantia nigra** (Figure 2–11). It is connected to the striatum via its own neural circuit. The neural tract from the substantia nigra to the striatum contains a large number of neurons that produce the neurotransmitter dopamine. Many neurons of the striatum are dependent on dopamine for proper functioning. If the levels of dopamine from the substantia nigra are lowered in the striatum, the results include muscular **rigidity**, **tremor**, gait disturbances, and difficulty initiating movement. This decrease in dopamine in the striatum can occur either as part of a disease process (e.g., Parkinson's disease) or through other means, such as an adverse effect of antipsychotic drugs that block the production of dopamine. The motor speech disorder associated with parkinsonism is called **hypokinetic dysarthria**, discussed in Chapter 8.

Another class of movement disorders, known as **hyperkinetic disorders**, is also identified with damage to the basal ganglia. The symptoms of these disorders can be dramatically different from the tight, restricted movements seen in parkinsonian-type disorders. Huntington's disease (also known as Huntington's chorea) is a good example of a hyperkinetic movement disorder. It is a fatal,

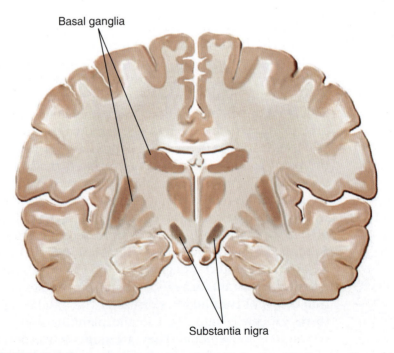

FIGURE 2–11. A coronal section of the brain showing the position of the substantia nigra in relation to the basal ganglia.

inherited disease that results in the progressive loss of neurons in the striatum and other areas of the brain. The symptoms of the disorder include rapid, involuntary movements of the extremities, face, and tongue. As the disease progresses, the movements increase in intensity and could begin to affect the muscles of the torso. Dementia and behavioral problems eventually become evident as well. The movements of the hands, arms, and legs in an individual with Huntington's disease have sometimes been described as "dancelike" and "graceful." Although accurate to some extent, such descriptions minimize the debilitating effects these involuntary movements have on an individual's voluntary movements. The motor speech disorder found in Huntington's disease and similar disorders is called **hyperkinetic dysarthria**, which is examined in Chapter 9.

Cerebellum

The cerebellum helps to regulate muscle tone, maintain balance, and coordinate skilled motor movements. It is attached to the back of the brainstem and lies just below the occipital lobe of the cerebrum (Figure 2–12). Its name, which literally means "little cerebrum," comes from early anatomists, who thought it was an additional, smaller brain. This erroneous conclusion is understandable because the cerebrum and cerebellum have a similar outward appearance. Like the cerebrum, the cerebellum has two hemispheres that are divided by a longitudinal fissure. Its surface also contains many convolutions and grooves—more, in fact, than are found on the cerebrum. Because of these numerous convolutions, the cerebellum has a surface area that is nearly 75% of that of the cerebral cortex.

Like the basal ganglia, the cerebellum also receives neural impulses of intended motor movements from the association cortex. In addition, it receives sensory input from the vestibular labyrinth of the inner ear and from visual, tactile, auditory, and proprioceptive sensory receptors located throughout the body, all of which give the cerebellum access to information about the body's balance, position, and posture. It is thought that the cerebellum takes the preliminary motor impulses from the association cortex and integrates them with the sensory information available to it. The cerebellum adjusts and refines the motor impulses according to the body's immediate circumstances and sends these processed motor signals to the primary motor cortex via the thalamus. However, not all of the motor output from the cerebellum goes to the thalamus. The cerebellum also has efferent neural tracts that indirectly synapse with descending extrapyramidal tracts (discussed below). Through these connections with the extrapyramidal motor

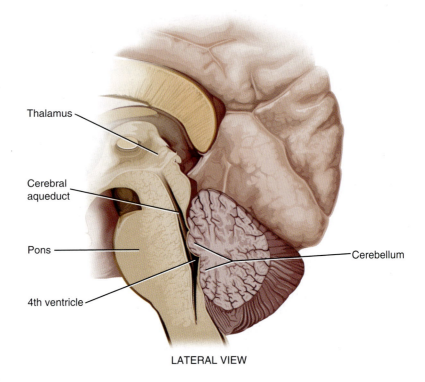

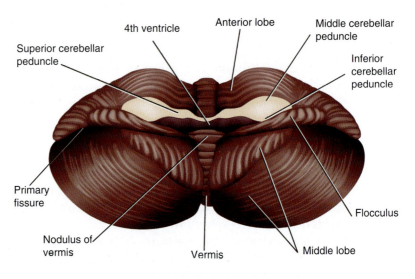

FIGURE 2-12. The cerebellum is attached to the posterior of the brainstem.

neurons, the cerebellum has a relatively direct influence on such motor activities as walking and maintaining posture.

Because of its many afferent and efferent connections with diverse parts of the nervous system, a cerebellum that is damaged can result in a variety of disorders. One of these is **ataxia**, which is a disturbance in the speed, range, and direction of movements. The muscle groups near the shoulders and pelvis might be particularly affected. The gait of an individual with ataxia is wide-based, lurching, and stumbling and is often described as having a "drunken" character. **Intention tremor** is also found with lesions of the cerebellar hemispheres. This type of tremor is observed only during the performance of voluntary movements, such as reaching for a glass of water. It is not present while an individual is at rest. Other disorders include involuntary oscillatory movements of the eyes (nystagmus), increased or decreased muscle tone, and disturbances of equilibrium. The motor speech disorder usually associated with cerebellar lesions is ataxic dysarthria, which is discussed in Chapter 7.

Thalamus

The **thalamus** is yet another important subcortical gray matter structure. Located deep to the basal ganglia and to the lateral sides of the third ventricle (Figure 2–13), the thalamus has been described as the doorway through which subcortical systems of the nervous system communicate with the cerebral cortex. It receives neural inputs of planned motor movements from both the basal ganglia and the cerebellum. Exactly what it does with these signals is not precisely understood. What is known, however, is that the thalamus has a vast amount of somatosensory information available to it. Practically every sensory impulse from the body passes through the thalamus on its way to the cortex. It is believed that the thalamus uses this sensory information to further refine the motor impulses from the basal ganglia and cerebellum.

Primary Motor Cortex

The primary motor cortex receives the neural motor impulses that have been processed, smoothed, and coordinated by the basal ganglia, the cerebellum, and thalamus. The neurons in the primary motor cortex have axons that are among the longest in the body; many extend all the way from the cortex to the lower portions of the spinal cord. These axons make up much of the descending

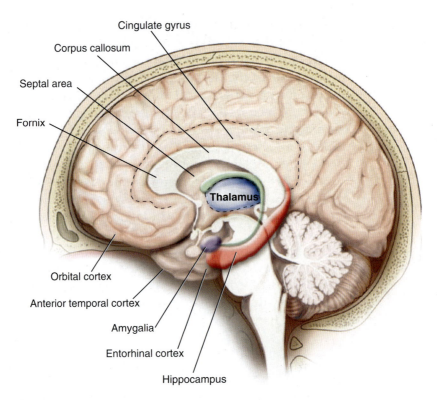

FIGURE 2–13. A lateral view of the thalamus in relation to the cerebrum.

motor tract called the **pyramidal system**. Direct electrical stimulation of the primary motor cortex has shown that its neurons are arranged in an inverted body scheme (Figure 2–14). When neurons near the bottom of the precentral gyrus are stimulated with an electrical probe, contractions occur in the muscles of the head and neck. In contrast, muscle contractions are observed in the leg and foot when neurons near the top of the gyrus are stimulated.

Direct electrical stimulation of the primary motor cortex also has revealed another important finding: Stimulation never elicits a complex, coordinated motor movement. Only simple muscle contractions are observed. This implies that the primary motor cortex is not the designer of purposeful, sequenced movements. If it were, electrical stimulation of its neurons would result in some type of complex movement pattern. The principal role of the primary motor cortex is thought to be to take voluntary movement patterns that are formulated elsewhere and transmit them to the cranial or spinal nerves via the tract of motor neurons called the pyramidal system.

However, it is too simplistic to think of the primary motor cortex as just a relay station for incoming movement patterns. It

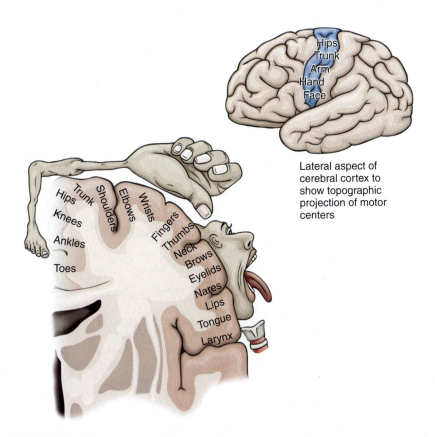

FIGURE 2-14. The neurons in the primary motor cortex are arranged in an inverted body scheme, with the neurons at the bottom of the gyrus being responsible for transmitting motor impulses to the neck and face muscles and the neurons at the top transmitting the impulses to the leg and foot muscles.

also has the ability to integrate information from other cortical areas into a planned movement. The **premotor area** and **supplementary motor area** both provide additional input to the primary motor cortex before a movement is initiated (Figure 2-15). These two cortical areas are located immediately anterior to the primary motor cortex, with the supplementary motor area extending over the top of the cerebral hemisphere and down into the longitudinal fissure. The neural signals contributed by these two areas are believed to exert further control over the final motor signals sent out by the primary motor cortex. The impulses from the premotor area seem to be especially important in visually guided movements, such as inserting a key in a lock. When this area is damaged, hand movements are notably clumsy. The influence of the supplementary motor area is a bit less definite. Neural signals from this area appear to facilitate the simultaneous use of both hands during complex sequences of movements.

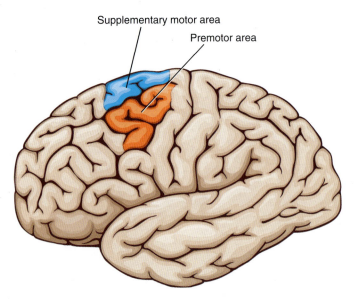

FIGURE 2-15. The premotor and supplementary motor areas play important roles in controlling and refining movements. The premotor area contributes to visually guided movements, and the supplementary motor area helps coordinate complex movements that involve the use of both hands.

Descending Motor Tracts

The descending motor tracts are the neural pathways carrying motor impulses that travel from the cortex to the brainstem and spinal cord. They are divided into two categories: the pyramidal system and extrapyramidal system. The functions of these two systems can be generalized by saying that the pyramidal system is responsible for carrying the impulses that control voluntary, fine motor movements, and the extrapyramidal system transmits impulses that control the postural support needed by those fine motor movements. For example, when someone is typing on a keyboard, it is the pyramidal system that carries the motor impulses that enable the person to make coordinated, independent finger movements on the keys. The extrapyramidal system, in turn, carries the impulses that keep the arms, shoulders, and back in a position that permits the fingers to move over the keyboard. Another generalization about these two systems is that the pyramidal system works at a conscious level, with the extrapyramidal system being more unconscious and automatic in its functions. As with any generalization, these are not absolutely true in every respect, but they do provide a good starting point for understanding the complex motor pathways that connect the higher centers of the brain to the muscles.

Pyramidal System

In the pyramidal system, most of the nerve fibers take a more or less direct path from the primary motor cortex to the brainstem or spinal cord, where they eventually synapse with cranial or spinal nerves. In fact, the pyramidal tract is sometimes called the **direct activation system** because of its relatively straight pathway from the cortex to the cranial and spinal nerves. Incidentally, the name *pyramidal* system comes from a point in the medulla (called the pyramids) where these descending fibers are compressed tightly together. By whatever name, this motor pathway is a key component of the motor system. Its fibers are divided into the corticospinal and corticobulbar tracts. The **corticospinal tract** is made up of axons that descend down from the cortex, through the **internal capsule**, the brainstem, and into the spinal cord (Figure 2–16). The axons terminate in the spinal cord, where many of them synapse with spinal nerves. The **corticobulbar tract** also is composed of axons descending from the cortex, but its axons terminate in the brainstem, where they synapse eventually with the cranial nerves. The term **bulbar** is a reference to an old name for the medulla, which once was known as the bulb. In summary, the pyramidal system consists of motor neurons that make a mostly direct course from the cortex to the spinal cord (corticospinal tract) or to the brainstem (corticobulbar tract).

Most axons of the pyramidal system have cell bodies that are located in the primary motor cortex. Some fibers of this system, however, also originate from the premotor cortex, the supplementary motor cortex, and the primary sensory cortex. Both corticospinal and corticobulbar fibers descend close to each other through the cerebrum. In the medulla, most corticospinal fibers cross the midline at a point called the pyramidal **decussation** and continue down the opposite side into the spinal cord. Beginning in the midbrain and continuing through the rest of the brainstem, the corticobulbar fibers gradually separate from the corticospinal fibers.

Unlike in the corticospinal tract, the fibers in the corticobulbar tract do not all cross the midline. They are distributed in a complex bilateral pattern before they synapse with the cranial nerves (Figure 2–17), which results in bilateral cortical **innervation** for most cranial nerves. This means, for example, that a stroke affecting the corticobulbar fibers in the left hemisphere will not paralyze most muscles served by the cranial nerves, because both the right and

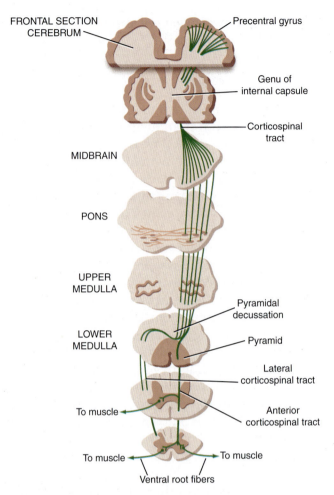

FIGURE 2-16. The corticospinal tract of the pyramidal system provides a more or less direct connection between the primary motor cortex (precentral gyrus) and the spinal nerves.

left cranial nerves will still receive motor innervation from the undamaged right hemisphere. The cranial nerves serving the muscles of the larynx, pharynx, palate, upper face, and jaw all receive this bilateral innervation. Keep in mind, however, that the muscles of the lower face and tongue primarily have **unilateral** innervation. These two parts of the head can be notably affected by unilateral cortical damage. Cranial nerve innervation of the head and neck muscles is discussed in greater detail in Chapter 4.

The pyramidal system is rudimental in lower animals such as mice and rats. In successively higher animals (dogs, monkeys, humans), it becomes increasingly larger and more sophisticated.

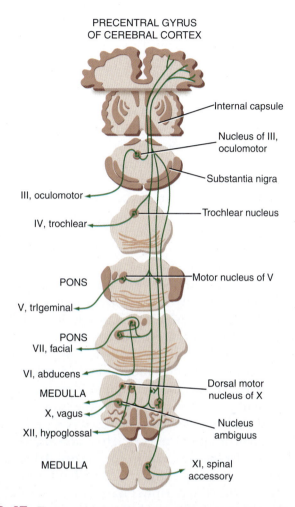

FIGURE 2-17. The corticobulbar tract of the pyramidal system connects the primary motor cortex (precentral gyrus) with most of the cranial nerves.

Damage to these fibers usually results in muscle weakness and rapid fatigue. Patients with injuries to the pyramidal system also report that increased mental concentration is needed to perform motor tasks that were previously accomplished with ease. In the motor speech system, unilateral damage to the pyramidal system results in a loss of fine motor movement in the articulators, a condition known as **unilateral upper motor neuron dysarthria** (see Chapter 6). However, the symptoms of pyramidal tract damage must be interpreted cautiously because other neural tracts are located close to the pyramidal fibers as they course through the cerebrum and brainstem. Damage that affects the pyramidal tract will almost always affect these other tracts as well, with results that complicate the clinical picture.

Extrapyramidal System

The extrapyramidal system is composed of a number of different, interconnected descending motor pathways. The term *extrapyramidal* simply refers to the motor tracts that are not part of the pyramidal system ("extra" to the pyramidal system). Many neurophysiologists do not use extrapyramidal when referring to these additional motor tracts because they think it inadequately depicts their varied functions. Some prefer to call it the **indirect activation system**, believing that this phrase better describes the system's complex, multiple interconnections. Others simply omit any single collective name and describe each descending motor pathway separately. Although recognizing these objections, this textbook uses the term *extrapyramidal* for this system because it is still used widely in clinical settings, and it does provide a broad, shorthand way to describe these motor tracts.

Four descending pathways of the extrapyramidal system are discussed here: the rubrospinal tract, reticulospinal tract, vestibulospinal tract, and tectospinal tract. Remember that each of these is similar to the pyramidal system in that they are neural motor pathways between the higher levels of the nervous system and the cranial or spinal nerves. They are different in that they originate in the brainstem, not in the cortex. They also are different in that they have many connections with other regions of the brain as they proceed to the peripheral nerves. For example, the cerebral cortex, the basal ganglia, and the cerebellum all have neural connections to the extrapyramidal system, through which these higher levels of the brain are able to directly influence the actions of the muscles innervated by the extrapyramidal tracts.

The **rubrospinal tract** originates in a group of neurons in the brainstem called the red nucleus (Figure 2–18). Its nerve fibers cross the midline shortly after leaving the red nucleus and continue down to the spinal cord. Because numerous rubrospinal fibers are mixed with pyramidal fibers and have synaptic connections in many of the same areas, it is thought that this tract might assist the pyramidal system in controlling voluntary movements.

The **reticulospinal tract** originates in the **reticular formation**, which is a group of cells coursing through the midbrain, pons, and medulla (Figure 2–19). The reticular formation has several important functions. In addition to being part of the extrapyramidal motor system, it has controlling effects on an individual's level of consciousness, blood pressure, respiration, and attention. The

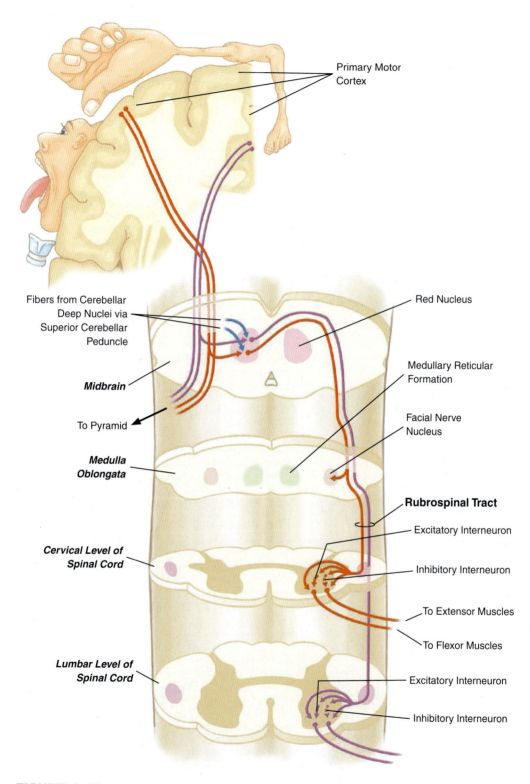

FIGURE 2–18. The rubrospinal tract—one of the tracts of the extrapyramidal system.

45

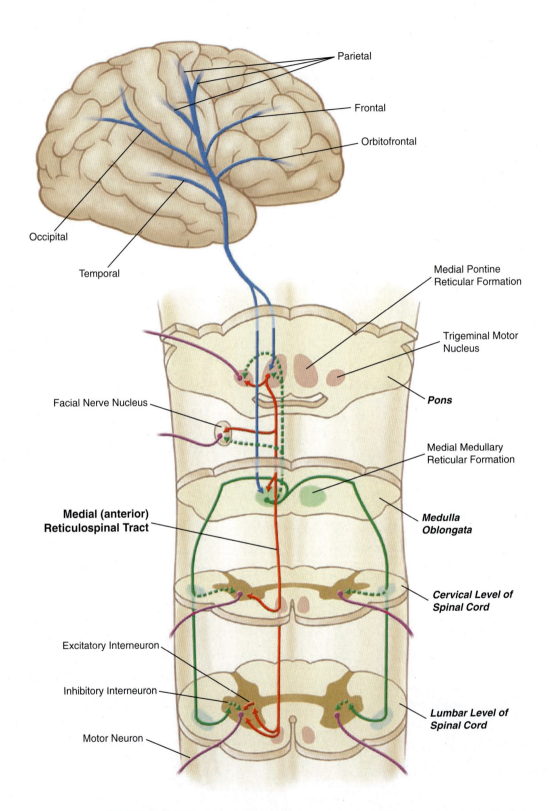

FIGURE 2–19. The reticulospinal tract (reticulospinal and corticoreticular pathways)—another tract of the extrapyramidal system.

fibers of the reticulospinal tract receive afferent input from many sources, including the motor and sensory cortices, the basal ganglia, the substantia nigra, and the red nucleus. Because of these varied inputs, the reticulospinal tract has an important influence on the spinal nerves. This tract is believed to be especially important in maintaining upright posture and the body's ability to turn toward external stimuli. It also might allow for some voluntary, gross motor movements, such as raising an arm or leg. Furthermore, the reticular formation and the reticulospinal tract contain "built-in" reflexive motor patterns that can operate without higher nervous system input. For example, this tract enables some infants born without a cerebrum to perform basic movements such as sucking, stretching, and yawning.

The final two extrapyramidal tracts have little to do with motor speech production, so we mention them only briefly. The vestibulospinal tract originates in the vestibular apparatus of the inner ear, courses through the pons and medulla, and terminates in the spinal cord. It helps the body maintain posture and balance. The last tract is the tectospinal tract. Its fibers originate in the midbrain and end in the cervical portion of the spinal cord. This tract receives many afferent inputs from the eyes and the visual cortex and, consequently, plays an important role in keeping the eyes and the head oriented to external stimuli.

It is useful to think of the extrapyramidal system as operating in parallel with the pyramidal system. This means that while the pyramidal system is transmitting fine motor neural impulses to the cranial and spinal nerves, the extrapyramidal system is simultaneously controlling the muscles that provide the postural support needed to accomplish those fine motor movements. Taken as a whole, the postural muscles innervated by the extrapyramidal system include those of the torso and the larger muscle groups of the arms and legs. The extrapyramidal system's influence on the cranial nerves and muscles of the speech mechanism is not completely understood. It is known that neurons in the reticular formation (the origin of the reticulospinal tract) have many synaptic connections with the cranial nerves. Through those connections, the extrapyramidal system influences the reflexes, muscle tone, and probably some voluntary movements of the speech mechanism.

Cranial and Spinal Nerves

Before discussing cranial and spinal nerves, the difference between upper and lower motor neurons needs to be examined. Various authors have used different criteria for defining upper motor neurons. For example, some say that upper motor neurons are only those in the pyramidal system. Others state that the definition should include all the motor neurons in the CNS. This textbook uses this second definition. **Upper motor neurons** are all the descending motor fibers coursing through the CNS that eventually make a synaptic connection to the motor neurons in the PNS. This includes the two pathways of the pyramidal system (the corticospinal and corticobulbar tracts) and the pathways of the extrapyramidal system (the rubrospinal, reticulospinal, vestibulospinal, and tectospinal tracts). To put it briefly, upper motor neurons are the motor fibers within the CNS. **Lower motor neurons**, in contrast, are the motor neurons in the cranial and spinal nerves. From a clinical standpoint, the distinction between these is important because damage to upper motor neurons results in symptoms that are usually quite different from those seen after damage to lower motor neurons. In general, upper motor neuron damage results in spasticity. The motor speech disorder associated with bilateral upper motor neuron damage is called **spastic dysarthria** (Chapter 5). Lower motor neuron damage results in muscle paralysis or paresis (weakness). **Flaccid dysarthria** (Chapter 4) is the result of damage to the lower motor neurons in the cranial nerves that innervate the muscles of speech production.

Cranial Nerve Nuclei

As stated previously, the cranial nerves are attached to the brainstem at points called the cranial nerve nuclei. Figure 2–20 shows that a cranial nerve's sensory and motor fibers separately branch out from the brainstem. The cell bodies of the sensory neurons are gathered outside the brainstem in a bundle called a cranial **ganglion**. The cell bodies of the lower motor neurons are grouped inside the brainstem. It is in that area within the brainstem that the lower motor neurons in the cranial nerves synapse with upper motor neurons from the pyramidal and extrapyramidal systems. If the complex interaction of neurotransmitters from upper motor neurons reaches a certain excitatory threshold, the upper motor neurons will transmit their motor impulses to the cranial nerve motor neuron, which will then transmit its own neural impulse directly to the muscle tissue it innervates.

Spinal Nerve Nuclei

The spinal nerves are attached to the spinal cord in a manner that is roughly similar to the attachments of the cranial nerves and brain-

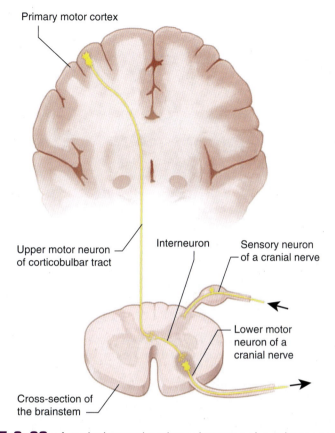

FIGURE 2–20. A typical neural pathway between the primary motor cortex and the lower motor neuron of a cranial nerve. The cell bodies of motor neurons in the cranial nerves are located within the brainstem at sites known as cranial nerve nuclei.

stem (Figure 2–21). The sensory and motor fibers branch from the spinal cord separately. As with the sensory fibers of the cranial nerves, a spinal ganglion contains the cell bodies of the sensory neurons. Spinal sensory fibers attach to the spinal cord on its **dorsal** (back) surface. A cross-sectional view of the spinal cord (Figures 2–21 and 2–22) shows that the center of the spinal cord contains an H-shaped region of gray matter. This spinal gray matter is composed of neuron cell bodies. The cell bodies of the lower motor neurons in the spinal nerves are located in the **ventral** (front) horn of the spinal gray matter. This is where the spinal nerves' lower motor neurons synapse with the pyramidal system, extrapyramidal system, and sensory neurons. From the ventral horn, the motor axons of the spinal nerves project out to the muscles they innervate (Figure 2–23). Again, the interplay of neurotransmitters from the upper motor (and

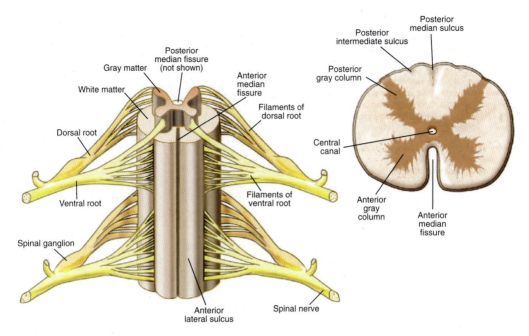

FIGURE 2–21. Motor neurons in spinal nerves branch off from the anterior portion of the spinal cord (inside the ventral roots).

also sensory) neurons at their synaptic connections with the spinal lower motor neurons determines whether a neural impulse will be transmitted to a muscle.

Neuromuscular Junction

Finally, the neural impulse arrives at the place where a muscle actually contracts to cause a movement. The **neuromuscular junction** is the point where the axons of lower motor neurons make synaptic connections with muscle cells (Figure 2–24). At the end of a motor neuron axon, there are many small terminal branches that synapse with the membrane of a muscle cell. Each of these small branches makes a synaptic connection with only one muscle cell. When the neural impulse traveling down the axon reaches the terminal branch, the neurotransmitter acetylcholine is released by the axon into the microscopic gap between the axon and the muscle cell. This neurotransmitter binds to special receptors in the membrane of the muscle cell. When enough acetylcholine is present in the muscle cell receptors, an electrochemical impulse occurs throughout the muscle cell, which then causes the contraction of the muscle fiber.

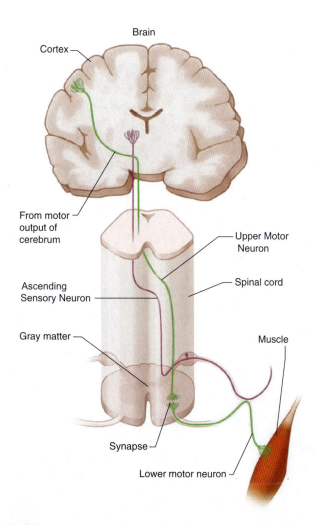

FIGURE 2-22. The cell bodies of motor neurons in the spinal nerves are located in the ventral horns of the spinal cord gray matter. The cell bodies of sensory neurons in the spinal nerves are located just outside the spinal cord.

With its numerous terminal branches, a single axon is able to cause contractions in many individual muscle cells. The actual number of muscle cells innervated by an axon varies according to the amount of fine motor control needed by a body part. A single axon may innervate many hundreds of individual muscle cells in large muscle groups or just a few cells in the muscles that perform intricate movements, depending on how much control of the movement is necessary. In the thigh, for example, a neural impulse from one axon will cause the simultaneous contraction of many muscle cells, which is appropriate, as the thigh is seldom called on to make small, discrete movements. However, in the face or fingers,

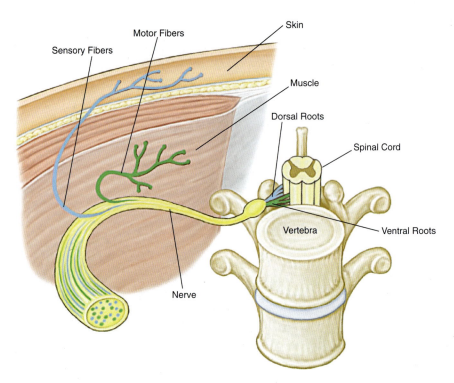

FIGURE 2-23. Spinal nerves transmit motor impulses to the skeletal muscles and sensory impulses from the skin, joints, and other areas of the body.

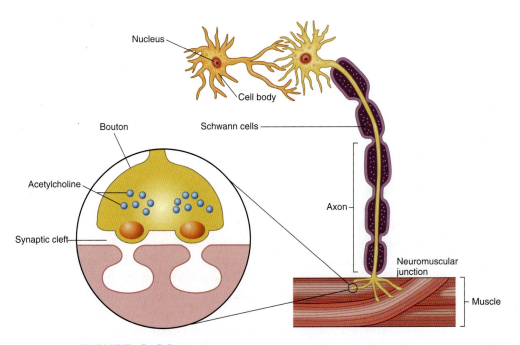

FIGURE 2-24. Lower motor neurons make synaptic connections with muscle tissue at the neuromuscular junction.

one axon will control only a handful of muscle fibers, resulting in greater cortical control over the contractions of those muscles. This difference in the number of muscle fibers innervated by a single axon is called the **innervation ratio**.

As stated at the beginning of this chapter, understanding the motor system is an important part of making the correct diagnosis of a motor speech disorder, as well as developing an appropriate treatment plan. If damage in any part of the motor system affects the muscles of speech production, the result can be a motor speech disorder. The particular motor speech disorder that occurs depends on which part of the motor system is damaged. Each of the upcoming chapters of this textbook examines one of the dysarthrias and apraxia of speech. Significant parts of the chapters are devoted to explaining how these disorders are linked to damage to specific parts of the motor system.

Summary of the Motor System

- The motor system is an important and very complex component of the nervous system. It is responsible for controlling all volitional movements.
- The motor system is composed of many parts, including the primary and association cortex, the basal ganglia, the cerebellum, the thalamus, the pyramidal and extrapyramidal tracts, and the neuromuscular junction. Either directly or indirectly, all of these components of the motor system communicate with each other through highly complex pathways within the nervous system.
- Damage at any level of the motor system can result in a movement disorder. When the damage affects the muscles of speech production, the result can be a motor speech disorder.

Study Questions

1. What is the cerebral cortex, and why is it important?
2. What are cranial nerve nuclei, and where are they located?
3. Describe the difference between tracts and nerves.
4. Describe the association cortex and its importance in formulating a movement.

5. How are the functions of the primary cortex different from the functions of the association cortex?
6. What roles do the basal ganglia and cerebellum play in the creation of a movement?
7. How is it known that movements do not originate in the primary motor cortex?
8. What is the difference between the pyramidal and extrapyramidal tracts?
9. Describe the anatomical distinction between lower and upper motor neurons.
10. What happens at the neuromuscular junction?

Chapter 3

Evaluation of Motor Speech Disorders

Goals of a Motor Speech Evaluation

Speech Production Components and Disorders
- Respiration
- Phonation
- Resonance
- Articulation
- Prosody

Standardized Tests for Dysarthria

Standardized Tests for Apraxia of Speech

Conducting a Motor Speech Evaluation
- Muscle Strength
- Speed of Movement
- Range of Movement
- Accuracy of Movement
- Motor Steadiness
- Muscle Tone

Instructions for the Motor Speech Evaluation
- Background Information and Medical History
- Face and Jaw Muscles at Rest and During Movement
  - *Explanation of Specific Tasks*
- Tongue at Rest and During Movement
  - *Explanation of Specific Tasks*
- Velum and Pharynx at Rest and During Movement
  - *Explanation of Specific Tasks*
- Laryngeal Function
  - *Explanation of Specific Tasks*

Auditory-Perceptual Evaluations of the Motor Speech Mechanism
- Phonatory-Respiratory System
  - *Explanation of Specific Tasks*
- Resonation System
  - *Explanation of Specific Tasks*
- Combined Systems (Phonation, Respiration, Resonation, and Articulation)
  - *Explanation of Specific Task*
- Stress Testing of the Motor Speech Mechanism
- Testing for Nonverbal Oral Apraxia
  - *Explanation of Specific Task*
- Testing for Apraxia of Speech
  - *Explanation of Specific Tasks*
- Analysis of Connected Speech

Summary of the Evaluation of Motor Speech Disorders

Study Questions

Appendix 3–1: Motor Speech Examination

Most beginning clinicians find evaluating and diagnosing motor speech disorders to be a challenging task for several reasons. First, it can be difficult to distinguish among the dysarthrias because many of the speech characteristics of one dysarthria will be present in one or more of the other dysarthrias. For example, imprecise consonants and harsh vocal quality are characteristics of every one of the dysarthrias. Second, an accurate diagnosis requires clinicians to listen very carefully to determine which of their patients' speech errors are most characteristic of a suspected motor speech disorder. Clinicians usually develop this skill with experience, which beginning clinicians will not have yet acquired. Finally, a detailed knowledge of the human motor system is an invaluable asset in determining which speech errors are most important in making a correct diagnosis.

It takes a concerted effort to learn about the motor system because it is such a complex organization of nerve cells and nervous system structures. However, when a clinician learns the parts and functions of the motor system, the many symptoms of motor speech disorders become less confusing. In short, the successful evaluation of motor speech disorders requires clinicians to match what they hear in a patient's speech with what they know about the functioning of the human motor system.

For beginning clinicians, the primary challenge is to become familiar with how speech varies from one motor speech disorder to another. Inexperienced clinicians need to learn what makes flaccid dysarthria different from spastic dysarthria, what makes ataxic dysarthria different from hypokinetic dysarthria, and so forth. Fortunately, the evaluation and diagnosis of motor speech disorders can be accurate if beginning clinicians learn the characteristics of motor speech disorders, become familiar with the neuromuscular bases of these disorders, and acquire hands-on practice in a clinical practicum.

There are two basic methods of evaluating motor speech disorders: instrumental and perceptual analysis. **Instrumental analysis** uses sophisticated devices to objectively measure the components of speech production.

For example, nasal and oral airflow during speech can be measured precisely by computerized instruments. Other instruments can accurately detect changes in voice onset time, atypical formant frequencies in vowels, subtle loudness variations, and many additional aspects of speech production. In contrast, in the perceptual analysis method of assessment, the examiner uses his or her ears to detect motor speech disorders. The value of the perceptual analysis method is that the ear is the ultimate judge of whether there is problem with an individual's speech. If a motor speech disorder cannot be detected by ear, is there actually a disorder that needs to be treated?

This textbook concentrates on the perceptual analysis method of evaluating motor speech disorders for several reasons. Although the importance of instrumental assessment of these disorders is without question, most practicing clinicians do not have access to such devices, and they must rely primarily on what their ears tell them. Furthermore, instrumental assessment is described in great detail in other sources. Readers wishing to learn more about instrumentation in the assessment and treatment of motor speech disorders should refer to a text such as Clinical Management of Sensorimotor Speech Disorders, Second Edition *(McNeil, 2009).*

Goals of a Motor Speech Evaluation

In many ways, the goals of a motor speech evaluation are no different from the goals of any speech-language evaluation. Haynes and Pindzola (2011) said that a speech-language evaluation is done to understand a patient's problem and to establish the beginning level of treatment. This certainly applies to a motor speech evaluation. During a motor speech evaluation, the clinician collects relevant background information about a patient and then asks the patient to perform numerous tasks to assess the function of his or her motor speech system. Once this information is collected, the clinician should have a good description and understanding of the patient's speech abilities. With this knowledge, the clinician also has a baseline against which to compare the effects of any treatment.

Duffy (2020), Swigert (2010), and others have suggested specific questions that clinicians should ask themselves during a motor speech evaluation. This list of questions is designed to lead clinicians to a correct diagnosis (Duffy, 2020). In fact, it is not an exaggeration to say that the primary purpose of a motor speech evaluation is to obtain the information necessary to answer these questions. If a clinician can answer each of the following questions with a detailed, informed, and accurate response, the evaluation will be nearly complete:

1. Is there a problem with the patient's speech?
2. If there is a problem, what is the best way to describe it?
3. Does the problem seem to be the result of a neurologic disorder?
4. If it seems to be neurologic in origin, did it appear suddenly or slowly?
5. Is the problem related strictly to speech production, or is it more of a problem with language, such as aphasia?
6. If it is a problem of speech production, do most of the problems seem to be related to the sequencing of phonemes (i.e., apraxia of speech)?
7. If there are no phoneme sequencing errors, what are the characteristics of the patient's speech errors and any associated motor problems?

The last two questions lead to the final steps in a motor speech evaluation. Question 6 asks whether the patient's speech disorder is dysarthria or apraxia of speech. Question 7 asks which type of dysarthria might be present. If clinicians are able answer these seven questions with confidence, they will likely make an accurate diagnosis.

Speech Production Components and Disorders

Speech does not just happen. It is dependent on the coordinated interactions of five components (or processes) that are essential for normal speech production—respiration, phonation, resonance, articulation, and prosody. These five components must work together and be combined smoothly for speech to be produced normally. When one or any combination of the five is affected by a neuromotor disturbance, the result will be a motor speech disorder, either dysarthria or apraxia of speech.

Dysarthria is a speech production deficit that results from neuromotor damage to the PNS or CNS. This damage could affect any of the five components of speech production. Dysarthria is not a language disorder, like aphasia, or a cognitive disorder, like dementia. Likewise, dysarthria is not a result of an abnormal anatomical structure (e.g., cleft palate), a sensory loss (e.g., deafness), or a psychological disturbance. It is strictly a speech production disorder caused by neuromotor damage. There are actually a number of different types of dysarthria, with each having its own characteristics. Table 3–1 lists the causes and some of the more obvious characteristics of the various dysarthrias.

Apraxia of speech also is a motor speech disorder. It is a deficit in the ability to create accurate phoneme sequences that have the correct timing and placement of articulatory movements. It often results in distorted articulation and prosody. Although it is the result of CNS damage, the movement problem in apraxia of speech is not caused by muscle weakness or slowness. As with dysarthria, apraxia of speech is neither a language or cognitive disorder, nor the result of an anatomical, sensory, or psychological disorder. It is a disorder in the ability to time-sequence the motor commands needed to move the articulators smoothly and accurately from one position to another during the production of voluntary speech.

As already mentioned, when any of the five components of speech production are affected by a neuromotor disorder, dysarthria or apraxia of speech will result. (Whether it is one or the other depends on where the disorder occurs in the nervous system. Apraxia of speech is nearly always associated with damage to the left hemisphere of the brain. Dysarthria, in contrast, can be caused by damage to many parts of the nervous system.) Because the five components of speech production play such important roles in motor speech disorders, each is discussed separately.

Respiration

The primary function of **respiration** is to exchange oxygen from the atmosphere for carbon dioxide from cells in the body. By exchanging these gases, respiration maintains life. Respiration also is essential for speech production. It provides the subglottic air pressure that is needed to set the vocal folds into vibration. Speech production depends on a full, steady supply of air—especially for connected speech. If the air supply is not full or steady, speech production is affected. For example, if the nerves that innervate the respiratory muscles are damaged, those muscles will be weak and might not be able to move as much air into and out of the lungs

TABLE 3–1 The Primary Etiologies and Characteristics of the Various Dysarthrias

Type of Dysarthria	Caused By	Primary Characteristics
1. Flaccid	Damage to the cranial nerves, spinal nerves, or the neuromuscular junction.	Muscle weakness that can result in imprecise consonants, breathy phonation, hypernasality, shallow breath support, and abnormal prosody.
2. Spastic	Bilateral damage to the upper motor neurons of the pyramidal and extrapyramidal systems; often caused by brainstem strokes.	Spasticity and weakness in the speech musculature that results in harsh or strained-strangled phonation, imprecise consonants, hypernasality, and abnormal prosody.
3. Unilateral Upper Motor Neuron	Unilateral damage to upper motor neurons.	Imprecise consonants are the most common characteristic. There may be irregular articulatory breakdowns or harsh vocal quality in some patients.
4. Ataxic	Damage to the cerebellum or the neural tracts that connect the cerebellum to the rest of the central nervous system.	Problems controlling the timing and force of speech movements, resulting in speech that often has a "drunken" quality. Imprecise consonants, distorted vowels, irregular articulatory breakdowns, and abnormal prosody.
5. Hypokinetic	A reduction of dopamine in part of the basal ganglia. Parkinsonism is the most common cause of this dysarthria.	A reduction in the range and speed of speech movements. Harsh or breathy phonation, imprecise consonants, and abnormal prosody. In some patients, there is an increased rate of speech.
6. Hyperkinetic	Often associated with damage to the basal ganglia, but in some conditions the cause is unknown.	Involuntary movements that interfere with normal speech production. Unexpected inhalations and exhalations, irregular articulatory breakdowns, and abnormal prosody.
7. Mixed	Neurological damage that extends to more than one portion of the motor system.	Any combination of the characteristics of the six pure dysarthrias. For example, a patient with parkinsonism could have a brainstem stroke that might result in a hypokinetic-spastic mixed dysarthria.

as they normally would. Therefore, nerve damage means less air for speech production, which limits the affected individual's ability to speak in anything but short phrases. In addition, respiratory deficits that reduce the amount of air available for speech can also cause reduced loudness and breathy voice quality.

Phonation

Phonation is the production of voiced phonemes through vocal-fold vibrations in the larynx. Normal phonation is dependent on the complete **adduction** of the vocal folds and enough subglottic air pressure to set the vocal folds to vibrating. Just the right amount of tension needs to be present during the adduction of the vocal folds to produce a clear phonation. Neuromotor damage to the nerves that innervate the vocal-fold adductor muscles can have several effects on speech production. In conditions such as flaccid dysarthria, the damage could cause weak or incomplete adduction. This weakness results in phonations that have a breathy or harsh quality. In conditions such as spastic dysarthria, the damage can cause the adduction to be too tight, which results in the phonation having a strained-strangled quality. Neuromotor damage to the laryngeal muscles also might reduce the ability to change pitch or loudness during phonation.

Resonance

Resonance is the proper placement of oral or nasal tonality onto phonemes during speech. This is accomplished by the raising and lowering of the velum. Oral resonance is produced when the velum is raised and closes off the nasal cavity from the vocal air stream, which sends the sounds through the oral cavity. Nasal resonance is produced when the velum is lowered and the oral cavity is blocked by the lips or tongue, thereby directing the entire air stream out through the nose. The key factor in this process is the movement of the velum. The muscles in the velum need to respond quickly to the different resonance requirements of the phonemes being produced during speech. When the nerves innervating these velar muscles are damaged, the muscles could be weakened or their movements slowed. Weak or slow velar muscles cannot raise the velum completely to separate the nasal cavity from the vocal air stream during the production of nonnasal speech phonemes. The resulting speech will have a hypernasal quality because nasal resonance is being applied to phonemes that ordinarily have only oral resonance.

Articulation

Articulation is the shaping of the vocal air stream into phonemes. This shaping is accomplished in different ways. The air stream may be blocked for stop and affricate phonemes, tightly restricted for fricative phonemes, slightly restricted for semivowels, or relatively unrestricted for vowels. The shaping of the air stream happens at various points along the vocal tract. It also is accomplished by different structures within the vocal tract, known as **articulators**. Correct articulation requires the articulators to perform movements that have the appropriate timing, direction, force, speed, and placement for any given phoneme. By any measure, accurate articulation is the result of a very complex series of movements.

Unfortunately, neuromotor damage often affects the articulators. When this damage affects the muscles of the lips, tongue, jaw, velum, or vocal folds, articulation is impaired. The degree of impairment depends on the severity of the damage and on which articulators are affected most severely. The articulation errors that can be heard after neuromotor damage include imprecise consonants, distorted vowels, inappropriate silences, and irregular articulatory breakdowns.

Prosody

Prosody is the melody of speech. In most instances, prosody uses stress and intonation to convey meaning. **Stress** is accomplished by changing the pitch, loudness, and duration of syllables within words to give those words added importance or to clarify meaning. **Intonation** is the use of pitch changes and stress to communicate, for example, whether an utterance is a question, assertion, or exclamation. Adding prosody to an utterance is not a simple task. Accurate and clear prosodic features of a message require the coordinated participation of phonation, respiration, resonance, and articulation. For example, to increase the loudness of a syllable or word, an increased exhalation of air from the lungs is coordinated with a simultaneous tensing of the vocal folds. To change pitch, the vocal folds lengthen or shorten, which is accomplished by the simultaneous actions of several laryngeal muscles. To increase the duration of a syllable, the articulators are held in their position for a moment longer than usual in coordination with a prolongation of phonation. The interactions of all of these vocal tract structures must be precise or prosody will sound abnormal.

Given that prosody is so dependent on the complex interaction of the other components of speech production, it should be easy to understand that neuromotor damage can affect prosody in a number of ways. For example, if the damage causes weakness or slowness in the muscles of respiration and phonation, the strength of these muscles and the timing of their contractions will be impaired. The resulting speech could have a monopitch and monoloud quality. If the damage causes involuntary movements of the vocal-tract muscles, the involuntary movements will interfere with voluntary speech movements. The resulting speech might have irregular pitch variations, sudden increases or decreases in loudness, and prolonged intervals between syllables or words.

Standardized Tests for Dysarthria

Compared to other adult communication disorders (e.g., aphasia), there are relatively few published standardized tests for dysarthria (Hegde & Freed, 2022). One potential reason for this is the wide availability of detailed, informal dysarthria assessment tools inside a number of textbooks. Duffy (2020), Hegde and Freed (2022), and Yorkston et al. (2010) each include complete assessment tools for dysarthria in their chapters on assessment of motor speech disorders. Nevertheless, the stand-alone standardized tests that are available do provide a few special features that are not found in the textbook-based assessments.

- **Frenchay Dysarthria Assessment-2** (Enderby & Palmer, 2008)—First published in 1983, the Frenchay Dysarthria Assessment-2 is unique in that it is the only published test that aids in the differential diagnosis of the various dysarthrias and provides information on intelligibility. Moreover, this test also suggests which elements of the client's speech most affect intelligibility, something that can assist in developing treatment goals. The client's performance on a variety of tasks (reflexes, respiration, lips and tongue at rest and during movement, velopharyngeal closure, laryngeal function, and intelligibility for words, sentences, and conversation) is rated on a 9-point scale. The administration time is reasonably short. The authors report good intra- and interrater reliability and validity. Normative data are provided for ages 12 to 97 and for clients with specific types of dysarthria.

- **Assessment of Intelligibility of Dysarthric Speech** (Yorkston & Beukelman, 1981)— This test is a widely used standardized assessment of intelligibility. It examines single-word and sentence intelligibility of speakers with dysarthria. It also provides data on speaking rate. For the single-word assessment task, clients are asked to randomly read 50 words while being audiotaped. Later, a naive listener judges the client's productions for intelligibility by listening to the audio recording. By determining the total number of words spoken and the total number that were correctly understood by the listener, a percentage of intelligible words is easily calculated. A similar procedure is used for assessing sentence intelligibility. The client randomly reads 22 sentences, ranging in length from 5 to 15 words, while again being audiotaped. The naive listener then transcribes the words in the sentences while listening to the recording, and thereby provides a percentage of words that were understood correctly. The rate of speech is calculated by dividing the time it takes to read the sentences into the total number of words spoken. The Assessment of Intelligibility of Dysarthric Speech is also able to provide estimates of severity and communication efficiency (i.e., how close the client's speech is to normal speech).

- **The Speech Intelligibility Test for Windows** (Beukelman et al., 2007)—This test is an updated version of the Computerized Assessment of Intelligibility of Dysarthric Speech (Yorkston et al., 1984). Like the Assessment of Intelligibility of Dysarthric Speech, the Speech Intelligibility Test for Windows provides measures of single-word and sentence intelligibility, rate of speech, and communication efficiency. The calculation of scores is done automatically by the computer program, allowing for a quick determination of intelligibility percentages and rate of speech. In addition, the program is able to determine a percentage of correct vowels and consonants (including specific scores for stops, fricatives, affricates, semi-vowels, nasals, and pressure consonants). Interjudge reliability of this test is good.

- **The Dysarthria Impact Profile** (Walshe et al., 2009)—This self-report questionnaire examines the patient's perception of how dysarthria affects his or her life. Such information can be valuable in planning the course of treatment because patients might have unrealistic perceptions about their condition. It is possible that a patient with a moderate to severe dysarthria might think the disorder is quite mild. Conversely, another patient might feel that the severity is high, when family and friends actually describe it as mild. In either case, the patient's misperceptions are likely to affect the course of treatment and complicate successful communication in natural settings. In a situation where a patient's reports of communication success or failure vary significantly from those of family and friends, the Dysarthria Impact Profile might be a useful part of the assessment. The test is divided into four sections: (a) The Effect of Dysarthria on Me as a Person, (b) Accepting My Dysarthria, (c) How I Feel Others React to My Speech, and (d) How Dysarthria Affects My Communication With Others. Typical statements to be rated include, "I rely on others to talk for me whenever possible," and "I don't care what other people think of my speech." Responses are recorded on a 5-point scale, ranging from *strongly agree* to *strongly disagree*. The administration time is approximately 15 min.

Standardized Tests for Apraxia of Speech

The only standardized, norm-referenced assessment of apraxia of speech is the **Apraxia Battery for Adults-Second Edition** (ABA-2; Dabul, 2000). It is designed to diagnose apraxia of speech in adolescents and adults, as well as measure severity. Compared to the first edition, the ABA-2 includes more difficult items for detecting mild apraxia of speech and has updated norm data (49 normal individuals and 40 with apraxia). It also includes suggestions for treatment planning, recognizing atypical profiles, and tracking changes in speech production over time. The administration time is short, only about 20 min. The test manual includes psychometric data for reliability, content validity, criterion-related validity, and construct validity. No data are reported for intrajudge reliability, interjudge reliability, or test–retest reliability. The ABA-2 contains six subtests:

- Diadochokinetic Rate—The client is asked to say the syllable combinations "puh-tuh," "tuh-kuh," and "puh-tuh-kuh" for 3 s over three trials. The clinician records how many repetitions are produced on each trial, with the highest number recorded as a "Best Trial."
- Increasing Word Length—The client is asked to repeat three words of increasing length (e.g., thick–thicker–thickening). The clinician scores the productions on a scale of 0 to 2.
- Limb Apraxia and Oral Apraxia—The client is asked to perform hand and arm movements (e.g., "Show me how you

make a fist") and nonverbal oral movements (e.g., "Stick out your tongue"). The client's responses are scored on a scale of 0 to 5.

- Latency Time and Utterance Time for Polysyllabic Words—The client is asked to name pictures; the clinician records how long it takes from the initial presentation of the picture to the beginning of the utterance (latency time) and how long it takes to say the target word or words (utterance time).
- Repeated Trials Test—The client is asked to repeat target words three times. The clinician counts the number of errors in each production and then compares the number of errors in the first and third productions, scoring a minus if there are fewer errors in the first attempt compared to the third, scoring a plus if there are more in the first compared to the third, and scoring a zero if there is no difference.
- Inventory of Articulation Characteristics of Apraxia—The clinician obtains and analyzes speech samples from the client (see the following paragraph).

The final subtest of the ABA-2 (Inventory of Articulatory Characteristics of Apraxia) asks the clinician to obtain several speech samples by asking the client to describe a picture, read aloud, and count to 30. Based on these three samples, the clinician determines the presence or absence of 15 speech behaviors. If 5 or more of them are present in the sample, the client could have a diagnosis of apraxia of speech:

1. Exhibits phonemic anticipatory errors
2. Exhibits phonemic perseverative errors
3. Exhibits phonemic transposition errors
4. Exhibits phonemic voicing errors
5. Exhibits phonemic vowel errors
6. Exhibits visible/audible searching
7. Exhibits numerous off-target attempts at the word
8. Errors are highly inconsistent
9. Errors increase as phonemic sequence increases
10. Exhibits fewer errors with automatic speech than volitional speech
11. Exhibits marked difficulty initiating speech
12. Intrudes schwa sound between syllables or in consonant clusters

13. Exhibits abnormal prosodic features
14. Exhibits awareness of errors and inability to correct them
15. Exhibits expressive-receptive gap

The behaviors on this list are reflective of the traditional characteristics of apraxia of speech, but some researchers have questioned whether all the items have the ability to differentiate apraxia of speech from those found in other speech and language disorders, such as the literal paraphasias in fluent aphasia. For example, Pierce (1991) reported that only three of these (difficulty initiating speech, intrusion of the schwa, and abnormal prosody) are observed primarily in apraxia of speech; most of the others can be seen in clients with either apraxia of speech or fluent aphasia. McNeil et al. (2009) went even further and suggested that only the intrusion of the schwa and abnormal prosody are exclusively seen in individuals with apraxia of speech. All the remaining items are observed exclusively in cases of fluent aphasia (anticipatory, perseverative, and transposition errors; very inconsistent errors) or in either disorder (the remaining nine items). Until these questions are resolved with further research, clinicians using the full ABA-2 to diagnose apraxia of speech might want to interpret the results with caution or confirm the test's findings with additional assessments. Some researchers, however, have used selected subtests of the ABA-2 as part of their own nonstandardized assessment protocols to diagnose apraxia of speech or estimate severity. For example, Wambaugh et al. (2013) used the ABA-2's Increasing Word Length and Repeated Trials subtests, along with a discourse task, a consonant production probe, a sentence repetition task, and a multisyllabic word repetition task to help determine the presence of apraxia of speech.

Although it is not a commercially published standardized test like the ABA-2, the Apraxia of Speech Rating Scale (ASRS) also is available (Strand et al., 2014). For the ASRS, the clinician administers a variety of spoken language tasks that are designed to evoke speech errors typically found in apraxia of speech: short conversation, picture description, word repetition, prolonged vowel, alternate motion rate (AMR), sequential motion rate (SMR), and sentence repetition. A patient's performance on these tasks is then matched to 13 characteristics of apraxia of speech and rated on a 5-point scale ranging from 0 (*not observed*) to 4 (*severe*). The 13 characteristics are similar to those described by Wambaugh et al. (2006a), which are examined in Chapter 11. A unique aspect of the ASRS is that it accommodates the co-occurring presence of either dysarthria, aphasia, or both. The ASRS has been refined several times since its first introduction, and Duffy et al. (2023) reported good reliability and validity for the latest version of the ASRS. However, Hybbinette et al. (2021) cautioned that clinicians without extensive experience with apraxia of speech might have difficulty achieving adequate inter- and intrajudge reliability when scoring it.

Conducting a Motor Speech Evaluation

The following pages contain a complete, detailed review of the motor speech examination found at the end of this chapter (Appendix 3–1). The tasks on this examination were collected and adapted from a variety of sources, including the Marshfield Clinic Motor Speech Examination (unpublished), Darley et al. (1975), and Wertz et al. (1991). When conducting this motor speech examination, the clinician is assessing the components of a patient's motor speech system.

Respiration, phonation, articulation, resonance, and prosody are all evaluated using these tasks. However, a clinician also should be careful to assess more than just the five components of speech production. As the evaluation is administered, the clinician needs to constantly assess the patient's muscle strength, speed of movement, range of motion, accuracy of movement, motor steadiness, and muscle tone. These neuromuscular processes are the foundation of all voluntary movement in the body. Darley et al. (1975) called these six processes the "salient features" of neuromuscular function. Each of these salient features makes its own contribution to normal speech production. If any of these are defective, the motor speech system will be affected adversely. Moreover, the nature and degree of a defect can provide important information for making a correct diagnosis, which is why the features need to be examined carefully during a motor speech examination.

Muscle Strength

If a muscle within the motor speech mechanism does not have adequate strength, it might not be able to perform its speech production tasks adequately. Decreased muscle strength anywhere in the motor speech mechanism can affect respiration, articulation, resonance, phonation, and prosody. Muscle strength is assessed in numerous sections of this book's motor speech evaluation protocol. For example, a patient is asked to press his or her tongue against a tongue blade or asked to count out loud from 1 to 100 (a task known as "stress testing" the speech mechanism).

Speed of Movement

Accurate speech requires very rapid muscle movements. The tongue and vocal folds, in particular, make many rapid movements during the production of even a short utterance. Reduced speed of movement is a common characteristic of most dysarthrias; however, one dysarthria, hypokinetic dysarthria, could have increased speed of movement. Speed of movement is assessed through tasks that concentrate on AMR and SMR. AMR tasks move the articulators through a single series of rapid back-and-forth movements, such as repeating "puh, puh, puh" or "tuh, tuh, tuh" as rapidly as possible. SMR tasks, in contrast, move the articulators repeatedly through a quick sequence of movements, such as repeating "puh, tuh, kuh" as many times as possible on one breath of air. Both AMR and SMR tasks are included in the protocol.

Range of Movement

Range of movement is how far the articulators can travel during the course of a movement. Instances of reduced range of movement include an inability to fully open the jaw or completely adduct the vocal folds. Darley et al. (1975) and Duffy (2020) both mentioned that prosody, especially, could be affected by reduced range of movement in the articulators. Range of movement is assessed most directly in the first portion of the protocol, during which the patient is asked to extend or hold the articulators in various positions.

Accuracy of Movement

Clear speech production requires accurate movements by the articulators. An accurate movement is one in which strength, speed, range, direction, and timing are precisely coordinated (Darley et al., 1975). If any of these are out of sync, the result can be an inaccurate movement, causing such problems as a distorted consonant or intermittent hypernasality. The AMR and SMR tasks are good for assessing the accuracy of movement, as are conversational speech and spoken paragraph reading.

Motor Steadiness

Motor steadiness is the ability to hold a body part still. There are several disorders in which involuntary movements prevent motor steadiness, the most common of which is tremor. These involuntary contractions can affect the laryngeal musculature and lead to a tremulous vocal quality during speech. Other disorders can cause larger, more obvious, involuntary movements that interfere with all voluntary movements. In the protocol in Appendix 3–1, motor steadiness is assessed by tasks that require a patient to hold a position or prolong a vowel. A breakdown in motor steadiness will reveal itself in an inability to maintain a still position or to produce a prolonged vowel that is smooth and steady.

Muscle Tone

Normal muscle tone is the small, constant amount of muscle contraction that is always present, even when a muscle is fully relaxed. Muscle tone maintains a muscle in a "ready-to-move" condition and allows for quick movement when necessary. Damage to the nervous system can either decrease or increase muscle tone, depending on where the damage occurs. Both circumstances can have detrimental effects on movement. Decreased muscle tone is associated with muscle weakness or paralysis. Increased tone is associated with muscle spasticity or rigidity. In the Appendix 3–1 protocol, abnormal muscle tone can be inferred by listening to the patient's speech or by looking at the affected body parts.

Instructions for the Motor Speech Evaluation

Because most readers of this textbook probably have not administered many motor speech evaluations, the following pages offer a step-by-step explanation of what each task is assessing. When appropriate, an explanation of the importance of a task is provided. The entire evaluation takes between 30 and 40 min to administer, depending on the capabilities of the patient. When this much time is not available, it is possible to use the short version of the examination. (By performing only the items in **bold type** on the form, the administration time is cut to about 15 min, while still sampling the patient's abilities in most of the examination's subsections.) Once the evaluation is completed, the clinician will have fully assessed and described the patient's speech production abilities. From the information collected about the patient, the clinician should be able to make an accurate diagnosis of any motor speech disorder that might be present.

Background Information and Medical History

This first portion of the evaluation usually is completed without too much difficulty. The information can be obtained from the patient, family members, other medical professionals, and medical records. It is important to be as thorough as possible when collecting this information because it can provide many clues leading to a correct diagnosis. For example, slow development of the problem could indicate a progressive neurologic disorder. On the other hand, a rapid onset might suggest that an acute condition caused the disorder, perhaps a stroke. Medical records can provide important information on the patient's medical history, possible site of lesion, and current status of the problem. Rosenbek et al. (1989) recommended that the following information be obtained from medical records:

- The primary and secondary medical diagnoses, along with descriptions of the major symptoms.
- The date when the condition was first noted, sometimes called the "date of onset."
- Information on the site of a lesion (i.e., the place in the nervous system where the damage has occurred).
- Earlier instances of nervous system damage.
- Evidence of limb involvement, such as weakness, involuntary movements, or motor sequencing problems (limb apraxia).
- Information on the patient's visual acuity, including any evidence of visual-field deficits.
- Information on the patient's hearing acuity.

If the patient is being interviewed for this section, you should first provide a brief overview of the assessment tasks and their purpose. Such an introduction might relieve the patient's anxiety regarding the assessment and help to ensure his or her full participation in the tasks. During this initial interview, you can also learn much about the patient's awareness of and reaction to the problem. Some individuals might recognize that their speech is different, yet they are not worried about it. Others might appear to be very troubled by a problem that is so mild as to be imperceptible to most listeners. Such information is valuable in making recommendations for treatment.

Face and Jaw Muscles at Rest and During Movement

This section of the evaluation examines the muscles of the patient's face. You are looking for any abnormal muscle tone or strength, asymmetrical facial features, and restricted range of movement. Most of these tasks assess the functioning of the facial cranial nerve (VII), because it provides motor innervation to the facial muscles. The trigeminal cranial nerve (V) is examined during the tasks that require jaw movements.

Explanation of Specific Tasks

1. Is the mouth symmetrical? Here the examiner is looking for any signs of lower-face paralysis or weakness, which can cause one side of the mouth to droop lower than the other. Be aware, however, that a small amount of mouth asymmetry is normal and does not necessarily indicate a neuromuscular disorder.
2. Can the examiner force the lips open? On this task, the examiner is checking for muscle strength. Of course, the side of the mouth that is drooping will almost always be the weaker side. This will be the side that one should be able to force open more easily with the fingers.
3. Does the face have an expressionless, mask-like appearance? This task checks for one of the more obvious symptoms of parkinsonism (see Chapter 8). Individuals with parkinsonism frequently have a reduced ability to express emotion through their facial expressions. Individuals with moderate and severe parkinsonism might consistently show a blank facial expression, no matter what their internal emotional state might be.
4. When the patient looks up, is there wrinkling on both halves of the forehead? This task assesses the possible site of neurologic damage. If the damage has occurred, for example, to the right facial cranial nerve (VII) near where it branches out from the brainstem, the entire right half of the affected side of the face will be weakened or paralyzed. In this situation, when the patient looks up, the skin of the right side of the forehead will not wrinkle, because the forehead muscles on that side of the face will not contract

normally. If, however, the damage has occurred to either the left or right tract of the upper motor neurons, muscles of both sides of the forehead will most likely show movement, with only the lower face showing evidence of weakness or paralysis. This is because the upper branch of the facial cranial nerve that serves the forehead muscles receives bilateral innervation from the upper motor neurons, but the lower branch serving the lower face receives only unilateral innervation from the upper motor neurons. The innervation of the facial muscles is explained in more detail in Chapter 4.

5. Is the patient's smile symmetrical? This task and the next two look at voluntary movement of the lower face muscles. The examiner is checking for any evidence of weakness or reduced range of motion. In addition, you need to check for signs that the patient is groping for the correct position to accomplish this task. If groping is present, it could be evidence of a nonverbal oral apraxia. In such a case, be sure to administer the portions of the protocol covering apraxia. Apraxia of speech is covered in Chapter 11.

6. Is the patient able to pucker his or her lips? This task assesses muscular strength and range of movement of the orbicularis oris muscles of the lips. Weakness on one side of the mouth could result in an asymmetrical puckering of the lips.

7. Is the patient able to puff out his or her cheeks and hold the air in the oral cavity as you squeeze the cheeks? Here the examiner is assessing the strength of the lips and the velum to maintain an airtight seal. Weakness at either end will result in leakage of air out of the mouth or the nose when pressure is applied to the patient's cheeks. Look closely at the lips as you squeeze the cheeks to determine whether that is where air is escaping. If you are confident that the lip seal is tight, any leakage is probably occurring at the velopharyngeal port. The function of the velum is assessed on several additional tasks later in the protocol.

8. Does the jaw hang loosely? If so, this would suggest significant bilateral damage to the trigeminal cranial nerve (V), which innervates the jaw muscles. However, bilateral damage is not common. Typically, damage affects only one side. When the damage is on only one side of the jaw, the muscles on the unaffected side will provide more than enough strength to hold the jaw in a normal position.

9. Does the jaw deviate to one side when the mouth is wide open? This task checks for unilateral damage to the

trigeminal cranial nerve. When the jaw muscles on one side of the face are weaker than on the other, the jaw might deviate to the weaker side when the mouth is opened widely.

10. Is the patient able to move the jaw to the right and left? An inability to do this suggests bilateral weakness of the jaw muscles. However, hesitations or groping on this task also might indicate a nonverbal oral apraxia.

11. Is the patient able to keep the jaw closed while the examiner attempts to open it? This task assesses the strength of the muscles that elevate the jaw, primarily the masseter and temporalis. The examiner's ability to manually open the jaw suggests bilateral weakness in these muscles—possibly the result of bilateral damage to the trigeminal cranial nerve.

12. Is the patient able to keep the jaw open while the examiner attempts to close it? This task examines the muscles that open the jaw. These muscles are the digastricus, mylohyoid, and geniohyoid. If you can manually close the jaw while the patient attempts to keep it open, bilateral weakness of these muscles is indicated.

Tongue at Rest and During Movement

The tongue is one of the key articulators. Impairments to its structure or function can have significant effects on the articulation of speech sounds. It is especially important to evaluate the tongue at rest and during movement. Both positions can provide important diagnostic information. Most of the assessment tasks in this section examine the function of the hypoglossal cranial nerve (XII), which innervates the intrinsic and extrinsic muscles of the tongue. If groping tongue movements are noted in any of these tasks, be sure to complete the apraxia section of the evaluation.

Explanation of Specific Tasks

1. Does the size of the tongue appear normal at rest? When damage occurs to lower motor neurons (e.g., those in the cranial nerves), the muscles normally innervated by those neurons will shrink because of atrophy. If there is unilateral damage to the hypoglossal nerve, the half of the tongue on the damaged side can take on a furrowed, shrunken appearance. When this damage occurs to both the left and right hypoglossal cranial nerves, the muscle atrophy will affect the whole tongue, leaving the entire tongue shrunken.

2. Is the tongue symmetrical at rest? If damage to the hypoglossal cranial nerve (XII) is restricted to only one side, the resulting atrophy will be restricted to that same side. The tongue will consequently have an asymmetrical appearance, with the unaffected side looking normal and only the other side demonstrating the atrophy.

3. Are **fasciculations** present when the tongue is at rest? Fasciculations are small involuntary movements that may occur in a muscle when motor innervation has been lost through damage to lower motor neurons. If fasciculations are present after damage to the hypoglossal cranial nerve, you will see small, nonrhythmic dimpling along the surface of the tongue, or you might see subtle "wormlike" movements of the entire tongue.

4. Does the tongue remain still while at rest? In addition to fasciculations, other conditions can result in involuntary movements when the tongue is supposedly at rest. Hyperkinetic movement disorders such as chorea and dystonia could cause the tongue to involuntarily protrude, retract, rotate, and move side to side. Hyperkinetic movement disorders are discussed in Chapter 9.

5. Is the patient able to protrude the tongue completely? This assesses range of motion for the posterior fibers of the genioglossus muscle, which protrudes the tongue, and the vertical and transverse intrinsic muscles, which give the tongue its "pointed" shape when protruded. If there is bilateral weakness of these muscles, the tongue can be protruded only a limited distance, if at all. If the weakness is unilateral, the protruded tongue will deviate to the affected side. This deviation to the affected side is the result of unequal contractions of the left and right sides of the genioglossus muscle in the tongue. The contractions of the unaffected side of this muscle will overcome the weakened contractions on the other side of the muscle, thereby causing the tongue to point to the affected side. You can check the strength of tongue protrusion by having the patient push the tongue against a tongue blade held firmly in front of the mouth.

6. Can the patient keep the tongue tip at midline while the examiner pushes the tongue to the left and right? This task checks the strength of several tongue muscles, including the genioglossus, superior longitudinal, and inferior longitudinal muscles.

7. Is the patient able to touch the upper lip with the tongue tip? Here you are assessing the range of motion of the

tongue protrusion muscles (genioglossus, vertical, and transverse intrinsic muscles) and the superior longitudinal muscle, which elevates the tongue tip.

8. Can the patient keep the tongue tip pressed against the inside of the cheek as the examiner pushes the cheek inward? This is an examination of strength for a number of tongue muscles, primarily the longitudinal muscles. The tongue tip will deviate to the left or right with simultaneous contraction of either the left or right superior and inferior longitudinal muscles, respectively. Unilateral weakness in these muscles is evident through comparison of the amount of outward force the tongue is able to apply to either the right or left cheek.

9. Can the patient move the tongue from side to side? This task examines range of motion for the superior and inferior longitudinal muscles. These muscles are used to lateralize the tongue from one corner of the mouth to the other. Reduced lateral tongue movement to one side of the mouth will reveal unilateral weakness of these muscles.

Velum and Pharynx at Rest and During Movement

This section of the evaluation looks at the structure and function of the velum and pharynx. Most of the muscles in these structures are innervated by the vagus cranial nerve (X). It is difficult to obtain much in-depth information about these structures in this portion of the examination because they are difficult to see clearly. In truth, you are only able to look for the most obvious anatomical and functional deviations. Additional information about the velum and pharynx can be obtained in later sections of this examination.

Explanation of Specific Tasks

1. Does the velum rise symmetrically each time the patient says /a/? Have the patient repeat /a/ four or five times. Make sure there is a brief pause between each production. This will allow the velum to return to its resting position after each /a/, giving you a better opportunity to observe the full range of velar movement. A normally functioning velum and pharynx work together to close the velopharyngeal port during the production of nonnasal sounds. You should see the entire velum rise promptly just before phonation. At the

same time, the sides and back of the upper pharynx should move slightly inward to meet the rising velum.

In cases of moderate to severe bilateral weakness of the velum and pharynx, you should be able to observe reduced speed and range of motion of these structures when the patient repeats /a/. However, these reductions can be difficult to detect visually when there is mild bilateral weakness. When there is unilateral muscular weakness of the velum and pharynx, the unaffected side should demonstrate nearly normal movement. The impaired side will show little or no movement. The uvula will be pulled toward the stronger, unaffected side as that side of the velum rises.

2. Is there a pharyngeal gag **reflex** when the back wall of the pharynx is touched? The gag is a protective reflex. Its purpose is to clear the upper pharynx of an obstruction that might threaten to block the airway. Testing this reflex assesses the neuromuscular loop that starts with the sensory nerves in pharyngeal muscles and tissue. When the sensory nerves in the pharynx are stimulated by the touch of a foreign object, they send a sensory impulse through the glossopharyngeal cranial nerve (IX) to the brainstem. From the brainstem, a motor impulse is sent directly to the pharyngeal and velar muscles via the vagus cranial nerve (X), which causes those muscles to contract rapidly. Damage to any portion of this loop leads to a decreased or absent gag reflex. Note, however, that many individuals without neurologic damage are quite insensitive to pharyngeal stimulation and do not readily demonstrate a gag reflex.

Laryngeal Function

The function of the larynx cannot be observed directly. To actually observe the actions of the larynx, you need instrumentation, such as a laryngeal mirror or a flexible nasoendoscope. However, some procedures indirectly assess laryngeal function. The following three tasks evaluate the strength and range of movement of the laryngeal adductor and abductor muscles. Other tasks later in the evaluation assess phonation, which is a key function of the larynx.

Explanation of Specific Tasks

1. Is the patient able to produce a sharp cough? This task assesses the strength of vocal-fold adduction. Producing a

sharp cough requires tight vocal-fold adduction for building up subglottic air pressure. When adduction is weak, the cough will have a soft, breathy quality because the adductor muscles are not strong enough to hold air in the lungs. In some instances, this task also assesses the adequacy of the respiratory system. If the respiratory muscles are not strong enough to provide a forced exhalation of air, the resulting cough also will have a soft, breathy quality. The next step of this evaluation presents a procedure for determining whether a breathy cough is the result of laryngeal or respiratory weakness.

2. Can the patient produce a sharp **glottal stop**? In this task, the patient is asked to produce an abrupt glottal stop (or a forceful grunt), to assess the strength of vocal-fold adduction. Duffy (2020) recommended this procedure to help determine whether a weak cough is the result of inadequate vocal-fold adduction or poor breath support. If a patient who produces a weak cough can bring the vocal folds together with enough force to make a sharp glottal stop, then he or she has sufficient adductor muscle strength to close the **glottis** tightly. This would suggest that a weak cough is the result of poor breath support, not adductor muscle weakness.

3. Is **inhalatory stridor** present? If abductor muscle paralysis prevents the vocal folds from being abducted completely, inhalatory stridor— a breathy wheeze that can be heard during inhalation—could be present. This vocal-fold abductor paralysis may be caused by unilateral or bilateral damage to the vagus cranial nerve. In severe cases, the stridor is actually a phonation on inhalation. Although stridor might be evident on quiet breathing, most patients will need to take a quick, deep breath before it will be noticeable.

Auditory-Perceptual Evaluations of the Motor Speech Mechanism

In most cases, the ear is the best instrument for evaluating deficits of the motor speech mechanism. A clinician with an experienced ear can often make a quick, accurate diagnosis based only on the acoustic characteristics of a patient's speech. The importance of developing a sharp ear for the assessment of motor speech disorders cannot be overstated. After all, what a listener hears provides the ultimate judgment of whether speech production is defective.

Accordingly, most of the remaining evaluation tasks rely on a clinician's perceptual analysis of a patient's speech.

Phonatory-Respiratory System

It is logical to assess the phonatory and respiratory components of the speech mechanism at the same time because normal phonation is so dependent on an adequate supply of subglottic air pressure. In this protocol section, the clinician will determine the length of time the patient can prolong an /a/. Listen critically to the quality, pitch, and loudness of the patient's phonation, because each of these characteristics can provide much useful diagnostic information.

Explanation of Specific Tasks

1. "Take a deep breath and say /a/ as long, steadily, and clearly as you can." This task assesses both the adequacy of breath support and vocal-fold adduction for phonation. If there is too little breath support, there will be inadequate subglottic air pressure to prolong the /a/ for 15 s. If the vocal folds are not adducted fully, excess amounts of air will escape from the larynx during phonation. This wastes subglottic air and lessens the length of the phonation. To determine whether a reduced length of phonation is the result of poor breath support or incomplete vocal-fold adduction, check the results from the previous section of the evaluation, which provided for assessment of the adequacy of vocal-fold adduction.

2. Is there a latency period between the signal to say /a/ and the initiation of phonation? If there is a delay, it could be the result of weakness in the phonatory-respiratory system. It could also be the result of a problem of sequencing the motor movements needed to produce the /a/. Such sequencing difficulties are characteristic of apraxia, which is assessed in greater detail later in the evaluation.

3. Quality, pitch, and loudness of phonations can be evaluated. In a normal phonation, the vocal quality is steady, even, smooth, and clear. The presence of hypernasality indicates inadequate velopharyngeal closure. Breathiness can indicate incomplete vocal-fold adduction during phonation. Harshness is an abnormal vocal quality that is caused by the friction of air being passed through vocal folds that are almost fully adducted. **Diplophonia** is the simultaneous production of two pitch levels during phonation. In motor

speech disorders, it is usually the result of unilateral vocal-fold paralysis.

Pitch can be affected by motor speech disorders. It might be too low, as in spastic dysarthria and several of the hyperkinetic dysarthrias. There could be a tremor in the phonations, which is present in such disorders as essential voice tremor, one of the hyperkinetic dysarthrias. Pitch breaks are sudden shifts in pitch during phonation. These are heard most often in flaccid and spastic dysarthria.

Loudness can be affected by motor speech disorders. The involuntary movements in hyperkinetic dysarthria can cause excessive loudness variations during phonations. Poor respiratory support or inadequate phonation can cause decreased loudness, perhaps most often heard in flaccid and hypokinetic dysarthria.

Resonation System

This portion of the evaluation assesses velopharyngeal function. Weakened or paralyzed velar muscles result in incomplete velopharyngeal closure, which is heard perceptually as hypernasality. In motor speech disorders, hypernasality is most frequently a symptom of flaccid or spastic dysarthria. Hyponasality, the counterpart of hypernasality, is rarely present in the speech of individuals with dysarthria or apraxia of speech. Because other tasks in this motor speech evaluation have already evaluated elements of the resonatory system (velar movement and hypernasal voice quality), the findings of the following two tasks should be combined with the results of the previous tasks to arrive at the most accurate assessment of the patient's velopharyngeal function.

Explanation of Specific Tasks

1. "Take a deep breath and say /u/ for as long as you can." On this task, ask the patient to prolong the high, back vowel /u/, which usually maximizes velopharyngeal closure. While the patient says /u/, hold a small mirror first under one nostril and then under the other. Nasal emission of air during this phonation will be revealed as fogging of the mirror. You should disregard any momentary fogging of the mirror at the very beginning or end of the phonation. However, the mirror should remain clear during the middle of the phonation.

2. "This time I'm going to squeeze your nose. Don't let it bother you." Here the clinician makes a perceptual judgment of whether hypernasality is present during the prolongation of /u/. By alternately squeezing and releasing the nostrils while the patient is producing /u/, you are intermittently stopping any nasal airflow during phonation. If there is hypernasality, you will hear a difference in resonance as the patient's nose is squeezed and released.

Combined Systems (Phonation, Respiration, Resonation, and Articulation)

AMR is an assessment of a patient's ability to move the articulators rapidly yet smoothly in a repetitive motion. It also is known as the diadochokinetic rate. AMRs are a key evaluation task for motor speech disorders. They provide valuable information on the speed and rhythm of syllable production. AMRs are very important in a motor speech evaluation because individuals with different types of dysarthria typically perform differently on this task.

- Individuals with flaccid and spastic dysarthria usually have slow and regular AMRs.
- Individuals with ataxic and hyperkinetic dysarthria often have slow and irregular AMRs.
- Some individuals with hypokinetic dysarthria have AMRs that are more rapid than normal. In certain individuals with this dysarthria, the AMRs are said so quickly that their articulation of the phonemes is blurred.

By carefully analyzing the patient's AMR performance, one can often obtain important diagnostic information about the patient's dysarthria.

Explanation of Specific Task

"Take a deep breath and say 'puh, puh, puh' as long, as fast, and as evenly as you can." After saying these directions, be sure to demonstrate for the patient how the syllables should be produced. To obtain an accurate count of the patient's AMRs, it is important to always use some type of instrumentation during this task, either a computer, a tape recorder, or some other recording device. Even experienced clinicians have difficulty timing and counting syllable repetitions if the patient's performance is not recorded. In this task, you are primarily listening for the speed and rhythm of the productions, but loudness, pitch, and articulation also are important. For example, excessive variations in syllable loudness are typical of ataxic and hyperkinetic dysarthria; blurred articulation can be a characteristic of hypokinetic dysarthria.

SMR is a task that assesses a patient's ability to move the articulators in a rapid, smooth sequence of motions. Typically, SMRs are more difficult to perform accurately than AMRs. This task is often useful in bringing out the symptoms of apraxia of speech. It is not unusual to have individuals with apraxia of speech complete the AMR task successfully but be unable to complete even the first attempt at the SMR sequence. (This is not to suggest, however, that all individuals with apraxia of speech are able to complete the AMR task successfully; many have difficulty with both tasks.) Some of the errors individuals with apraxia of speech might demonstrate on the SMR task include delays in beginning the task, phoneme substitutions, incorrect sequencing of syllables, and articulatory groping for the correct phoneme placement.

"Now I want you to make those three sounds together." As with the AMRs, it is important to record the patient's trials on the SMR task to obtain an accurate syllable count. One should also be sure to demonstrate for the patient how the syllables should be produced.

Stress Testing of the Motor Speech Mechanism

This task screens for **myasthenia gravis**, a disorder that causes rapid fatigue of the muscles during a sustained motor activity (see Chapter 4). To test for myasthenia gravis, ask the patient to count quickly from 1 to 100. Listen for a relatively rapid deterioration of articulation, resonance, or phonation while the patient is counting. Typically, there will be a recovery of muscle function after a rest period, but performance will decline if the muscles again are taxed in a sustained activity.

Testing for Nonverbal Oral Apraxia

Apraxia is a disruption in the ability to voluntarily sequence complex movements accurately. It is not the result of muscle weakness, reduced range of motion, or a cognitive inability to plan the target movement. Apraxia is a problem in timing and accuracy of a complex movement that has already been planned by the higher centers of the brain. Two types of apraxia affect the speech musculature: nonverbal oral apraxia and apraxia of speech. Nonverbal oral apraxia is a disruption in the sequencing of oral movements that are nonverbal, sometimes described as "vegetative movements." Examples of nonverbal oral movements include smiling, puckering the lips, protruding the tongue, and biting the lower lip. Individuals with this type of apraxia will demonstrate hesitations, groping, and revisions when attempting to perform nonverbal oral movements. It is possible for someone to have nonverbal oral apraxia but not have apraxia of speech. It is also possible for someone to have apraxia of speech but not nonverbal oral apraxia. Usually, however, these two types of apraxia are co-occurring disorders—if one is present, so is the other.

Explanation of Specific Task

"Now I want you to do some things." These tasks assess the patient's ability to perform voluntary nonverbal oral movements. Do not demonstrate the desired movement for the patient immediately after reading the command. Wait until the patient has attempted the task independently before demonstrating the movement. The patient's performance is graded on an 11-point scale, which ranges from a prompt response to no oral movement. Such a scoring system allows the clinician to obtain a much more detailed picture of a patient's performance than a simple right or wrong scoring. You should become familiar with the 11 points before administering this portion of the evaluation.

Testing for Apraxia of Speech

Apraxia of speech, a disruption in the timing and accuracy of voluntary movements for speech production, is the other type of apraxia that can affect the speech musculature. Individuals with apraxia of speech often demonstrate pauses and distortions when they are attempting to speak, especially when trying to say multisyllabic words. These errors can include a slow rate of speech, abnormal prosody, groping to position the articulators correctly, and distorted phonemes. Interestingly, both automatic and emotional speech can be relatively free of apraxic errors, which means that such verbal tasks as counting, uttering an expletive, or replying to a social greeting might be produced more accurately. Apraxia of speech is discussed in more detail in Chapter 11.

Explanation of Specific Tasks

1. "Say these words for me." This task has the patient repeating or reading a list of words. The list starts with a two-syllable word and progresses to a complex sequence of increasingly

longer words that all start with the same consonant–vowel–consonant (CVC) syllable. It should be extremely difficult for an individual with apraxia of speech to complete this list without numerous sequencing errors. Not only are most of the words multisyllabic, most of them also are low-frequency words, meaning that they do not occur often in everyday conversations. Patients with apraxia usually have more difficulty pronouncing low-frequency words than high-frequency words.

2. "Now these." Individuals with apraxia of speech typically have little difficulty producing single-syllable words with a simple CVC construction in which the initial and final consonants are identical. Words of this type are included in the evaluation for two reasons. First, the patient should find them to be a successful change of pace from the difficult previous task. Second, the words provide a strong indication of severity if the patient makes many apraxic errors on these words. Because these words should be fairly easy for most individuals with apraxia of speech, a patient who has difficulty with them is probably severely affected by the apraxia.

3. "Now repeat these sentences after me." The sentences on this task should be difficult for individuals with apraxia of speech. These items are uncommon sentences that contain numerous multisyllabic words. They should evoke some apraxic errors in most individuals suspected of having apraxia of speech.

4. "Count from 1 to 20." Because this is an overlearned, automatic verbal task, many individuals with apraxia of speech should be able to complete it with far fewer errors than they will demonstrate on the next task.

5. "Now count backward from 20 to 1." Most individuals with apraxia of speech will make multiple errors on this task, if they can complete it at all. Although they are producing the same words as in the prior task, counting backward is not an overlearned verbal activity. Consequently, this should be a difficult task for most patients with apraxia of speech.

Analysis of Connected Speech

In this final portion of the evaluation, the clinician should have the patient read one of the standard reading passages such as the Grandfather passage or the Rainbow passage. To ensure an accurate analysis of the patient's connected speech, it is very important to obtain a good quality audio or video recording of this task. Rate the characteristics of the patient's speech according to the questions listed at the end of the examination (Darley et al., 1975). A complete analysis of connected speech should provide much of the information needed to distinguish one dysarthria from another.

Summary of the Evaluation of Motor Speech Disorders

- Evaluating motor speech disorders can be a challenging task for inexperienced clinicians. There are numerous elements of speech production that must be assessed to make a proper diagnosis. The clinician needs to evaluate a patient's respiration, phonation, resonance, articulation, and prosody during a motor speech examination.
- Instrumentation and perceptual analysis are the two primary methods of assessing motor speech disorders. Most clinicians use perceptual analysis to make their diagnosis. With this method, clinicians use their eyes and ears to determine whether a motor speech disorder is present in a given patient.
- In addition to evaluating the elements of speech production (e.g., respiration, phonation, etc.), a complete motor speech examination will examine the six processes that are the foundation of all voluntary movements: muscle strength, speed of movement, range of movement, accuracy of movement, motor steadiness, and muscle tone.
- At the most basic level, a motor speech examination allows a clinician to fully describe a patient's speech production abilities. With this complete description of the patient's abilities, the clinician should be able to logically answer pertinent questions about the patient's deficits and arrive at a correct diagnosis.

Study Questions

1. What are the two basic methods of evaluating motor speech disorders?
2. According to Haynes and Pindzola, what are the two goals of any speech-language evaluation?
3. What are the five components of speech production?

4. Define dysarthria.
5. Define apraxia of speech.
6. What are Darley, Aronson, and Brown's salient features of neuromuscular function, and why are they important?
7. Name two evaluation tasks that assess tongue strength.
8. What are AMRs and SMRs, and why are they important?
9. What might inhalation stridor indicate?
10. Why might an individual with apraxia of speech have difficulty counting backward from 20 to 1?

Appendix 3-1

Motor Speech Examination

Patient's Name:

Date of Examination:

Patient's Age:

Neurologic Diagnosis:

Relevant Personal Information:

Medical History:

INSTRUCTIONS: Answer each item <u>yes</u> or <u>no</u> and indicate the degree of impairment as follows:

- 0 = no impairment
- 1 = mild impairment
- 2 = moderate impairment
- 3 = severe impairment

Also be sure to answer all other questions in the space indicated.

I. STRUCTURAL-FUNCTIONAL SPEECH MECHANISM EXAMINATION

	Yes	No	Degree

A. Facial Musculature at Rest: CN VII

  1. Is mouth symmetrical? ___ ___ ___

  If no, describe: _____

  _____

  2. Can patient resist examiner's attempt to force lips open? ___ ___ ___

  3. Are eyes open? ___ ___ ___

  4. Are eyes partially closed? ___ ___ ___

  5. Is facies rigid or masked? ___ ___ ___

  6. Is there wrinkling of forehead (when looking up without moving head?) ___ ___ ___

  7. Is nose symmetrical? ___ ___ ___

  If no, describe: _____

  _____

B. Facial Musculature During Voluntary Movement: CN VII

  1. Is smile symmetrical? ___ ___ ___

  If no, describe: _____

  _____

  2. Is groping present?+ ___ ___ ___

  3. Can patient pucker the lips? ___ ___ ___

  If no, describe: _____

  _____

  4. Is groping present?+ ___ ___ ___

  5. Can patient puff out cheeks and maintain lip seal when pressure is applied? ___ ___ ___

  If no, describe: _____

  _____

C. Mandibular Musculature at Rest: CN V

  Does mandible hang lower than normal? ___ ___ ___

+Any groping should be followed up with the complete apraxia battery.

	Yes	No	Degree

D. **Mandibular Musculature During Voluntary Movement: CN V**

   1. When mouth is open as widely as possible, is there deviation to one side? ____ ____ ____

   If no, describe: _____

   _____

   2. Is groping present?+ ____ ____ ____

   3. Can patient move mandible voluntarily to the right or left? ____ ____ ____

   4. Can patient resist examiner's attempt to open lower jaw when teeth are clenched? ____ ____ ____

   5. Can patient keep mouth wide open as examiner attempts to force it closed? ____ ____ ____

E. **Tongue Musculature at Rest: CN XII**

   1. Is tongue normal in size? ____ ____

   If no, describe: _____

   _____

   2. Does tongue lie midline? ____ ____

   If no, describe: _____

   _____

   3. Is tongue symmetrical in shape? ____ ____

   If no, describe: _____

   _____

   4. With tongue resting atop edges of lower incisor teeth, is fasciculation observable? ____ ____

   5. Does tongue remain at rest? ____ ____

   If no, describe: _____

   _____

F. **Tongue Musculature During Voluntary Movement: CN XII**

   1. Can patient protrude tongue completely? ____ ____ ____

   If no, describe range and deviation: _____

   _____

*Any groping should be followed up with the complete apraxia battery.

	Yes	No	Degree

2. Is groping present?+

3. With tongue protruded, can patient resist examiner's attempt to force tongue to other side?

4. With tip of tongue, can patient resist examiner's attempt to force tongue to one side or other?

5. With tip of tongue, can patient touch:

    upper lip?

    alveolar ridge?

    If no, describe: _____

_____

6. With tongue in cheek, can patient resist examiner's effort to force tongue inward?

7. Can the patient move the tongue from side to side?

    If no, describe: _____

_____

G. The Velum and Pharynx at Rest and During Movement: CN X

    1. Does the velum rise symmetrically each time the patient says /a/?

    If no, describe: _____

_____

    2. Is there a gag reflex when the back wall of the pharynx is touched?

H. The Function of the Larynx: CN X

    1. Is the patient able to produce a sharp cough?

    2. Can the patient produce a sharp glottal stop?

    If no, describe: _____

_____

    3. Is inhalatory stridor present?

    If yes, describe: _____

_____

II. ACOUSTIC MOTOR SPEECH EXAMINATION

                                                                                   Yes   No   Degree

A. Phonatory-Respiratory System:

1. <u>Directions to patient</u>: "Take a deep breath and say /a:/ as long, steadily, and clearly as you can."

   a. Duration: **Trial 1:** _____

                     Trial 2: _____

                     Trial 3: _____

                     Average: _____

   (average is 15 s for adults & 10 s for school-aged children)

   b. Latency: Is there a latency period between signal to say /a:/ and initiation of phonation?   ____ ____ ____

   c. Quality:

       Steady and even   ____ ____ ____

       Smooth and clear   ____ ____ ____

       Hypernasality   ____ ____ ____

       Breathiness   ____ ____ ____

       Harshness   ____ ____ ____

       Diplophonia   ____ ____ ____

   d. Pitch

       Too high   ____ ____ ____

       Too low   ____ ____ ____

       Normal   ____ ____ ____

       Tremor   ____ ____ ____

       Pitch breaks   ____ ____ ____

   e. Loudness

       Excessive loudness   ____ ____ ____

       Inadequate loudness   ____ ____ ____

       Normal loudness   ____ ____ ____

   f. Describe Abnormalities: _____

   _____

	Yes	No	Degree

B. Resonatory System:

1. **Directions to patient**: "Take a deep breath and say /u:/ for as long as you can." Hold a (laryngeal) mirror beneath one nostril and then the other.

   Leakage from (L. R. Both) nostrils. ____ ____ ____

2. <u>Directions to patient</u>: "Now I want you to do the same thing, but this time I'm going to squeeze your nose. Don't let it bother you; just keep the /u:/ going."

   Change in resonance when occluding (L. R. Both) nostrils. ____ ____ ____

   Connected speech without nasal. ____ ____ ____

C. Combined Systems (Phonatory, Respiratory, Resonatory, and Articulatory)

   1. <u>A</u>lternate <u>M</u>otion <u>R</u>ate (diadochokinetic)

      <u>Directions to patient</u>: "Take a deep breath and say (e.g. /pʌpʌpʌ/) as long, and as fast, and as evenly as you can."
      Demonstrate.

      Is AMR slow? ____ ____ ____
      Is AMR excessively fast? ____ ____ ____
      Is AMR dysrhythmic? ____ ____ ____
      Is AMR uneven in loudness? ____ ____ ____
      Is AMR uneven in pitch? ____ ____ ____
      Is there a tremor? ____ ____ ____
      Is there equal spacing between syllables? ____ ____ ____
      Is there blurring (lack of differentiation between syllables)? ____ ____ ____
      Is there hypernasality? ____ ____ ____
      Is there nasal emission? ____ ____ ____
      Is there restriction in amplitude of motion of lips and jaw? ____ ____ ____
      Are there imprecise or distorted consonants? ____ ____ ____

Indicate rate per 5-s intervals on this table:

	/pʌ/	/tʌ/	/kʌ/	/pʌtʌkʌ/
Trial 1				
Trial 2				
Trial 3				
Average				

Average rate for /pʌ/ and /tʌ/ is about 30–35 repetitions for 5 s; /kʌ/ is somewhat slower.

2. <u>S</u>equential <u>M</u>otion <u>R</u>ate

    Directions to patient: "Now I want you to make those three sounds, 'puh,' 'tuh,' and 'kuh' together."

    Demonstrate. <u>Note</u>: Record the results (per 5-s trial) on the table above.

                    Yes No Degree

    a. Is patient able to move smoothly from syllable to syllable? ___ ___ ___

    b. Are sounds blocked, transposed, or omitted? ___ ___ ___

    If yes, describe: _____

    _____

3. Stress Testing of the Motor Speech Mechanism (screening for myasthenia gravis)

    Instruct the patient to count rapidly (approximately two numbers per second) at least up through 100.

    Demonstrate 1 through 10.

    Is there audible deterioration of phonation or articulation? ___ ___ ___

    If yes, describe: _____

    _____

III. TESTING FOR NONVERBAL ORAL APRAXIA

A. Tests for Nonverbal Oral Apraxia

<u>Directions to patient</u>: "Now I want you to do some things. Listen closely and do everything as completely and as well as you can. Are you ready?"

RESPONSE	TEST ITEM	GRADED RESPONSE SCALE
_____	1. **Stick out your tongue.**	1. Accurate and immediate response with no hesitation.
_____	2. Show me how you blow out a match	
_____	3. Show me your teeth.	2. Accurate after trial-and-error searching movement on command.
_____	4. **Round your lips.**	
_____	5. Touch your nose with the tip of your tongue.	3. Crude, defective in amplitude, accuracy, or speed on command.
_____	6. Bite your lower lip.	
_____	7. **Show me how you whistle.**	4. Partial response (an important part missing) on command.
_____	8. **Lick your lips all around.**	
	9. Clear your throat.	5. Same as (1) after demonstration.
_____	10. Move your tongue in and out.	6. Same as (2) after demonstration.
_____	11. Click your teeth together once.	7. Same as (3) after demonstration.
_____	12. Show me how you smile.	8. Same as (4) after demonstration.
_____	13. **Click your tongue.**	
_____	14. Chatter your teeth as if cold.	9. Perseverative response.
_____	15. Touch your chin with the tip of your tongue.	10. Irrelevant response.
_____	16. Show me how you cough.	11. No oral performance.
_____	17. **Puff out your cheeks.**	
_____	18. Wiggle your tongue from side to side.	
_____	19. Pucker your lips	
_____	20. **Alternately pucker and smile.**	

IV. TESTING FOR APRAXIA OF SPEECH (ORAL VERBAL APRAXIA)

<u>Directions to patient</u>: "Say those words for me." If patient is unable to repeat to verbal stimuli, present words as printed on cards. As patient reads or repeats the following, tape-record and transcribe errors.

1. slowpoke _____
2. conference _____
3. **Tahiti** _____
4. dressmaker _____
5. Annapolis _____
6. kindergarten _____
7. **condominium** _____
8. industrial revolution _____
9. Winnie-the-Pooh and Tigger too _____
_____
10. **stiff – stiffer – stiffening** _____
_____
11. base – baseball – baseball cap_____
_____
12. **fan – fancy – fantastic – fashionable** _____
_____
13. glow – glowing – glistening – glamorously _____
_____
14. rid – riddle – ridicule – ridiculous _____
_____

"Now these."

mime _____	shush _____
George _____	dude _____
pipe _____	tent _____
babe _____	**Nan** _____

"Please repeat these sentences for me."

1. **The beautiful girl was dancing.** _____

2. **Open this birthday present first.** _____

3. **The stranger walked into the store.** _____

4. **The birdwatcher saw a Norwegian Blue parrot.** _____

"Count from 1 to 20." Note: Indicate pauses for breath by a slash (/) after the appropriate number.

1 _____	2 _____	3 _____	4 _____	5 _____
6 _____	7 _____	8 _____	9 _____	10 _____
11 _____	12 _____	13 _____	14 _____	15 _____
16 _____	17 _____	18 _____	19 _____	20 _____

"Now count backward from 20 to 1."

20 _____	19 _____	18 _____	17 _____	16 _____
15 _____	14 _____	13 _____	12 _____	11 _____
10 _____	9 _____	8 _____	7 _____	6 _____
5 _____	4 _____	3 _____	2 _____	1 _____

V. CONNECTED SPEECH SAMPLE

Have the patient read "My Grandfather" or another standard reading passage and rate the following questions. If the patient has difficulty reading, show a standard picture such as the Cookie Theft to evoke at least 1 min of ongoing speech. If necessary point out neglected features of the picture by asking, "What's happening here?"

	Yes	No	Degree
1. Are vowels and consonants produced clearly?	___	___	___
2. Is the patient's rate of speech too slow? Or is it too fast?	___	___	___
3. Does the patient show inappropriate silent intervals between words?	___	___	___

	Yes	No	Degree
4. Does the patient show hypernasality?	___	___	___
5. Is nasal emission present?	___	___	___
6. Does the patient vary loudness normally?	___	___	___
7. If not, is there evidence of monoloudness?	___	___	___
8. Is there evidence of tremor in the patient's voice?	___	___	___
9. Does the patient show abnormal pitch variations?	___	___	___
10. Does the patient's voice have a harsh vocal quality?	___	___	___
11. Does the patient's voice have a strained-strangled vocal quality?	___	___	___
12. Does the patient's voice have a breathy vocal quality?	___	___	___
13. Does the patient speak in abnormally short phrases?	___	___	___
14. Are there moments of involuntary inhalation or exhalation?	___	___	___
15. Is inhalatory stridor present?	___	___	___
16. Does the patient use normal stress on the appropriate syllables or words?	___	___	___
17. If not, is there a reduction in normal stress?	___	___	___
18. Or is there excess and equal stress?	___	___	___

Chapter 4

Flaccid Dysarthria

Definitions of Flaccid Dysarthria

Neurologic Basis of Flaccid Dysarthria

Cranial Nerves of Speech Production
- *Trigeminal Nerve (V)*
- *Facial Nerve (VII)*
- *Glossopharyngeal Nerve (IX)*
- *Vagus Nerve (X)*
- *Accessory Nerve (XI)*
- *Hypoglossal Nerve (XII)*

Spinal Nerves

Causes of Flaccid Dysarthria

Physical Trauma
Brainstem Stroke
Myasthenia Gravis
Guillain-Barré Syndrome
Polio
Other Causes of Flaccid Dysarthria

Speech Characteristics of Flaccid Dysarthria

Resonance
Articulation
Phonation
Respiration
- *A Problem of Respiration or Phonation?*

Prosody

Key Evaluation Tasks for Flaccid Dysarthria

Treatment of Motor Speech Disorders

Treatment of Flaccid Dysarthria

Damage to the Trigeminal Cranial Nerve (V)

Damage to the Vagus Cranial Nerve (X)
- *Treatments for Resonance Deficits*
- *Surgical and Prosthetic Treatments*
- *Velar Strengthening and Nonspeech Exercises*
- *Behavioral Approaches for Mild Hypernasality (Modification of Speech)*
- *Treatments for Phonation Deficits*
- *Treatments for Prosodic Deficits*

Damage to the Facial (VII) and Hypoglossal (XII) Cranial Nerves
- *Traditional Articulation Treatment*
- *Treatments for Respiratory Weakness in Flaccid Dysarthria*

Summary of Flaccid Dysarthria

Study Questions

Each of the next seven chapters of this textbook examines one motor speech disorder. Each discusses the neurologic basis for the disorder, the most common causes, the various speech characteristics, and the available treatment options. This chapter examines flaccid dysarthria, a dysarthria associated with damage to lower motor neurons. Chapters 5 and 6 cover spastic dysarthria and unilateral upper motor neuron dysarthria, respectively. Both of these dysarthrias are identified with upper motor neuron damage. Chapters 7, 8, and 9 discuss ataxic, hypokinetic, and hyperkinetic dysarthria, respectively. These three dysarthrias are associated with damage to some of the most complex areas of the brain. Ataxic dysarthria is caused by damage to the cerebellum. Most cases of hypokinetic and hyperkinetic dysarthria result from dysfunction in the basal ganglia. Chapter 10 examines mixed dysarthria, which is caused by damage to multiple areas of the nervous system. Chapter 11 discusses apraxia of speech. Although not a dysarthria, apraxia of speech is classified as a motor speech disorder. It is most often associated with damage to the left frontal lobe of the brain.

Definitions of Flaccid Dysarthria

Most published definitions of flaccid dysarthria (sometimes called neuromuscular dysarthria) emphasize at least two specific characteristics of this disorder. First, they mention that flaccid dysarthria is caused by impairments of the lower motor neurons in the cranial or spinal nerves. This is important because it shows that this dysarthria is the result of damage to the PNS. Second, most definitions include a statement indicating that individuals with flaccid dysarthria have weakness in the speech or respiratory musculature, which results in the distinctive qualities of this motor speech disorder. The following two definitions highlight the major characteristics of flaccid dysarthria:

> [Flaccid dysarthria is] associated with lower motor neuron damage. The lesions may be in the motor neurons of the brainstem or spinal

cord, in the peripheral nerves leading from those motor neurons to the muscles of the head and neck and respiratory system, or at the neuromuscular junction where the peripheral nerve makes contact with the muscle. Breathiness, hypernasality, and imprecise consonants are among the frequent voice and speech problems noted with this form of dysarthria. (Weismer, 2007, p. 67)

[A] motor speech disorder with neuropathology of damage to the motor units of the cranial or spinal nerves that supply speech muscles (lower motor neuron involvement); speech problems caused mostly by muscle weakness and hypotonia. (Singh & Kent, 2000, p. 84)

Neurologic Basis of Flaccid Dysarthria

As mentioned, flaccid dysarthria is caused by damage to motor neurons of the PNS. These motor neurons are commonly known by two different names. They sometimes are called lower motor neurons because they are part of the PNS. The term *lower* distinguishes these motor neurons of the PNS from the motor neurons of the CNS, which are called upper motor neurons. Figure 4–1 illustrates the relationship between lower and upper motor neurons. These motor neurons are also sometimes known as the **final common pathway** because they are the last and only "road" that the neural impulses from the upper motor neurons can travel to reach the muscles. Flaccid dysarthria can be caused by any disorder that disrupts the flow of neural impulses along the lower motor neurons that innervate the muscles of respiration, phonation, articulation, prosody, or resonance.

Cranial Nerves of Speech Production

There are six pairs of cranial nerves that play a vital role in speech production: trigeminal, facial, glossopharyngeal, vagus, accessory, and hypoglossal. These six pairs of nerves are sometimes called the "cranial nerves of speech production." They are important because the lower motor neurons inside these nerves transmit motor impulses from the upper motor neurons to the muscles used in speech production. Normal speech production requires that these cranial nerves transmit their motor impulses accurately. If a cranial nerve is damaged, the motor impulses it sends to the muscles are likely to be distorted or perhaps even stopped completely. In either case, the damage to the cranial nerve will affect

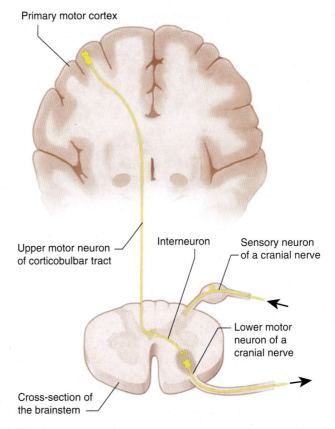

FIGURE 4–1. Upper motor neurons transmit motor impulses within the central nervous system and ultimately send these impulses to the lower motor neurons in the cranial or spinal nerves.

the accurate production of speech. Many different processes can harm the cranial nerves used in speech production. For example, a brainstem stroke can injure a cranial nerve by disrupting the flow of blood to the cell bodies of its lower motor neurons. Likewise, a growing tumor can compress a cranial nerve to such a degree that its function is compromised. Viral or bacterial infections can damage the tissue of the nerve directly. Physical trauma can injure a cranial nerve, such as when a fractured bone compresses or cuts the nerve. Surgical accidents also might cause damage—a slip of a scalpel can nick or completely sever one of these nerves.

If any of these conditions involve the cranial nerves of speech production, the result can be flaccid dysarthria. However, not all injuries to these cranial nerves cause every characteristic of flaccid dysarthria. The specific characteristics of this dysarthria depend on which nerve or combination of nerves is damaged. Damage to a branch of the vagus nerve can cause hypernasal speech, one of the most common characteristics of flaccid dysarthria. Damage to the hypoglossal nerve can cause distorted productions of lingual consonants, another common characteristic of this dysarthria. Damage to both the vagus and hypoglossal nerves can result in speech that is hypernasal and has distorted consonants. Accordingly, the following sections of this chapter examine each of the six cranial nerves involved in speech production, with particular emphasis placed on the consequences of injury to these nerves.

Trigeminal Nerve (V)

The trigeminal nerve is attached to the brainstem at the level of the pons. As it courses out from the brainstem, it divides into three main branches: ophthalmic, maxillary, and mandibular (Figure 4–2). The most important of these for speech production is the mandibular branch, which innervates the masseter, pterygoid, mylohyoid, and other mandibular muscles that elevate and lower the jaw. It also innervates the tensor veli palatini muscle in the velum. When this muscle contracts, it makes the soft palate stiffer and also helps open the eustachian tube.

Unilateral damage to the trigeminal nerve can result in weakness or paralysis in the jaw and velar muscles that are on the same side as the damage. In such cases, an individual's jaw might deviate toward the affected side when it is opened.

Over time, the gradual loss of tissue in the affected jaw muscle (muscular atrophy) could cause a slightly asymmetrical facial appearance. Fortunately, unilateral damage to the trigeminal nerve seldom affects speech production significantly because the jaw and velar muscles on the unaffected side of the body are usually strong enough to compensate for the weakened muscles on the affected side.

However, bilateral damage to the trigeminal nerve can have a very serious effect on articulation. (Bilateral damage means that the trigeminal nerve branching out from the left side of the brainstem and the one branching out from the right side of the brainstem both have been injured or impaired.) If the bilateral damage is severe, affected individuals cannot raise their jaw sufficiently to produce most consonant and vowel phonemes, especially those requiring bilabial, linguadental, or linguapalatal contact. Furthermore, their rate of speech is often slowed by this reduced ability to elevate the jaw.

Facial Nerve (VII)

The facial cranial nerve branches out from the brainstem just below the trigeminal nerve (Figure 4–3). As it courses to the muscles of the

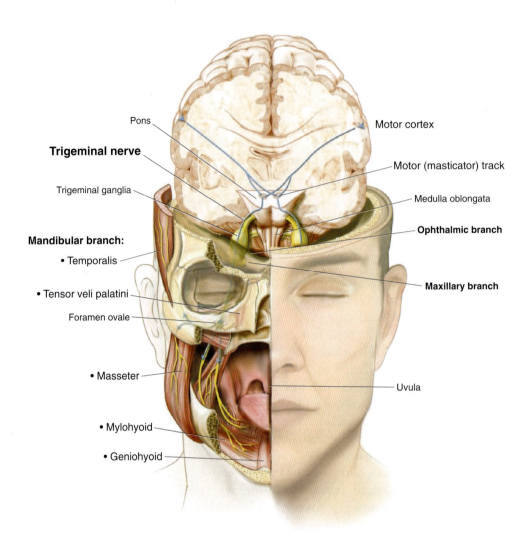

FIGURE 4–2. The trigeminal nerve has three main branches: ophthalmic, maxillary, and mandibular. The mandibular branch provides lower motor neuron innervation to the jaw muscles.

face, it divides into two major branches. For the most part, the cervicofacial branch innervates the muscles of the lower face through its buccal, lingual, and mandibular subbranches. The temporofacial branch innervates the muscles of the upper face through its temporal and zygomatic subbranches. Damage to the facial nerve can affect the muscles of the entire face on the same (**ipsilateral**) side as the lesion if it occurs above the point where the facial nerve divides into its cervicofacial and temporofacial branches. In such cases, all the muscles on the same side of the face as the damage will demonstrate some degree of weakness or paralysis. The result

4. FLACCID DYSARTHRIA   **105**

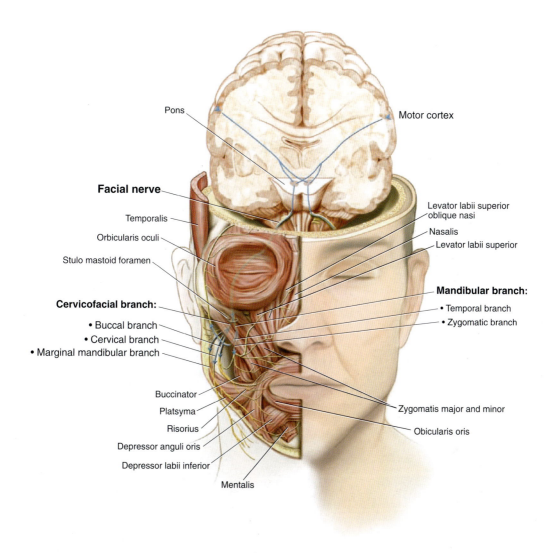

FIGURE 4–3. The major branches of the facial nerve.

of this facial nerve damage most likely will be drooping of the eyelid, mouth, cheek, and other structures on the affected side of the face. If the facial nerve damage occurs to just one of these branches, only the muscles innervated by that branch will be affected. For example, if the damage affects only the cervicofacial branch, the muscles of the lips will be affected, and the production of bilabial or labiodental sounds could be distorted.

Upper Motor Neuron Innervation of the Facial Nerve There is a difference in how the upper motor neurons of the corticobulbar tract innervate the lower motor neurons in the two branches of the

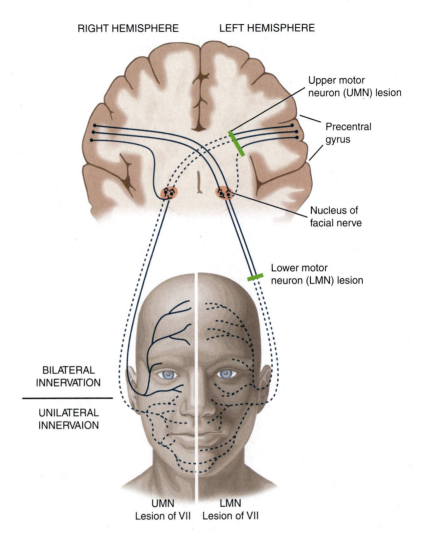

FIGURE 4–4. A unilateral lesion to the upper motor neurons that innervate the facial nerve will just affect the muscles of the lower face because that branch of the facial nerve only receives unilateral upper motor neuron innervation. In contrast, the branch of the facial nerve serving the upper face receives bilateral upper motor neuron innervation. Therefore, lower motor neuron lesions will affect all muscles below the point of damage.

facial nerve (Figure 4–4). The branch of the facial nerve that serves the upper face receives bilateral upper motor neuron innervation from both the right and left corticobulbar tracts. This means, for example, that unilateral damage to the right corticobulbar tract will not result in weakness or paralysis in the upper part of the left side of the face because the left corticobulbar tract also innervates this branch of the facial nerve. As a result, the upper face will still receive some upper motor neuron innervation despite the damage to the right corticobulbar tract. Consequently, there will be fairly normal contractions of all the muscles in the upper part of the face on both sides.

However, upper motor neuron innervation is different for the branch of the facial nerve serving the muscles of the lower face. This branch of the facial nerve receives only unilateral upper motor neuron innervation from the opposite (**contralateral**) side of the brain. Because of this unilateral innervation, right corticobulbar tract damage will result in weakness or paralysis on the left side of the lower face. Conversely, left corticobulbar tract damage will result in weakness or paralysis on the right side of the lower face.

In summary, unilateral upper motor neuron damage in one cerebral hemisphere will result in nearly normal upper face movements of the eyebrow, forehead, and eyelids on both sides of the face. However, movements of the cheek and mouth on the side of the face opposite to the site of the lesion will be notably weak, and these two parts of the lower face will probably have reduced range of motion. The type of dysarthria that can result from unilateral upper motor neuron damage is known as unilateral upper motor neuron dysarthria, discussed in Chapter 6.

Glossopharyngeal Nerve (IX)

This cranial nerve originates in the brainstem at the medulla (Figure 4–5) and courses out to the pharynx, where it innervates the stylopharyngeus and superior pharyngeal constrictor muscles. These muscles assist in the elevation and opening of the upper pharynx. Eliciting the gag reflex is one way to assess the function of this cranial nerve. The full importance of the glossopharyngeal nerve for speech is difficult to determine because damage to it also usually will affect the vagus nerve, a cranial nerve that definitely makes significant contributions to speech production. Nevertheless, the glossopharyngeal nerve probably plays a role in speech resonance and phonation by shaping the pharynx into the appropriate positions needed to produce various phonemes correctly.

Vagus Nerve (X)

The vagus nerve is one of the most important cranial nerves for speech production (Figure 4–6). Its origin is in the brainstem at the medulla, just below the glossopharyngeal cranial nerve, and it courses out from the medulla in close proximity to the glossopharyngeal and accessory cranial nerves. The vagus nerve is very long and has many branches serving such varied parts of the body as the larynx, intestines, heart, and velum, to name but a few. Three

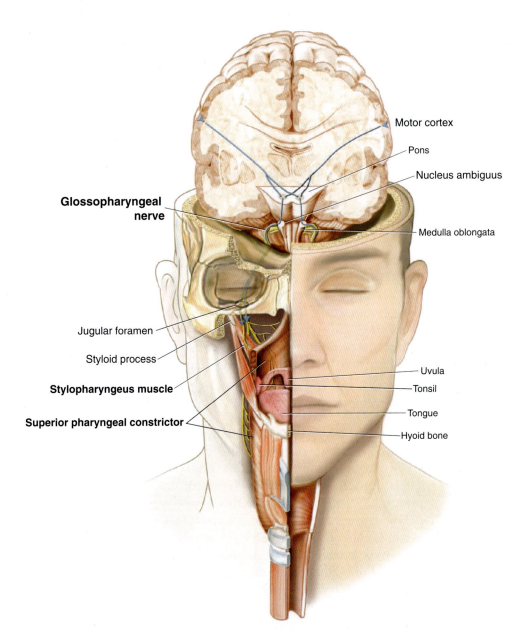

FIGURE 4–5. The glossopharyngeal nerve branches off from the brainstem just above the vagus nerve and courses out to the pharynx and tongue.

branches of the vagus nerve have special importance for motor speech production: the pharyngeal branch, the external superior laryngeal nerve branch, and the recurrent nerve branch.

Pharyngeal Branch The pharyngeal branch of the vagus nerve provides motor innervation for many muscles of the pharynx,

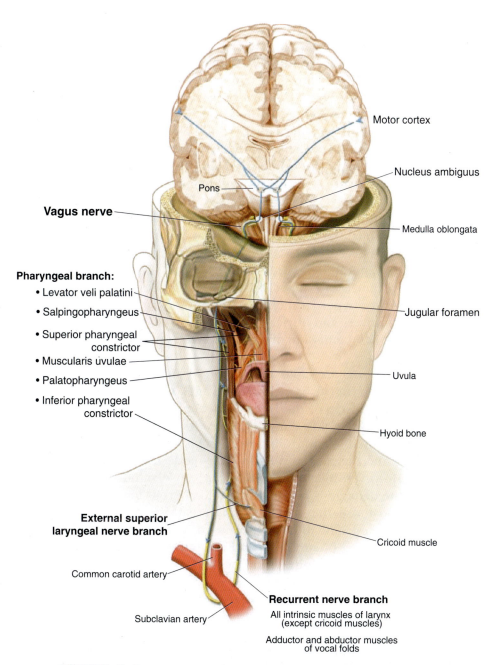

FIGURE 4-6. The many branches of the vagus nerve are amazingly complex. The recurrent nerve and the superior laryngeal nerve branches innervate the intrinsic muscles of the larynx. The pharyngeal branch (the pharyngeal plexus) innervates many muscles of the pharynx and velum.

including the musculus uvulae, levator veli palatini, salpingopharyngeus, palatopharyngeus, and the superior and middle pharyngeal constrictor muscles. Damage to the pharyngeal branch of the vagus nerve can affect the movement of the velum. For instance, unilateral damage to this branch can result in the affected side of the velum hanging visibly lower than the other side. In most cases, unilateral damage usually does not result in hypernasal speech because the velar muscles on the unaffected side usually will be able to raise the velum sufficiently to ensure adequate velopharyngeal closure on nonnasal phonemes.

However, bilateral damage to the pharyngeal branch of the vagus nerve can have a very significant effect on resonance. (Remember, bilateral damage means that both the left and right branches of a nerve have been injured in some manner.) When the damage is bilateral, nearly all the muscles of the velum will demonstrate weakness or paralysis. The result will be speech with moderate to severe hypernasality. In addition, the pressure consonants (stops, fricatives, and affricates) might be weak and distorted because of the nasal emission of air through the unsealed velopharyngeal port.

External Superior Laryngeal Nerve Branch The external superior laryngeal branch of the vagus nerve innervates the cricothyroid muscle of the larynx. This muscle helps to stretch and tense the vocal folds during speech. As a consequence, this muscle is essential in controlling vocal pitch. Unilateral damage to this nerve branch usually results in only modest difficulty in varying pitch. However, bilateral damage can cause significant problems. When the damage is bilateral, the cricothyroid muscle's ability to stretch and tense the vocal folds is greatly reduced. In such cases, an affected individual's voice might exhibit decreased loudness and increased breathiness, and the individual could have notable difficulty in changing vocal pitch.

Recurrent Nerve Branch This branch of the vagus nerve gets its name from the "double-back" route it travels from the brainstem to the larynx. The recurrent nerve branches from the vagus nerve after it leaves the cranium and then courses down near the heart before turning upward, traveling up along the trachea until it finally reaches the larynx. The recurrent nerve supplies the motor innervation to all the intrinsic muscles of the larynx except the cricothyroid muscle, which is innervated by the external superior laryngeal nerve. The recurrent nerve is a vital contributor to phonation because it supplies the motor innervation for all the adductor and abductor muscles of the vocal folds.

Unilateral damage to the recurrent nerve will cause the vocal fold on the affected side to be fixed in the paramedian position, which means that the fold is halfway between being fully adducted or fully abducted. An individual with unilateral vocal-fold paralysis will have breathy phonation and decreased vocal loudness. Bilateral damage to the recurrent nerve can fix both vocal folds in the paramedian position. When both vocal folds are in this position, they probably will still be close enough together to permit phonation on exhalation. However, this phonation will be very breathy and hoarse. Phonation on inhalation (inhalatory stridor) also might be evident because the vocal folds are fixed in this position during inhalation as well as exhalation.

Accessory Nerve (XI)

The accessory nerve is unique in that it is not a "pure" cranial nerve. It also contains neurons that branch out from the spinal cord. The cranial neurons of this nerve originate in the medulla just below the vagus nerve (Figure 4–7). In fact, many of its motor neuron axons merge with the vagus nerve shortly after they leave the medulla. These cranial motor neurons from the accessory nerve, working in conjunction with the vagus nerve, help innervate the intrinsic muscles of the velum, pharynx, and larynx. The spinal components of the accessory nerve supply motor innervation for the sternocleidomastoid and trapezius muscles. Because the neurons of this cranial nerve are so closely integrated with those of the vagus nerve, it is practically impossible to separate the functions of the two. In nearly all instances, damage to the cranial components of the accessory nerve will affect the vagus nerve as well and vice versa.

Hypoglossal Nerve (XII)

The hypoglossal cranial nerve originates in the medulla and courses to the tongue (Figure 4–8). This cranial nerve provides the motor innervation for all the intrinsic and most of the extrinsic muscles of the tongue. Unilateral damage to the hypoglossal cranial nerve results in weakness or paralysis in the half of the tongue that is on the same side as the nerve damage. If the damage is severe enough, the tongue muscles on the damaged side will eventually atrophy, leaving that half of the tongue shrunken. Furthermore, when the tongue is protruded, it will deviate toward the affected side because only half of the posterior genioglossus muscle is being contracted. Bilateral damage to the hypoglossal nerve will result in overall weakness of the tongue, reduction in the range of tongue movement, and muscle atrophy on both sides of the tongue.

As with the branch of the facial nerve that innervates the lower face, the hypoglossal cranial nerve primarily receives unilateral

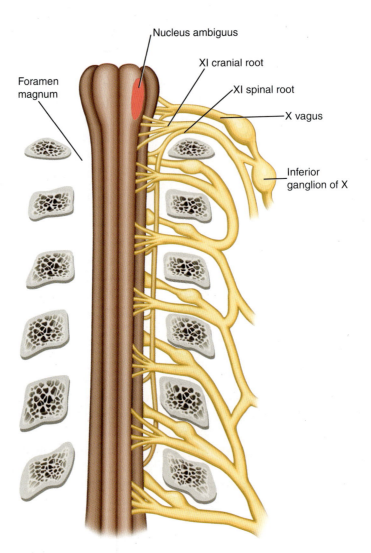

FIGURE 4–7. The cranial root and spinal roots of the accessory nerve.

innervation from the upper motor neurons. This means, for example, that most of the innervation for the right hypoglossal nerve comes only from the upper motor neurons of the corticobulbar tract that are in the left hemisphere of the brain. Damage to those left upper motor neurons will result in weakness in the right side of the tongue. Conversely, damage to the right upper motor neurons will result in weakness in the left side of the tongue.

Imprecise articulation is the primary characteristic of an individual with hypoglossal nerve damage. In cases of unilateral damage, the articulatory distortion will probably be mild because the unaffected side of the tongue can usually compensate for the weakened movements of the impaired side. Bilateral damage, however, can

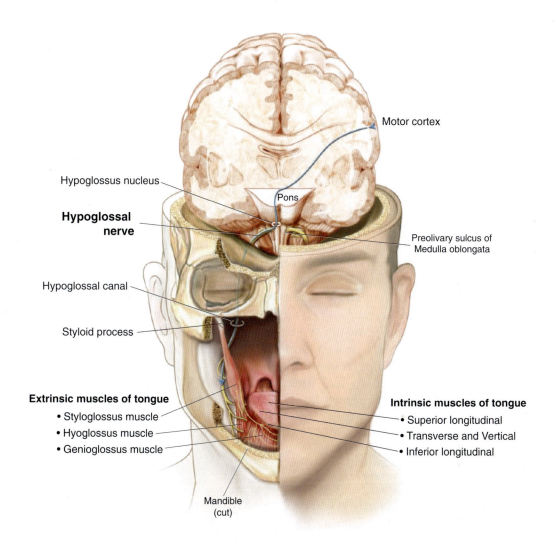

FIGURE 4–8. The hypoglossal nerve innervates all the intrinsic and most of the extrinsic tongue muscles.

have a much more significant effect on articulation. In these cases, phonemes requiring elevation of the tip or back of the tongue will be notably distorted (Duffy, 2020). Slow lingual movements also will be evident.

Spinal Nerves

The spinal nerves originate along the length of the spinal cord, from the cervical and thoracic sections down to the lumbar region. Many of the spinal nerves serve an important role in motor speech production because they provide the motor innervation for the muscles of respiration. One of the most important nerves of respiration is the phrenic nerve—a spinal nerve that originates from the cervical section of the spinal cord and provides the motor innervation of the diaphragm. The other muscles of inhalation and exhalation are innervated by the spinal nerves that originate along the cervical and thoracic portions of the spinal cord.

Damage to the cervical and thoracic spinal nerves can affect respiration and, thereby, can affect speech. In most instances, however, the damage must be quite widespread before a significant impairment of respiration will be evident. An exception to this is injury to the phrenic nerve, which can paralyze the diaphragm and result in significantly weakened inhalation. Individuals with impaired respiratory abilities might demonstrate decreased speech loudness as a result of reduced subglottic air pressure. Furthermore, these individuals could demonstrate shortened speech phrasing because of the reduced amount of air available for phonation. This shortened phrasing would almost certainly affect the prosody of their speech as well. Individuals with impaired respiration also might attempt to speak in longer phrases than their air supply will allow, resulting in a breathy or strained vocal quality toward the end of an utterance (known as "speaking on residual air").

Causes of Flaccid Dysarthria

Flaccid dysarthria can be caused by anything that disrupts the flow of motor impulses along the cranial or spinal nerves that innervate the muscles of speech production. Several conditions that damage lower motor neurons were briefly mentioned earlier in this chapter, such as brainstem stroke, tumors, and so forth. In the following paragraphs, the conditions that can cause flaccid dysarthria are examined in more detail.

Physical Trauma

Surgical trauma, head injury, and neck injury are common causes of flaccid dysarthria. Duffy (2005) indicated that these injuries caused 31% of flaccid dysarthria cases at the Mayo Clinic during a 23-year period—the highest percentage of all reported causes of this dysarthria. This high occurrence probably should not be surprising, given that physical damage leading to flaccid dysarthria can occur anywhere along the course of lower motor neurons, from the cell bodies in the brainstem to the neuromuscular junction.

Some of the surgical procedures that can lead to inadvertent damage to the cranial nerves of speech production include carotid endarterectomy (the removal of plaque deposits in a carotid artery), cardiac surgery, the removal of head and neck tumors, and dental surgery. In most of these cases, a cranial nerve is cut accidentally because of its proximity to the surgical site. Head and neck trauma resulting from motor vehicle accidents, blows to the head, and falls also can damage the cranial nerves of speech production. Broken bones from this type of trauma can compress or cut one of these cranial nerves. It also is possible that the rotational forces of such trauma can twist or stretch a nerve enough to cause damage. In any of these instances, the ability of the cranial nerve to carry motor impulses will be impaired, resulting in weakness or paralysis in the muscles innervated by the nerve.

Brainstem Stroke

Flaccid dysarthria can be caused by a stroke, which is more frequently called a **cerebrovascular accident** (CVA) by medical professionals. A stroke occurs when blood flow to the brain is interrupted because an artery breaks or is blocked. In either case, brain tissue is damaged from the lack of blood flow and the disruption of the neurons' metabolic processes. As with all other parts of the brain, the brainstem is rich with arterial blood flow, and when a stroke occurs in one of the brainstem arteries, the neurons served by that artery can be destroyed.

A brainstem stroke can affect the cranial nerves directly because the cell bodies of lower motor neurons (the cranial nerve nuclei) are located within the brainstem. When the blood supply to these cell bodies is blocked, many of the neurons will eventually die. This damage will impair the ability of the cranial nerves to transmit motor impulses to the muscles. The degree of impairment depends on the number of lower motor neurons that are lost to a stroke. If only a few neurons are affected, the resulting impairment of motor innervation might be minimal. If many of a cranial nerve's motor neurons are affected, numerous muscles innervated by that cranial nerve will be weakened or paralyzed.

It also is very possible for a single brainstem stroke to damage more than one cranial nerve. If the stroke is large enough to damage the cells in more than one cranial nerve nucleus, it will affect more than one cranial nerve. In fact, the damaging stroke does not have to be all that massive before it will affect more than one cranial nerve. Many cranial nerve nuclei are in close proximity in the brainstem. For example, the cranial nerve nuclei of the glossopharyngeal, vagus, and accessory nerves are quite close to each other in the brainstem. A single brainstem stroke in that area could affect the lower motor neurons in all three of those cranial nerves.

Myasthenia Gravis

Myasthenia gravis is a rare disease that affects the neuromuscular junction—the point where lower motor neurons synapse with muscle tissue. The primary symptom of this condition is the rapid fatigue of muscle contractions, with recovery occurring after a period of rest. Myasthenia gravis is caused by antibodies that block and, to a lesser extent, damage the parts of muscle tissue (the acetylcholine receptors) that receive the neurotransmitter acetylcholine from the lower motor neurons (Figure 4–9). The reception of acetylcholine at the muscle is what triggers a muscular contraction. When too many of these receptors are blocked, the muscle is not able to use enough acetylcholine for a full contraction. Consequently, the muscle cannot maintain the strength of its contractions over time, and the result is rapid fatigue and weakness. With rest, the muscle can make more efficient use of the acetylcholine, and stronger contractions will occur once again, but only for a short time.

There are several ways in which myasthenia gravis may progress in affected individuals. In about 51% of patients, the initial complaint is about eye muscle weakness that causes double vision or drooping of the upper eyelid. About 16% of patients have oral-pharyngeal weakness as the first symptom, which can cause flaccid dysarthria

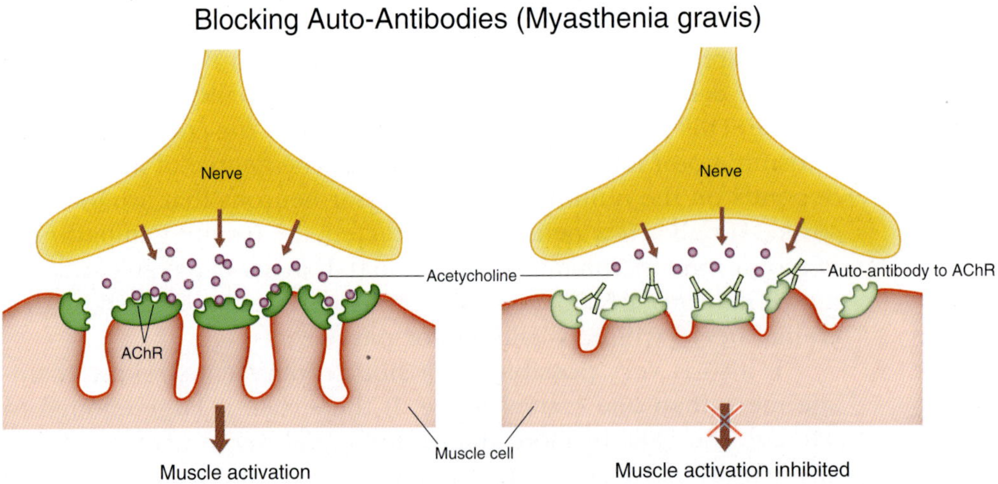

FIGURE 4–9. In myasthenia gravis, immune system antibodies impede the transmission of acetylcholine from lower motor neurons by blocking neurotransmitter receptors in muscle tissue.

or dysphagia. In some patients the condition eventually spreads to the limbs and trunk, causing a generalized myasthenia gravis.

Specific drugs can aid in the diagnosis of this disorder. An injection of Tensilon or similar anticholinesterase medications can almost immediately improve muscle contractions by prolonging the presence of acetylcholine in the neuromuscular junction, thereby providing more time for the neurotransmitter to be absorbed by the muscle. A patient with suspected myasthenia gravis will show rapidly improved muscle strength while the drug is present in the neuromuscular junction.

Effective medical treatments for myasthenia gravis are available. For example, immunosuppressant drugs are often used to inhibit the antibodies, which can minimize the blockage of acetylcholine receptors. Plasmapheresis can produce short-term benefits during acute attacks by filtering the antibodies from the blood. Some patients can benefit from the surgical removal of the thymus gland, which contains the lymphocytes that produce the antibodies (Dresser et al., 2021; Lazaridis & Tzartos, 2020).

Speech-language pathologists typically do not treat the speech deficits caused by myasthenia gravis, but they can be helpful in referring suspected cases to medical doctors for appropriate care. In a motor speech examination, myasthenia gravis is tested by having the patient count from 1 to 100 or read a long paragraph. If the disease is affecting the speech muscles, the patient will show a gradual onset of flaccid dysarthria during the prolonged speaking task, demonstrating hypernasality, decreased loudness, breathy voice quality, and imprecise articulation.

Guillain-Barré Syndrome

Guillain-Barré syndrome results in the progressive inflammatory loss of the myelin sheath around axons (Figure 4–10). The exact cause of this disorder is undetermined, but it frequently occurs after certain infections or immunization. The demyelination usually occurs in the PNS and tends to affect motor neurons more than sensory neurons. The progression can be quite rapid, often developing over a period of days or a few weeks. The peak of severity is often reached in about 2 weeks. This is in striking contrast to some of the better known progressive neurologic disorders, such as Parkinson's disease, which typically progress over a period of months or years.

In severe cases, Guillain-Barré syndrome can result in a near total paralysis of the entire body. Symptoms of weakness and numbness in the limbs are common early in this disorder, especially in the

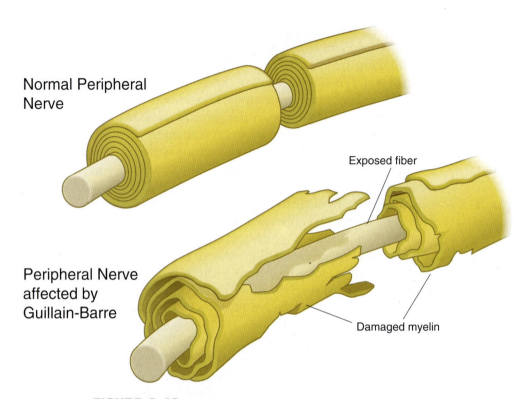

FIGURE 4–10. Guillain-Barré syndrome is an immune system disorder that causes damage to the myelin sheath around axons, primarily in the peripheral nervous system.

legs. Other early symptoms include flaccid dysarthria and dysphagia once the demyelination affects the cranial nerves. The recovery rate from Guillain-Barré syndrome is usually high, but 3% to 10% of affected individuals die during the acute stages of the disorder, often from either respiratory failure, blood pressure instability, or heart arrhythmia (Leonhard et al., 2019). Typical recovery occurs over a period of weeks or months. However, persons with the most severe cases might not fully recover and will always have some permanent weakness. For example, Shahrizaila et al. (2021) reported that 20% of Guillain-Barré patients have difficulty walking without assistance 1 year after onset. Speech-language pathologists can be involved with these patients during several stages of the disorder's progression. By monitoring changes in swallowing and speech intelligibility during the initial onset of symptoms, speech-language pathologists can make recommendations for oral feeding and for augmentative and alternative communication in those cases where speech becomes unintelligible. Speech-language pathologists might also be involved in the later recovery phase as swallowing improves and oral feeding gradually becomes possible again.

Polio

Polio is an infectious viral disease that attacks the cell bodies of lower motor neurons. Although vaccines have reduced the incidence of this disease greatly, unvaccinated individuals can become infected after close contact with a recently vaccinated child (Wiederholt, 2000). Polio most frequently affects the cervical and thoracic spinal nerves, often resulting in isolated respiratory weakness. When respiratory weakness occurs, the motor speech symptoms can include labored inhalation during speech, shortened speech phrases, speaking on residual air, and decreased loudness. Unfortunately, a polio infection is not always restricted to the spinal nerves. It also can affect the cranial nerves. In about 10% to 15% of polio cases, the virus can damage the lower motor neurons in the trigeminal, facial, glossopharyngeal, and vagus nerves (Duffy, 2020), resulting in weakness in the muscles innervated by those nerves.

Other Causes of Flaccid Dysarthria

Many additional disorders can cause flaccid dysarthria; this is a summary of just a few of them. A **tumor** growing in or near the brainstem can compromise a cranial nerve's ability to transmit its neural impulses to muscles. Tumors occurring along the course of a cranial nerve's pathway, such as in the neck or in any orofacial structure, also can affect the nerve's functioning. **Muscular dystrophy** is a disease that causes a progressive degeneration of muscle tissue. It can result in weakness in many muscles served by the cranial nerves, such as the tongue, face, and pharynx. **Progressive bulbar palsy** is a disorder that can affect both upper and lower motor neurons, although it often is present only in the lower motor neurons. When the lower motor neurons are affected, progressive bulbar palsy can cause flaccid dysarthria. When it is present in both sets of motor neurons, it can result in a mixed dysarthria, usually of the flaccid-spastic type (see Chapter 10).

Speech Characteristics of Flaccid Dysarthria

This section examines the typical speech characteristics of flaccid dysarthria. The effects of flaccid dysarthria on resonance, articulation, phonation, respiration, and prosody are discussed. It is important to remember, however, that not all individuals with flaccid dysarthria will demonstrate deficits in each of these areas, although some will. Furthermore, the severity level within each area will not necessarily be the same for any two patients. Individual variations in motor speech deficits are common for all the dysarthrias, even when the affected individuals share the same type of dysarthria. Because of these variations, it is important to look for clusters of symptoms when trying to diagnose a particular type of dysarthria. Once a cluster of symptoms has been identified, determine which type of dysarthria it most closely represents. This holds true for the diagnosis of any motor speech disorder, not just flaccid dysarthria.

Resonance

In their landmark study of dysarthria, Darley et al. (1969a, 1969b) examined the abnormal speech characteristics of 30 subjects with flaccid dysarthria. Table 4–1 ranks these subjects' nine most prominent speech errors. **Hypernasality** was the most noticeable error. It was present in the speech of 25 of the 30 subjects. Hypernasality is certainly an important diagnostic marker for flaccid dysarthria. Although it is not unique to flaccid dysarthria, it tends to be more noticeable in this type of dysarthria as compared with the other dysarthrias. Other resonance-related problems in flaccid dysarthria include **nasal emission** due to incomplete velopharyngeal closure, **weak pressure consonants** caused by decreased intraoral air pres-

TABLE 4–1 Most Common Speech Production Errors in 30 Individuals With Flaccid Dysarthria

Rank	Speech Production Errors
1	Hypernasality
2	Imprecise consonants
3	Breathiness (continuous)
4	Monopitch
5	Nasal emission
6	Audible inspiration
7	Harsh voice quality
8	Short phrases
9	Monoloudness

Note: From "Clusters of Diagnostic Patterns of Dysarthria," by F. L. Darley, A. E. Aronson, and J. R. Brown; 1969, *Journal of Speech and Hearing Research*, 12, p. 251. Copyright 1969 by American Speech-Language-Hearing Association. Reprinted with permission.

sure, and shortened phrases, which are the result of wasted air that escapes through the nasal cavity during speech. All of these resonance deficits primarily reflect bilateral damage to the pharyngeal branch of the vagus nerve because it innervates most of the muscles of the velum. Watch the PluralPlus Flaccid Dysarthria Case 1 video for an example of significant hypernasality in a patient with flaccid dysarthria following a head injury.

Articulation

Imprecise consonant production was the second most prominent abnormal speech characteristic of flaccid dysarthria reported by Darley et al. (1969a, 1969b). There can be a large range of severity for misarticulated phonemes in individuals with flaccid dysarthria, from only a mild distortion to complete unintelligibility. Damage to the facial and hypoglossal nerves is usually cited as a reason for these problems with the production of consonant phonemes (Duffy, 2020). Bilateral damage to the facial nerve can have a significant effect on the production of bilabial and labiodental phonemes, as well as of consonants and vowels requiring lip rounding. Bilateral damage to the hypoglossal nerve will likely result in misarticulations of phonemes requiring the elevation of the tongue, especially the tongue tip. For example, a damaged hypoglossal nerve can affect the production of the linguadental and linguapalatal phonemes, such as /j/ and /l/. In severe cases of bilateral hypoglossal nerve damage, the production of the linguavelar phonemes also will be impaired. Watch the PluralPlus Flaccid Dysarthria Case 2 video for an example of imprecise consonants in connected speech secondary to a brainstem stroke.

Damage to the trigeminal nerve also can affect articulation. As mentioned previously, bilateral damage to this nerve can result in difficulty elevating the jaw sufficiently to bring the articulators into contact with each other. Without proper jaw elevation, it might be impossible for an affected individual to accurately produce any of the consonants and most of the vowels. Such an individual might need to elevate the jaw by hand or use a device known as a "jaw sling" before intelligible speech is possible.

Phonation

Another common abnormal speech characteristic of flaccid dysarthria is **phonatory incompetence** (Darley et al., 1969a, 1969b). This term refers to the incomplete adduction of the vocal folds during phonation. It is caused by damage to the recurrent branch of the vagus nerve, which provides motor innervation to almost all of the intrinsic muscles of the larynx. Injury to this cranial nerve can leave the vocal-fold adductor and abductor muscles weak or paralyzed. If the adductor muscles are primarily affected, the vocal folds will not meet with enough strength to produce a clear phonation. The result will be phonation that has a **breathy voice quality**, which can almost sound like a whisper in severe cases. If the abductor muscles are primarily affected, the vocal folds will not be able to fully abduct during inhalation. When **abduction** is incomplete, there can be an audible inhalatory stridor.

As with hypernasality, phonatory incompetence is an especially valuable confirmatory sign for the diagnosis of flaccid dysarthria. It can be quite prominent in cases of flaccid dysarthria, to a degree that is not found in the other dysarthrias (Duffy, 2020). Moreover, the combined presence of hypernasality and phonatory incompetence is the strongest confirmatory sign that flaccid dysarthria is the correct diagnosis.

Respiration

Weakened respiration might or might not be a component of flaccid dysarthria. If the cervical and thoracic spinal nerves responsible for innervating the diaphragm and the intercostal muscles are damaged, the result can be decreased inhalation or impaired control of exhalation during speech. In either instance, the affected individuals will not have adequate amounts of subglottic air pressure for speech. Without enough subglottic air, the speech of individuals with flaccid dysarthria could demonstrate reduced loudness and shortened phrase length. Their speech might have a strained vocal quality if they speak on residual air to prolong the length of their phrases. Reduced loudness, shortened phrase length, and strained vocal quality will affect prosody. In addition, Darley et al. (1975) mentioned that individuals with weakened respiration also might demonstrate monoloudness and monopitch.

A Problem of Respiration or Phonation?

Many individuals with flaccid dysarthria inhale frequently while speaking, which can adversely affect the prosody of their speech. Although frequent inhalations are usually easy to identify, it is sometimes difficult to determine whether the problem is one of air wastage because of poor laryngeal valving or reduced **vital capacity** because of weakened respiration. In either case, the affected individual will probably demonstrate reduced loudness, shortened phrase length, and strained vocal quality in conversational speech. But how is a clinician to determine whether the problem is one of respiration or phonation? Duffy (2020) described a simple procedure to help determine which is the most likely cause of this problem.

1. Ask the individual to produce a good cough; listen to how sharp it sounds. A breathy, feeble cough might indicate weakness in the vocal-fold adductor muscles, inadequate respiration, or perhaps both.

2. Then ask the individual to produce a hard glottal stop; again listen to how sharp it sounds. Producing a hard glottal stop requires firm closure of the vocal folds but little respiratory effort. Consequently, the individual who produces a breathy cough and a sharp glottal stop might be demonstrating poor respiration. In turn, a breathy cough and a weak glottal stop might indicate that the cause of the air supply problem is either weak laryngeal closure or a combination of weak laryngeal and respiratory functioning.

Prosody

Individuals with flaccid dysarthria might demonstrate speech that has **monopitch** and **monoloudness**. Darley et al. (1969a, 1969b) noted both of these prosodic errors in their subjects with flaccid dysarthria. It is likely that these qualities are primarily the result of weakened laryngeal muscles that are unable to make the many fine vocal-fold adjustments needed for normal pitch and loudness variations. For example, if the cricothyroid muscle is weakened by damage to the superior laryngeal branch of the vagus nerve, it might not be able to tense and stretch the vocal folds sufficiently to produce normal changes in pitch and loudness. Incidentally, monopitch and monoloudness are not unique to flaccid dysarthria; they can appear in a number of other dysarthrias, such as spastic and ataxic dysarthria. Consequently, the presence of monopitch and monoloudness are not definite diagnostic markers for flaccid dysarthria, unlike the co-occurrence of hypernasality and phonatory insufficiency.

Key Evaluation Tasks for Flaccid Dysarthria

The following assessment tasks in Appendix 3–1 might be particularly useful in detecting key characteristics of flaccid dysarthria (Hegde & Freed, 2022):

- Vowel prolongation can produce the breathy voice quality that is typical of phonatory incompetence as well as the respiratory weakness that can shorten the length of the client's production of the vowel.
- Alternate motion rates can evoke the slow production of phonemes that is common in this dysarthria.
- Connected speech during conversation or while reading aloud can evoke a client's monopitch and monoloud prosody, shortened phrases, articulation distortions, and hypernasality.
- A speech stress test (counting 1–100) is needed in suspected cases of myasthenia gravis.
- There are a number of physical symptoms and speech errors that are more characteristic of flaccid dysarthria than of the other dysarthrias. When any of the following characteristics are noted during the motor speech assessment in Appendix 3–1, the client might have flaccid dysarthria:
  - Diminished or absent oral reflexes (e.g., gag reflex)—this contrasts with the hyperreflexes that can be present in spastic dysarthria.
  - Muscle atrophy in the muscles of the speech mechanism—atrophy is the result of lower motor damage (which also is the cause of flaccid dysarthria).
  - As previously noted, the combination of hypernasality and phonatory incompetence is a strong indicator of flaccid dysarthria.
  - Inhalatory stridor (audible phonation during inhalation) suggests laryngeal weakness that is often associated with flaccid dysarthria.
  - Diplophonia is more often associated with flaccid dysarthria than any other dysarthria.

Treatment of Motor Speech Disorders

Before examining the treatment of flaccid dysarthria, it is important to discuss a few general details about managing motor speech disorders. Recent reviews of the dysarthria treatment literature have mostly agreed that the behavioral interventions done by speech-language pathologists can have positive outcomes, but the nature of these treatments makes it difficult to draw definitive conclusions about which procedures provide the best outcomes (Chiaramonte et al., 2020; Finch et al., 2020; Gandhi et al., 2020; Mitchell et al., 2017). Variability of treatment structure, intensity, duration, and other factors make direct comparisons of procedures difficult and hinder the determination of which techniques are most effective. Because therapy for motor speech disorders is such a highly individualized process, it can sometimes be a challenge to know which procedure is definitely best for a given patient. Clinicians improve their chances of success when they have a structured base on which to build their treatments.

A very traditional way of organizing treatment is to (a) use assessment data to identify the problems, (b) write goals to address those problems, (c) begin working with the patient using appropriate treatment tasks, (d) increase the complexity of the tasks as the patient improves, and (e) work toward generalizing improved speech into real-world settings. Although there is nothing wrong with this approach, it glosses over the importance of dealing with the patient's perceptions and expectations. For example, some patients are not aware that their speech is different. Others fear the possibility of failure. Still others are reluctant to participate fully in treatment once they realize how much work will be required. Experienced clinicians almost always develop their own methods to successfully address all of these varied components that are needed to successfully treat these disorders. Rosenbek (2017) described an overall structure for treating motor speech disorders that prioritizes the patient's needs, yet still uses a traditional orientation toward therapy. He divided his recommendations into six components:

Component One: Recognizing Differences—In the situation where patients show minimal awareness of how their speech sounds, Rosenbek recommended asking a series of questions about the patients' speech, such as "Has your spouse or children said they cannot understand you? Have other people commented on your speech? Do you agree with what they say about your speech?" These questions can be the starting place for enhancing the patients' knowledge of their speech and how others react to it. Sometimes awareness of deficits can be enhanced by letting patients hear a high-quality audio recording of their speech. This can be a potent tool for many patients. A related procedure is to let patients hear two recordings of their speech, once while successfully using a treatment technique (e.g., slowed rate of speech, overarticulation) and once without. The contrast between the two recordings can clearly highlight the speech problems for patients and also demonstrate that improvements are possible.

Component Two: Willingness to Change—Remarkably, some patients are not fully committed to changing their speech or engaging in treatment. Rosenbek said that for these patients, it is not enough for a clinician to just describe the therapeutic process and a probable outcome. Such patients might be lacking motivation, or they are only considering the possibility of committing to the treatment process. Still other patients might be apprehensive about participating in speech therapy because it is so very unfamiliar to them. In these situations, it often is useful to have a close family member or friend involved in the sessions. It can be very reassuring and motivating for reluctant patients to hear words of satisfaction, encouragement, and surprise from these important individuals while the initial steps of treatment are conducted.

Component Three: Setting Goals—Rosenbek made solid recommendations on how to create treatment goals. He said that clinicians need to create their goals in collaboration with their patients. Rather than just telling patients, "These are the goals for your therapy sessions," clinicians should talk to the patients about what troubles them most about their speech. Is it poor articulation, weak phonation, monotone prosody, or something else? Clinicians and patients should decide on their treatment goals only after they have agreed on what is most troublesome. Rosenbek also mentioned that creating the initial goals might take more than one session and that the goals might need to be adjusted during the course of treatment—once again in collaboration with patients.

Component Four: Talking Therapeutically—Talking therapeutically occurs when patients speak carefully and intentionally using the therapeutic procedure (or procedures) recommended by the clinician. In the early treatment sessions, patients usually talk therapeutically only for short amounts of time, perhaps just during structured drills. As patients become more practiced with the procedure, though, they are gradually required to talk therapeutically for the entire session, even during moments of chit-chat between therapy activities. Furthermore, talking therapeutically means that an utterance is not started until the spoken message is fully formulated in the patients' mind, and their body is ready to produce it (e.g., having a full breath of air). Rosenbek cautioned that sometimes patients will find that their first attempts at talking therapeutically will sound worse than their day-to-day dysarthric speech. For example, during a first attempt at overarticulation or slowed rate of talking, speech might sound exaggerated or distorted. Patients need to be reassured that these early steps of treatment gradually will be adjusted. As they get better at the tasks, the speaking requirements will be modified to provide them ultimately with the most natural speech possible.

Component Five: Learning to Listen, Evaluate, and Self-Correct—These are essential skills if patients are going to generalize what they have learned in the clinic room to outside settings. In other words, patients need to become their own clinicians. Rosenbek recommended that clinicians and patients create a 3-point self-evaluation scale to describe moments of talking therapeutically. A score of 1 on the scale is for an utterance that is shows no improvement over the first day of treatment. A 2 is given for an utterance that is improved but not as good as possible. A 3 is assigned for an utterance that is the best possible. Clinicians and patients also must agree on what is being judged during these self-evaluations (e.g., clear articulation of target consonants, slower rate, louder phonation). They then practice using the scale until they are comfortable with it. The final step is for a comparison of clinician and patient scores. If the two scores do not agree, a short discussion is necessary to determine why. When there is agreement on the scoring and the score is a 1 or 2, patients attempt self-corrections to make the utterance the best possible. If the agreed score is a 3, clinicians can give brief feedback on why the utterance was successful.

Component Six: Add Cognitive-Linguistic Load—This is an important part of working toward generalization. Rosenbek mentioned that dysarthric patients' speech accuracy declines in settings where there are more cognitive-linguistic demands, such as talking about complex subjects or in loud, distracting environments. To help patients maintain their treatment gains in these real-world circumstances, clinicians need to design treatment tasks that mimic those difficult environments. He recommended, for example, requiring faster or longer responses, introducing visual or auditory distractions, and formulating complex responses or questions. He suggested bringing family members or volunteers into the clinic room so that they can converse with patients during the sessions. During all of these tasks of increased cognitive-linguistic load, the expectation is that patients will consistently talk therapeutically. Nevertheless, it is probable that performance will decline to some degree as the communicative demands increase. When this happens, clinicians and patients must remind themselves that continued work on the production, evaluation, and self-repair of complex utterances in difficult settings is an essential part of enhancing generalization.

Treatment of Flaccid Dysarthria

The final section of each remaining chapter contains treatment ideas for one of the dysarthrias. Clinicians should know that these sections cover the most practical treatment tasks based on the author's experience; however, they are not exhaustive. No book of this kind can include every treatment idea for such a complex collection of disorders as dysarthria and apraxia of speech. There are additional treatment ideas in other textbooks and research articles. Clinicians are encouraged to search out other treatment options. Two textbooks in particular are recommended for their treatment ideas, as well as for their general examination of motor speech disorders:

- *Motor Speech Disorders: Substrates, Differential Diagnosis, and Management* (4th ed.; Duffy, 2020)
- *Management of Motor Speech Disorders in Children and Adults* (Yorkston et al., 2010)

As has been mentioned several times in this chapter, flaccid dysarthria is caused by damage to the lower motor neurons in six specific cranial nerves. The following treatment options for flaccid dysarthria are grouped according to which cranial nerve is damaged. Flaccid dysarthria is often the result of damage to more than one cranial nerve, so combinations of various treatments are appropriate in those cases. The recommended number of trials in these treatments is only a rough guideline. The needs of patients vary greatly. Some will not be able to complete the recommended trials; others might benefit from more than the recommended trials. Clinicians will need to adjust the treatment tasks according to the requirements and abilities of their patients.

Before examining the specific treatment tasks, a few words should be said about using nonspeech oral strengthening exercises to improve speech production. Muscular weakness is a common characteristic of many types of dysarthria (Solomon et al., 2017). Consequently, some clinicians assume that nonspeech oral strengthening exercises (e.g., pursing the lips, smiling, pressing the tongue against a tongue blade) should be part of a treatment plan. However, the value of these activities as a dysarthria treatment is open to question. Kent (2015), Maas (2017), and others reported that no definitive research shows that these exercises make significant contributions to the recovery of speech production in motor speech disorders. Kent (2015) described such evidence as "nascent" (p. 777). One of the objections to using strengthening exercises is the finding that oral and pharyngeal muscle contractions during nonspeech tasks are quite different from muscle contractions made during speech. Because this difference in muscular function is so profound, repetitive nonspeech strengthening exercises cannot significantly improve the very dissimilar muscle contractions used in speech. Related to this point is a comment by Marzouqah et al. (2023) in their review of 26 studies that examined oral and pharyngeal motor exercises following a stroke. Although they concluded that these tasks could be beneficial for sleep breathing disorders and facial paresis,

> [t]he speech function outcomes (e.g., sentence intelligibility) were not affected [by the exercises]. This was not surprising—the use of exercises to improve speech remains controversial as muscle engagement in speech requires speed, high precision, and coordination over strength, but the specific exercises and measures targeting and reflecting these types of outcomes are lacking. (p. 632)

So, until there is research showing that oral strengthening exercises for dysarthria are effective, the general rule for treating the speech errors of patients with oral weakness should be this: If improving speech production is the goal, treatment activities should concentrate directly on speech production.

Damage to the Trigeminal Cranial Nerve (V)

Unilateral damage to this cranial nerve typically has a negligible effect on speech production. Patients with this type of injury probably will not need significant amounts of treatment, if they need any at all. However, bilateral damage to the trigeminal nerve, although rare, can leave the jaw muscles very weak or, in severe cases, can cause an inability to close the jaw. A jaw sling is one way to compensate for bilateral trigeminal nerve damage. This prosthetic device is placed under the jaw and lifts it close to the maxilla. By adjusting the amount of supportive jaw elevation provided, appropriate articulatory contact can be provided for the lower lip and the tongue. Jaw slings can be obtained at medical supply businesses, as well as from companies specializing in products for speech-language pathologists.

Damage to the Vagus Cranial Nerve (X)

As mentioned previously, damage to the vagus nerve also usually affects the glossopharyngeal and accessory cranial nerves because these three cranial nerves branch out from the brainstem in very close proximity to each other. Moreover, it is often difficult to separate the functions of these cranial nerves because they innervate many of the same anatomical structures. Consequently, it is appropriate to assume that the tasks presented in this section also are suitable treatments for damage to the glossopharyngeal and accessory nerves.

Treatments for Resonance Deficits

Injury to the pharyngeal branch of the vagus nerve can result in weak, incomplete elevation of the velum, which could cause hypernasal resonance. The severity of the hypernasality depends partly on whether the damage to this nerve branch is unilateral or bilateral. Unilateral damage might result in only mild hypernasality because the unaffected pharyngeal nerve branch from the contralateral side continues to innervate the muscles on the other side of the soft palate. However, bilateral damage to the pharyngeal branch of the vagus nerve usually results in moderate to severe hypernasality because the muscles on both sides of the soft palate are either weakened or paralyzed.

Surgical and Prosthetic Treatments

Two procedures are used in the surgical treatment of **velopharyngeal incompetence**. The first is the **pharyngeal flap procedure**. In this procedure, a flap of tissue from the pharynx is surgically attached to the velum. As a result, much of the velopharyngeal port is closed by this attached flap of tissue. However, the sides of the flap are left loose to provide an opening between the oral and nasal cavities, which is important for nasal breathing and producing nasal speech sounds. The other surgical procedure used to treat hypernasality is called **posterior pharyngeal wall augmentation**. In this procedure, Teflon paste, hyaluronic acid (a natural substance used cosmetically to fill facial wrinkles), cartilage, or fat is injected into the pharynx at the point where the velum normally makes contact when it is elevated. The injection creates a bulge at that point on the pharynx and lessens the distance the velum must rise before velopharyngeal closure is completed. The effectiveness of these two procedures in individuals with dysarthria has been inconsistent. They have worked for some patients but not for others. Pharyngeal augmentation has had especially mixed results (Woo, 2012) and probably works best when velar incompetence is mild (Young & Spinner, 2022).

Because of these variable results, a prosthetic treatment called a **palatal lift**, essentially a dental retainer that has a rear extension that helps push upward on the velum, currently is used more frequently than either of the surgical treatments (Alfwaress et al., 2017; Light et al., 2001). Because of this upward push, the device can aid in the elevation of the velum during speech. Duffy (2020) and Yorkston et al. (2001) indicated that the palatal lift is the most successful treatment for serious resonance problems in individuals with dysarthria. However, these authors also mentioned the characteristics of individuals who are the best candidates for this prosthetic device:

- Hypernasality is their most serious speech production deficit.
- Their medical condition is stable and not deteriorating.
- They have enough teeth onto which the lift can be attached.
- They do not have a hyperactive gag reflex or significant oral spasticity.
- They have the patience and motivation to use the lift.
- They are able to insert and remove the device independently.

Given these criteria, it should be clear that a palatal lift is not appropriate for all patients. However, even motivated patients might need to adjust to wearing these devices. In some cases, they just need to get used to having the lift in their mouths. Others initially find that the lift does not aid in the closure of the velopharyngeal port as much as they would have hoped. Suggestions for fine-tuning velopharyngeal closure in those patients include Dworkin's (1991) recommendation of a series of increasingly difficult velum closure activities to improve the effectiveness of the palatal lift. Also, Ono et al. (2005) reported that a combination of self-monitoring and biofeedback using a See-Scape improved the intelligibility of their palatal lift patient during a 3-month course of treatment. The results showed improved velar closure in the patient's connected speech, which especially helped his production of pressure consonants. (A See-Scape is a simple yet sensitive airflow instrument that can show the escape of air through the nostrils.) Garhnayak et al. (2020) also successfully used a palatal lift in a 20-year-old patient with hypernasal speech.

A related oral device is a palatal augmentation prosthesis. Similar to a palatal lift in that it also clips onto the hard palate like a (thick) dental retainer, this device is designed to facilitate tongue-to-palate contact by shortening the vertical movement needed to make tongue–palate closure. It is used when tongue elevation is inadequate for normal speech or swallowing, such as after a partial glossectomy or stroke. Several studies have found that a palatal augmentation prosthesis can improve production of lingual-platal phonemes during speech and enhance oral-phase swallowing in individuals with tongue elevation deficits (Nagao et al., 2023; Yokoyama et al., 2022). Hirasaki et al. (2023) successfully combined a palatal lift and palatal augmentation into a single prosthesis for a patient with both hypernasal speech and significant dysphagia.

Velar Strengthening and Nonspeech Exercises

Numerous researchers agree that velar strengthening and stimulation procedures do little to improve velopharyngeal closure in most cases of flaccid dysarthria (Brookshire, 2015; Dworkin & Johns, 1980; Palmer & Enderby, 2007; Strand & Sullivan, 2001). Yorkston et al. (2001) found no evidence that pushing and pulling techniques, strengthening tasks, or blowing activities (using such items as whistles, bubbles, or cotton balls) can enhance velar function for speech. Although such tasks might seem logical, they are not recommended. Current research indicates that muscle contractions for nonspeech tasks are very different from contractions for velar closure during speech. As a result, there is little relationship between nonspeech velar movements and those during speech (Yorkston et al., 2001).

However, there is one velar strength-training procedure that has shown promise and has a research-based foundation (Kuehn, 1997). It uses the continuous positive airway pressure (CPAP) device that normally is used as a treatment for sleep apnea. A CPAP activity is different from the blowing exercises mentioned in the prior paragraph in that it provides resistance to velar movement during speech tasks. For this procedure, the patient wears a nasal mask that sends a continuous flow of air through the nasal cavity and into the upper pharynx. As the air flows downward through the velopharyngeal port, the patient engages in speech tasks requiring a variety of velar movements. As the patient speaks, the velum is forced to work against the resistance of the downward flowing air throughout the time the patient is speaking. This means that the velar muscles are being stressed while actually contracting for speech movements, which differs significantly from activities that stress nonspeech velar contractions. Although CPAP has been used with only a small number patients with dysarthria (Liss et al., 1994), it is worthy of further investigation.

Behavioral Approaches for Mild Hypernasality (Modification of Speech)

Some patients with hypernasality can minimize their resonance problem by modifying their speech. Clinical experience and expert opinion suggest that this can be useful in cases of mild hypernasality (Strand & Sullivan, 2001; Yorkston et al., 2001). It is not recommended for patients with moderate or severe resonance problems. These modification procedures include the following tasks:

- Reduce rate of speech—Reducing the rate of speech can increase intelligibility and lessen the perception of hypernasality in some individuals with flaccid dysarthria (Strand & Sullivan, 2001; Yorkston et al., 2010). Numerous activities can help in reducing the rate of speech (see Chapter 8). One that might be appropriate in cases of flaccid dysarthria is the use of finger or hand tapping to set the appropriate speaking rate. In this procedure, the patient speaks one word or syllable for every tap of the clinician's finger or hand. In general, slowing the rate in this manner increases intelligibility because it allows extra time for the articulators to reach their targets, thus resulting in more precise articulation of phonemes. The slower rate might decrease hypernasality because it can give a slow-moving velum extra time to fully and accurately close the velopharyngeal port during connected speech, which also promotes improved production of the pressure consonants.

- More open-position mouth during speech—Exaggerated jaw movements during speech can also lessen the perception of hypernasality (Picheny et al., 1985; Strand & Sullivan, 2001). Swigert (2010) recommended a sequence of steps that can increase the patient's ability to maintain a more open mouth while speaking. First, increase the patient's awareness of what is hypernasal speech. This can be accomplished through clinician modeling and by having the patient read sentences that have either many nasal phonemes or no nasal phonemes. Second, have the patient look in a mirror while repeating sentences that contain many open vowels. The patient should try to maintain exaggerated jaw movements while repeating the sentences. Third, the clinician can use negative practice to demonstrate the positive effects of an open-mouth posture. For example, instruct the patient to purposefully keep the mouth nearly closed during speech. With the mouth almost closed, the patient's speech should be noticeably more hypernasal as compared to when a wide-open posture is used. Instant replays of video or audiotape recordings could also be useful in helping the patient hear the difference in hypernasality between the open- and closed-posture speech.

- Increase loudness—The perception of hypernasality can sometimes be minimized by having the patient speak more loudly. Louder speech tends to mask the hypernasal resonance in individuals with flaccid dysarthria. Equally important, the louder speech can often increase intelligibility by simply making it easier for a listener to hear what is being said. Modeling appropriate loudness levels is a key component of this treatment. Visual feedback on loudness is also helpful for most patients. A sound pressure level meter (either as a stand-alone instrument or an app on a smartphone) can give patients a visual cue as to what the desired loudness should be.

Treatments for Phonation Deficits

Damage to the recurrent branch of the vagus nerve can cause significant problems of phonation because this branch innervates nearly all the intrinsic muscles of the larynx. Damage to this nerve branch usually results in breathy or harsh vocal quality, as laryngeal muscle weakness or paralysis prevents the vocal folds from fully adducting. There are several treatment tasks that can bring the vocal folds together more completely during phonation and could result in a clearer, more normal vocal quality.

- Effortful closure—Some patients can adduct their vocal folds more tightly by just consciously putting more physical effort into speaking more loudly. Not only can increasing loudness improve phonation, but it also might enhance the patient's intelligibility. McAuliffe et al. (2017) found that when their dysarthric speakers consciously spoke more loudly, listeners reported significant gains in intelligibility. A further analysis of their data showed that the physical effort of speaking more loudly actually improved the articulatory distinctiveness of vowels, which also contributed to improved intelligibility. Slowing the rate of speech also improved intelligibility but not as often as increased loudness. Interestingly, the improvements were not restricted to dysarthria type. Similar intelligibility improvements in dysarthric stroke and traumatic brain injury (TBI) patients have been noted using the Lee Silverman Voice Treatment, another effortful phonation procedure (Wenke et al., 2008; Youssef et al., 2015) that is discussed in Chapter 8.

When conscious effort is not enough to bring the vocal cords together more tightly, pushing and pulling procedures might help with adduction by providing an overall increase in muscle contractions in the torso and neck. Examples of these procedures include having a sitting patient push up on the arms of a chair while phonating an open vowel or having the patient pull up on the edge of a heavy table while prolonging a vowel. With enough time and practice, these procedures might help patients realize that they can produce more normal-sounding phonations when they apply greater physical effort (Ramig, 1995; Spencer et al., 2003).

- Holding breath—Holding a deep breath of air requires the ability to fully adduct the vocal folds. The tighter the adduction, the better the air will be held in the lungs. Ask the patient to inhale deeply and hold his or her breath. Use a small mirror under the nostrils to detect leaking air. Work to the point at which the patient can hold a breath for about 15 s over 10 consecutive trials. Be sure to give sufficient rest periods between the trials.

- Hard glottal attack—Some patients can demonstrate a better quality phonation when they begin an utterance with a hard glottal attack (Dworkin & Meleca, 1997; Spencer et al., 2003). Dworkin (1991) described a complete exercise for this procedure. The basic steps are to have the patient hold a deep breath, bear down, and attempt to phonate a tight /a/. This tight phonation should be modified into a more normal vocal quality as soon as possible to avoid the negative side effects of consistent hard glottal attacks during speech.

- Head turning and sideways pressure on the larynx—When there is unilateral weakness or paralysis of one vocal fold, phonation will be breathy because the weak fold will not be able to fully adduct to the midline of the glottis. With some patients, a more complete vocal fold adduction might be achieved either when the head is turned toward the affected side or when the larynx is pushed by hand from the affected side (i.e., pushed toward the unaffected side). In both instances, the weakened vocal fold can be brought closer to the opposite fold, thereby improving the quality of the phonation (Spencer et al., 2003).

Although it might seem unlikely that these two tasks would ever be useful in a real-world conversational setting, a recent clinical episode showed the benefit of the head-turning procedure. During the initial assessment of a brainstem stroke patient with unilateral vocal fold paresis, the clinician asked her to turn her head side-to-side while continuously speaking. Both the clinician and the patient noticed that the quality and loudness of her phonation was modestly better when her head was turned to the right. The clinician explained to the patient why this change in posture improved her speech, and nothing more was said about it. The patient, without telling the clinician, started modifying her home environment to take advantage of this technique. She and her husband changed their usual seating arrangements at home as well as in other settings so that he was more or less exclusively on her right side whenever they were talking. It was not until the patient was about to be discharged that she told the clinician how she had implemented the head-turning technique to her benefit. She reported that it allowed her husband to understand her better throughout the day, partly because of her improved phonation but also (she thought) because he could see her face fully when she was speaking. The use of environment management like this to enhance communicative effectiveness is something that should never be overlooked when treating dysarthria and related neurogenic disorders. Berry and Sanders (1983) were among the first to document how manipulating a patient's everyday environment can promote intelligibility. They recommended procedures such as sitting no more than 4 ft from the speaker, avoiding rooms with reverberant acoustics, turning off televisions and radios, looking directly at the speaker's face, and having the speaker start an utterance with a carrier phrase (e.g., "I want to tell you about . . . .").

Treatments for Prosodic Deficits

Damage to the exterior superior laryngeal branch of the vagus nerve can impair the function of the cricothyroid muscle, which helps vary vocal pitch by stretching and relaxing the vocal folds. Many clinicians and researchers recognize the importance of treating prosodic errors (Darley et al., 1975; Duffy, 2020; Dworkin, 1991; Yorkston, Hakel, et al., 2007). Problems with intonation, stress, and rhythm contribute significantly to the unnatural prosody found in most individuals with all types of dysarthria. The following prosody tasks would be appropriate for individuals with flaccid dysarthria.

- Pitch range exercises—Exercises of this type can be a useful starting place for work on intonation. Dworkin (1991) recommended that these exercises begin with an assessment of a patient's ability to perceive obvious pitch changes in the clinician's voice. If the patient is unable to make these distinctions, the prognosis is poor for improving the patient's pitch control. However, if the patient can tell the difference between the pitch changes, the exercises might help. First, have the patient prolong an /a/ at the lowest pitch and then at the highest pitch possible. Once the highs and lows have been established, the patient is asked to sing up and down this pitch range by dividing the range into about eight individual notes. In the final exercises, the patient reads printed sentences that have arrows written above and below key words indicating the normal pitch changes for those words. For example, an up arrow at the end of a question would indicate that the patient should raise the pitch on the final word.

- Intonation profiles—This task uses lines to show intonation changes in written sentences. Lines immediately below words indicate a flat intonation. Lines farther below words indicate a drop in pitch. Lines above words indicate a rise in pitch. These lines can be added easily to any written sentence, no matter whether it is a statement or a question. For most patients, it is usually best to start with short, simple sentences and progress to longer sentences. The ultimate goal is to have the patient take the pitch changes produced in this structured activity and begin to use them in conversational speech.

- Contrastive stress drills—These tasks are designed for the clinician to ask a question, with the patient answering it by adding stress on key words to convey the intended meaning of the answer (McHenry, 1998). For example, the clinician might ask the following question about a picture of a man playing football: "Is the man playing basketball?" The patient will answer, "No. The man is playing football." The clinician's next question might be, "Is the woman playing football?" The patient's answer to this question would be, "No, the man is playing football." A third question might be, "Is the man watching football?" The patient would answer, "No, the man is playing football." The length of the questions and the complexity of the pictures for this task can easily be varied to match the abilities of the patient.

- Chunking utterances into syntactic units—Duffy (2020) mentioned that some individuals with dysarthria need to learn to divide their utterances according to normal pauses within and between sentences. This is necessary because their dysarthria has limited the number of words they can produce on a single exhalation. To compensate for this limitation, the following task teaches the patient to inhale at the points in an utterance at which natural syntactic pauses occur. Examples of these natural pauses include after introductory clauses or phrases ("In the morning, [inhale] I went shopping at the store."), between clauses or phrases ("She went there, [inhale] but I missed her."), and between short sentences ("I saw the movie. [inhale] It was pretty good."). By inserting inhalations at points at which normal pauses occur in an utterance, individuals with flaccid dysarthria are often able to maintain a more natural rhythm in their speech. This rhythm is lost when the patient haphazardly places inhalations within an utterance (Britton et al., 2017).

Damage to the Facial (VII) and Hypoglossal (XII) Cranial Nerves

Damage to the facial nerve affects speech production primarily by decreasing lip strength and range of movement. This weakness and reduced range of lip motion results in distorted bilabial and labiodental phonemes. Damage to the hypoglossal nerve can cause weakness and reduced range of motion of the tongue, which results primarily in imprecise labial consonant productions. Traditional articulation drills are often recommended for the treatment of these errors (Yorkston et al., 2010).

Traditional Articulation Treatment

Traditional articulation treatment tasks concentrate directly on improving the articulation of phonemes. They include a number of principles that have been established components of traditional articulation treatment for many years. Repetitive practice, clinician feedback, and increasing the patient's awareness of articulation errors are all parts of these treatments. Because of the many creative methods of modifying and combining these treatment tasks, beginning clinicians should think of the following descriptions only as templates of how these activities might be implemented. For example, with some patients, it might be very appropriate to combine intelligibility drills and phonetic placement tasks into one treatment activity. Clinicians are encouraged to find which of these activities are best for their various patients.

- Intelligibility drills—First mentioned by Yorkston et al. (1988), intelligibility drills are tasks in which the patient is given a list of words or sentences to read. Then the clinician turns away from the patient so that he or she will only be able to understand the patient's speech if it is articulated clearly. By not looking at the target word list or at the patient's mouth, the clinician will depend entirely on the patient's articulation to understand the target word. If the clinician does not understand the target word, the patient needs to determine why the word was unclear and then try saying it again. If this second attempt fails, the clinician can look at the target word and give the patient specific feedback on why he or she could not understand the utterance (e.g., "I didn't know it was 'sleep' because I couldn't hear the 'p.' Try it again, and let me really hear the 'p' this time.").

- Phonetic placement—This procedure treats articulation errors by instructing patients on the correct position of the articulators before they attempt to produce a target sound. Phonetic placement can be especially valuable in that it educates patients on how certain speech sounds are produced. Many individuals with dysarthria realize they are producing speech sounds incorrectly, but they have little understanding of why their productions are in error. For example, phonetic placement can educate speakers with dysarthria about why their production of a /d/ actually sounds closer to a /z/ or a /p/ sounds closer to a /b/ and so forth.

- Exaggerating consonants—Also known as overarticulation, exaggerating consonants is a treatment procedure that teaches the patient to fully articulate all consonant phonemes. Darley et al. (1975) suggested that most patients need to concentrate especially on **medial** and final consonants because these are the sounds most likely to be poorly articulated in connected speech. The improvements in intelligibility can be dramatic when individuals with flaccid dysarthria fully articulate the medial and final consonants in words.

    Park et al. (2016) used exaggerating consonants as the basis of an intensive treatment program for dysarthria. Their patients had a variety of different types of dysarthria, caused by either traumatic head injury or stroke. The study used a small group repeated measures design to determine the effects of overarticulation (in combination with slower and slightly louder speech) on dysarthric patients' single word and sentence intelligibility. There were 16 treatment sessions (1-hr sessions, four times a week, for 4 weeks). The patients were first oriented to the treatment tasks so that they knew what was expected. The treatment sessions started with 10 min of prepractice where patients reviewed a random selection of the tasks that were to be used later in the session. The following

10 min required the patients to repeat 10 functional phrases five times each (e.g., "What are we doing tomorrow?"). The next 10 min had the patients repeating 10 service requests five times each (e.g., Where is the _____?"). During the final 30 min, the patients read aloud, described pictures, and engaged in conversation. Feedback during most of the sessions consisted of whether the patients' utterances were *clear* or *unclear*. Homework also was a part of the treatment procedure. The results showed that naive listeners noted improved conversational intelligibility in all patients compared to pretreatment samples. Many of the other outcome measures also were positive. This technique was adapted for telehealth applications in a small study with 15 participants receiving Be Clear treatment 4 days a week for 4 weeks. The results were modest yet promising (Whelan et al., 2022).

- Minimal contrast drills—These drills have the patient concentrate on producing pairs of words that vary by only one phoneme. The distinction between the words can be in the voicing (park–bark), manner of production (dime–mime), or place of production (sea–she) of consonants. The distinction also can be between vowels (man–men), but working on consonants does more to enhance intelligibility in most patients. These word pairs can be used alone, in phrases, or in sentences, depending on the needs of the specific patient.

Treatments for Respiratory Weakness in Flaccid Dysarthria

As mentioned earlier, when patients with flaccid dysarthria demonstrate insufficient breath support for speech, it is often difficult to determine whether the problem is the result of shallow respiration or the leakage of air at the larynx. When shallow respiration is suspected, there are several procedures that could maximize respiratory function in these individuals.

- Correct posture—Many patients have problems with postural support and frequently can be found sitting in their wheelchairs in a slumped position. Their poor postural strength could result in shallow breathing, which often affects phonation and prosody. The simplest strategy to address this problem is to ask the patient to sit more upright. For many patients, surprising improvements in respiration for speech can occur when they are sitting with their heads up and shoulders back (Britton et al., 2017; Horton et al., 1997). Although proper posture might be successful, reminders to the patient about sitting upright will probably be necessary. If the patient is unable to improve posture through cues from the clinician, prosthetic devices might be needed to maintain the correct position (Spencer et al., 2003).

- Compensatory prosthetic devices—An abdominal binder (girdle) that wraps around the waist can help provide the support needed for a patient to maintain a more upright posture (Watson & Hixon, 2001). Beyond just helping with posture, the binder also can help a patient exhale with more force while speaking, which could lessen monopitch prosody and improve overall intelligibility. However, some authors report that this device is only a temporary solution for posture problems. Rosenbek and LaPointe (1985) cautioned that prolonged use of such a device might eventually result in pneumonia because it restricts the patient's ability to fully inhale, although Britton et al. (2017) said that this difficulty can be minimized if the binder is carefully placed between the bottom edge of the rib cage (the costal margin) and the pubis. When placed correctly, the binder does not limit rib expansion while breathing.

- Duffy (2020) and Swigert (2010) both described another type of compensatory device, called an expiratory board, that can be used with individuals in wheelchairs. When a padded lap tray on the wheelchair is positioned next to the patient's abdomen, it can provide a rigid surface for the patient to lean on. By leaning forward against this pad while speaking, the patient will compress the abdomen and force the diaphragm upward, which could result in a more forceful exhalation for speech.

- Speaking immediately on exhalation—Some patients with flaccid dysarthria waste a significant amount of subglottic air by beginning their phonations shortly after they have started to exhale. By cueing the patients to begin phonating immediately on exhalation, they can use more of their available subglottic air pressure. Swigert (2010) suggested that the first step in this exercise is to have the patient place a hand on the abdomen and begin a simple /m/ phonation the moment the hand starts to move inward on exhalation. If necessary, the clinician can place his or her hand on the patient's hand to know when to cue the patient to begin the phonation.

- Cueing for complete inhalation—Sometimes breath support for speech can be increased just by reminding the patient to inhale fully before speaking. The clinician will probably need to give frequent reminders about this early in treatment. The ultimate goal is to have these deeper inhalations become a habitual part of the patient's conversational speech. To maximize the efficient use of subglottic air, it is often effective to combine the cues to inhale completely with reminders to speak immediately on exhalation.

Summary of Flaccid Dysarthria

- Flaccid dysarthria can be caused by any process that damages the lower motor neurons used in speech production. The lower motor neurons are found in certain cranial and spinal nerves.
- The cranial nerves of speech production are the trigeminal nerve (V), facial nerve (VII), glossopharyngeal nerve (IX), vagus nerve (X), accessory nerve (XI), and hypoglossal nerve (XII). The spinal nerves are important for speech production because they innervate the muscles of respiration.
- The speech characteristics of flaccid dysarthria include hypernasality, imprecise consonants, and a breathy voice quality.
- Some clinicians believe that the treatment of flaccid dysarthria should include nonspeech oral-motor exercises; however, it is more productive to work on strategies that concentrate directly on increasing the intelligibility of a patient's speech.

Study Questions

1. Define flaccid dysarthria in your own words.
2. Flaccid dysarthria can occur after damage to which part of the nervous system?
3. Why are lower motor neurons also known as the final common pathway?
4. What are the six cranial nerves of speech production?
5. Which cranial nerve innervates the intrinsic muscles of the larynx?
6. What role do the spinal nerves play in speech production?
7. How can a brainstem stroke cause flaccid dysarthria?

8. How can it be determined whether the poor breath support demonstrated by a patient with flaccid dysarthria is the result of weak respiration or poor laryngeal valving?
9. Why are muscle-strengthening exercises not recommended as a treatment for flaccid dysarthria?
10. What are the two surgical treatments for velopharyngeal incompetence?

Chapter 5

Spastic Dysarthria

Definitions of Spastic Dysarthria

Neurologic Basis of Spastic Dysarthria
   Role of Upper Motor Neurons in Spastic Dysarthria
   Significance of Bilateral Damage

Causes of Spastic Dysarthria
   Stroke
   Amyotrophic Lateral Sclerosis
   Traumatic Head Injury
   Multiple Sclerosis
   Other Causes of Spastic Dysarthria

Speech Characteristics of Spastic Dysarthria
   Articulation
   Phonation
   Resonance
   Prosody
   Respiration

Additional Characteristics of Spastic Dysarthria

Spastic Dysarthria Versus Flaccid Dysarthria

Key Evaluation Tasks for Spastic Dysarthria

Treatment of Spastic Dysarthria
   Treatment of Phonation Deficits
   Treatment of Articulation Deficits
      Stretching
      Traditional Articulation Treatments
   Treatment of Prosody Deficits
   Treatment of Resonance Deficits
      Surgical and Prosthetic Treatments
      Behavioral Treatments for Hypernasality

Summary of Spastic Dysarthria

Study Questions

Definitions of Spastic Dysarthria

Many definitions of spastic dysarthria state that it is caused by bilateral damage to upper motor neurons. This is one of the features that distinguishes between spastic and flaccid dysarthria, because the latter is caused by damage to lower motor neurons. Most definitions also state that the speech of an individual with spastic dysarthria is slow and effortful and has a harsh vocal quality. One of the following definitions also states that hyperactive and abnormal reflexes can be observed in some patients with this disorder.

> [Spastic dysarthria is] seen in association with damage to the upper motor neurons that convey nerve impulses from the motor areas of the cerebral cortex to the lower motor neurons originating from the bulbar cranial nerve nuclei. The resulting speech disturbance reflects the clinical signs of upper motor neuron damage, which include spastic paralysis or paresis of the involved muscles, hyperreflexia (e.g., hyperactive jaw-jerk), little or no muscle atrophy (except for the possibility of some atrophy associated with disuse), and the presence of pathological reflexes (e.g., sucking reflex). (Murdoch et al., 1997, p. 287)

> Spastic dysarthria is one of the most common types of speech dysarthrias and can be associated with various aetiologies, including cerebral palsy and traumatic brain injury. Spastic dysarthria is characterized by excessive nasalization, disordered speech prosody, imprecise articulation, and variable speech rate which often render the speech unintelligible. (Paja & Falk, 2012, p. 62)

Neurologic Basis of Spastic Dysarthria

Spastic dysarthria is a relatively common type of dysarthria, accounting for 7.3% of motor speech disorder cases seen at the Mayo Clinic (Duffy, 2013). The name *spastic dysarthria* might be a bit confusing to readers who are not familiar with the disorder. It is true that individuals with this disorder have the increased muscle tone of spasticity in various muscles of the vocal tract, but they also have weakness, reduced range of motion, and decreased fine motor control in many of these same muscles. As mentioned, the motor deficits in spastic dysarthria are caused by bilateral damage to the upper motor neuron tracts (Figure 5–1). A clear understanding of the upper motor neuron tracts is important for knowing why spas-

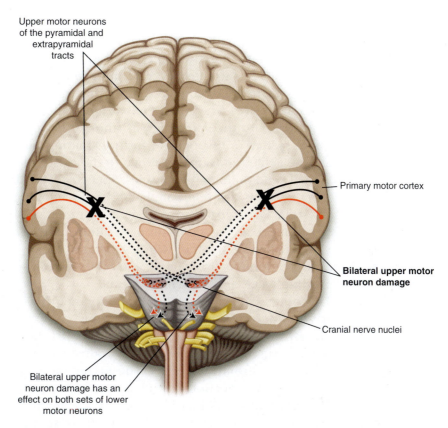

FIGURE 5–1. Spastic dysarthria is caused by bilateral upper motor neuron damage to the pyramidal and extrapyramidal systems.

tic dysarthria occurs. Therefore, this chapter begins with a review of the organization and function of the upper motor neurons.

Role of Upper Motor Neurons in Spastic Dysarthria

Whereas flaccid dysarthria is the result of damage to lower motor neurons, spastic dysarthria is caused by damage to upper motor neurons. Specifically, spastic dysarthria is caused by bilateral damage to both the pyramidal and extrapyramidal neural pathways that serve the speech mechanism. To better understand how damage to upper motor neurons can cause spastic dysarthria, a brief reexamination of the pyramidal and extrapyramidal systems might be helpful. First, remember that upper motor neurons are part of the CNS, and they originate in the cortex and brainstem. Second, remember that upper motor neurons are grouped into the pyramidal and extrapyramidal systems.

The upper motor neurons that are part of the pyramidal system originate principally in the primary motor cortex and course down more or less directly to the lower motor neurons, which, in turn, travel out to the muscles. The upper motor neurons in the pyramidal system are divided into those that travel from the cortex to the cranial nerves (the corticobulbar tract) and those that travel from the cortex to the spinal nerves (the corticospinal tract). The pyramidal system is responsible for transmitting neural impulses for discrete skilled movements down to the lower motor neurons, which then send them to the muscles. Speech is one of the discrete skilled movements that relies on the proper functioning of the pyramidal system. Damage to the parts of the pyramidal system serving the speech mechanism will result in weakness and slowness in the speech musculature. In other words, when the pyramidal system is damaged, the tongue, lips, velum, and other speech structures will demonstrate weak and slow movements.

The other collection of upper motor neurons is called the **extrapyramidal system**. It is an incredibly complex network of neural pathways. The upper motor neurons in the extrapyramidal system originate primarily in the brainstem, but also receive important input from the cortex. The extrapyramidal system has numerous interconnections throughout the brain, including the reticular formation and the red nucleus. If the pyramidal system is a direct pathway between the cortex and the lower motor neurons, then the extrapyramidal system is definitely an indirect pathway between the two. Ultimately, however, the upper motor neurons of the extrapyramidal system do synapse with lower motor neurons of the cranial and spinal nerves.

Overall, the extrapyramidal system is responsible for transmitting signals that maintain posture, regulate reflexes, and monitor muscle tone. The work of the extrapyramidal system is done in parallel with that of the pyramidal system—while the pyramidal system is transmitting its neural impulses for skilled movement to lower motor neurons, the extrapyramidal system is also transmitting its impulses for posture and muscle tone to the lower motor neurons. When these two systems are intact, their functions blend together remarkably well and allow us to accomplish complex movements effortlessly. When they are damaged, however, a number of problems can arise. As stated previously, damage to the pyramidal system will result in weak and slow skilled movements. In turn, damage to the motor neurons of the extrapyramidal system can result in weakness, increased muscle tone (spasticity), and abnormal muscle reflexes.

Spastic dysarthria can occur when there is damage to both the pyramidal and extrapyramidal systems that innervate the speech muscles. The co-occurrence of damage to both of these systems is not all that unusual because their neurons are close to each other throughout much of the CNS. In fact, because they are physically so close to each other, when one system is damaged the other system will almost always also be damaged. It is rare to find a stroke, head injury, tumor, infection, or other disorder that causes damage to only the pyramidal system or only the extrapyramidal system. In nearly all instances, the damage will extend to both systems.

Significance of Bilateral Damage

At this point, it should be clear that spastic dysarthria is the result of damage to the upper motor neurons of both the pyramidal and extrapyramidal systems. The final factor leading to spastic dysarthria is that the damage must be bilateral—the damage must affect both the left and right tracts of the pyramidal and extrapyramidal systems. If the damage is unilateral, the result will be a relatively mild motor speech disorder known as unilateral upper motor neuron dysarthria (see Chapter 6). Unilateral upper motor neuron dysarthria is not as serious as spastic dysarthria, because most of the cranial nerves serving the speech muscles (except the lower face and tongue) receive bilateral innervation from the upper motor neurons of the pyramidal and extrapyramidal systems. When the damage to the upper motor neurons is unilateral, the cranial nerves will still receive some innervation from the upper motor neurons on the opposite, undamaged side. As a result, most of the speech musculature will be affected relatively mildly, as in cases of unilateral upper motor neuron dysarthria. When the damage to upper motor neurons is bilateral, however, many more of the speech muscles are affected, and the result can be spastic dysarthria.

Because both the pyramidal and extrapyramidal systems are affected, the symptoms of this dysarthria are a combination of what would be expected if each system were damaged individually. Consequently, the speech production muscles of individuals with spastic dysarthria will show weakness, slow movements, **spasticity** (increased muscle tone), and perhaps abnormal reflexes. The weakness and slowness might be most evident in the movements of the tongue and lips, although they certainly can exhibit some spasticity as well. In general, the spasticity probably will be most noticeable in the laryngeal muscles. This spasticity usually will result in hyperadduction of the vocal folds. The spasticity also could affect the velum and cause incomplete velopharyngeal closure during the production of non-nasal phonemes.

Causes of Spastic Dysarthria

Any injury that causes bilateral damage to the upper motor neurons of the pyramidal and extrapyramidal systems can lead to spastic dysarthria. A number of disorders are capable of creating this type of damage to upper motor neurons. These include strokes, degenerative diseases, traumatic head injury, infections of brain tissue, and tumors. Because some of the conditions leading to spastic dysarthria are quite rare, the following sections concentrate on the most frequently encountered causes.

Stroke

Strokes are the most common cause of spastic dysarthria. Because of the specific areas that must be damaged (i.e., bilateral damage to both the pyramidal and extrapyramidal tracts), spastic dysarthria will occur only when two or more strokes occur in certain combinations or when a single stroke occurs in the brainstem. The following list highlights circumstances that need to take place before a stroke can cause spastic dysarthria:

- A single stroke can cause spastic dysarthria only when it occurs in the brainstem. This is because the neural fibers of both the right and left pyramidal and extrapyramidal systems are in very close proximity to each other in the brainstem. Consequently, a single stroke in the brainstem can be extensive enough to damage both the left and right upper motor neurons of these two systems.
- A single stroke in one of the cerebral hemispheres cannot cause spastic dysarthria because it will affect only the left or right pyramidal and extrapyramidal system, depending on the side on which the stroke occurs. It takes at least one stroke in each cerebral hemisphere to cause the bilateral upper motor neuron damage that leads to spastic dysarthria.
- A single stroke in one cerebral hemisphere can sometimes appear to cause spastic dysarthria. This can happen when a preexisting condition has previously caused damage to the upper motor neurons of the pyramidal and extrapyramidal systems in the opposite cerebral hemisphere. This damage could be an old stroke, head injury, tumor, or similar injury to the other hemisphere. Spastic dysarthria will happen only when the new stroke

in one hemisphere is combined with previous cerebral damage in the other hemisphere.

Amyotrophic Lateral Sclerosis

Degenerative neurologic diseases such as **amyotrophic lateral sclerosis (ALS)** can cause spastic dysarthria. ALS is a disease of unknown cause that results in the progressive degeneration of lower and upper motor neurons. It is a terminal disorder; the average life expectancy is 22 months from the time of onset. The course of ALS varies across individuals. Some initially have lower motor neuron involvement and demonstrate flaccid dysarthria, weakness in the arms and legs, and muscle atrophy. Other individuals primarily have upper motor neuron involvement in the early stages of the disorder. When the upper motor neuron damage is predominant, individuals with ALS could have spastic dysarthria, hyperactive gag and jaw reflexes, and swallowing disorders. In nearly all cases, however, the disease eventually involves both upper and lower motor neurons. Once both sets of motor neurons are affected, most individuals with ALS have a mixed dysarthria of the flaccid-spastic type. Mixed dysarthria is discussed in Chapter 10.

Traumatic Head Injury

A head injury can produce widespread damage to cortical, subcortical, and brainstem structures. In many head injuries, the damage is extensive because the whole brain is violently shifted within the cranium, which causes linear and rotational movements of the brain in relation to the movements of the skull. The consequences of this shifting can be stretched and torn axons, lacerated brain tissue, and blood vessel hemorrhage in numerous parts of the brain.

Because of this widespread damage to the brain, head injury can cause bilateral damage to the pyramidal and extrapyramidal systems. In such cases, the affected individuals could exhibit spastic dysarthria. It also is likely that a mixed dysarthria, such as flaccid-spastic or spastic-ataxic, will result from a head injury, given the extensive damage that occurs in this type of trauma.

Multiple Sclerosis

Multiple sclerosis is a suspected immunologic disorder that results in the inflammation or complete destruction of the myelin sheath covering axons. The amount of myelin affected by multiple sclerosis usually varies from millimeters to several centimeters along the length of a given axon. Multiple sclerosis can affect myelin just about anywhere within the CNS, including the cerebral hemispheres, cerebellum, brainstem, and spinal cord. When there is bilateral involvement of the upper motor neurons, spastic dysarthria might be one of the consequences of multiple sclerosis. However, given the many different areas of the CNS that can be affected by this disease, multiple sclerosis could result in other types of dysarthria, such as ataxic dysarthria or mixed dysarthria. The disorders that can result in a mixed dysarthria are discussed in Chapter 10.

Other Causes of Spastic Dysarthria

A number of additional disorders can cause spastic dysarthria. For instance, a brainstem tumor can affect upper motor neurons in a similar way to a single brainstem stroke. Because the pyramidal and extrapyramidal tracts are in such close proximity in the brainstem, a single brainstem tumor can compress or destroy the upper motor neurons from both hemispheres and perhaps cause spastic dysarthria. Another condition that can lead to spastic dysarthria is **cerebral** anoxia, brain damage from a lack of oxygen in the blood, such as what occurs when an individual stops breathing. As with all of the previously mentioned disorders, cerebral anoxia could cause spastic dysarthria because it is capable of producing widespread neural damage that extends to the upper motor neurons on both sides of the brain. Finally, viral or bacterial infections in cerebral tissue also are able to damage upper motor neurons bilaterally. Although these types of infections are sometimes restricted to specific portions of the brain, they also are capable of encompassing much larger areas and, thereby, can affect the upper motor neurons in both hemispheres.

Speech Characteristics of Spastic Dysarthria

As seen in the definitions of spastic dysarthria at the beginning of this chapter, individuals with this type of dysarthria demonstrate a number of different speech errors. Overall, the speech errors in this dysarthria are the result of spasticity, slowness, and weakness in the vocal-tract muscles. Articulation, phonation, resonance, and prosody are usually affected more than respiration, but each

TABLE 5–1	The Most Common Speech Production Errors in 30 Individuals With Spastic Dysarthria

Rank	Speech Production Errors
1	Imprecise consonants
2	Monopitch
3	Reduced stress
4	Harsh voice quality
5	Monoloudness
6	Low pitch
7	Slow rate
8	Hypernasality
9	Strained-strangled quality
10	Short phrases
11	Distorted vowels
12	Pitch breaks
13	Breathy voice (continuous)
14	Excess and equal stress

Source: From "Clusters of Diagnostic Patterns of Dysarthria," by F. L. Darley, A. E. Aronson, and J. R. Brown, 1969, *Journal of Speech and Hearing Research*, 12, p. 253. Copyright 1969 by American Speech-Language-Hearing Association. Reprinted with permission.

of these components of speech production can demonstrate the effects of the bilateral upper motor neuron damage. The following paragraphs examine how this damage affects these components. Much of the information in this section comes from Darley et al.'s (1969a, 1969b) examination of the speech errors of 30 subjects with spastic dysarthria. Table 5–1 lists the most noticeable errors in the speech of the subjects in that study. Watch the PluralPlus Spastic Dysarthria Case 1 and 2 videos demonstrating the speech difficulties in this disorder.

Articulation

Darley et al. found that articulation errors were very common in their subjects with spastic dysarthria. Imprecise consonant production was the most common articulation disorder in that study. It occurred in all 30 subjects with spastic dysarthria. The imprecise production of consonants in this dysarthria could be the result of several factors, including abnormally short voice onset time for voiceless consonants, incomplete articulatory contact, and incomplete consonant clusters (Hardcastle et al., 1985). Vowel distortions also can be heard in spastic dysarthria. (Note: Although imprecise consonants are heard frequently in spastic dysarthria, their occurrence is not especially helpful in establishing a diagnosis of spastic dysarthria because these errors are a common problem in every type of dysarthria.)

Phonation

Darley et al. found that **harsh vocal quality** was the most common phonatory error in their subjects with spastic dysarthria. Harsh vocal quality has a definite "friction-of-air" characteristic to it. This harshness occurs when air leaks through a partially open glottis during phonation. In cases of spastic dysarthria, a harsh vocal quality is believed to be caused by the purposeful partial abduction of the vocal folds (Duffy, 2020). By keeping the vocal folds partly abducted, individuals with spastic dysarthria are able to prevent the spastic muscle tone in their larynx from closing the glottis too tightly during speech. Consequently, they let some subglottic air leak through their tense, partly abducted vocal folds. The result is a harsh vocal quality.

A **strained-strangled vocal quality** also can occur in spastic dysarthria. A strained-strangled vocal quality is perceptually different from harshness. Whereas there is a breathy friction of air in harshness, a strained-strangled vocal quality is characterized by subglottic air that is being forced through a narrow, tightly constricted larynx. As with harsh vocal quality, a strained-strangled vocal quality is caused by spasticity of the laryngeal muscles, which can result in a tight hyperadduction of the vocal folds. Darley et al. (1969a, 1969b) found a strained-strangled vocal quality to be one of the most distinguishing speech errors of spastic dysarthria. It was more noticeable in this dysarthria than in any other. Its value as a diagnostic marker is tempered slightly, however, by the fact that it does not occur consistently in all cases of spastic dysarthria. It was present in only 20 of the 30 subjects in that study.

Low pitch is another phonatory characteristic that can appear frequently in spastic dysarthria. It is assumed that the low pitch in spastic dysarthria is a result of increased muscle tone in the larynx. As with a strained-strangled vocal quality, low pitch can be more apparent in spastic dysarthria than in any other dysarthria. However, from a clinical perspective, low pitch alone is probably not distinctive enough to be a consistent indicator of spastic dysarthria because it also can appear in several other dysarthrias.

Resonance

Hypernasality can occur often in spastic dysarthria. Darley et al. (1969a, 1969b) noted it in most of their subjects. It is caused by spasticity in the velar muscles, which slows and reduces the range of soft palate movement. The result is incomplete velopharyngeal closure during nonnasal speech sounds. The hypernasality associated with spastic dysarthria is generally not as severe as that in flaccid dysarthria; the difference between the two is a matter of degree. The hypernasality in spastic dysarthria, although noticeable to a listener, usually does not include nasal emission. In contrast, nasal emission frequently accompanies the hypernasality of flaccid dysarthria, especially in moderate to severe cases.

Prosody

There are several common prosody errors in spastic dysarthria. The first is monopitch intonation in connected or conversational speech. One of the most obvious characteristics of spastic dysarthria, monopitch is caused by an overall tenseness of the laryngeal muscles. When these muscles demonstrate this spastic tenseness, they have a reduced ability to contract and relax—just the opposite of what is needed normally to vary vocal pitch. For example, the contraction and relaxation of the cricothyroid muscle in the larynx can raise or lower pitch during speech by stretching or tensing the vocal folds. However, when this muscle's ability to contract and relax is restricted by spastic hypertonicity, variations in pitch will also be restricted, resulting in monopitch.

A second prosody error is monoloudness, a deficit in the ability to vary vocal intensity during speech. As with monopitch, monoloudness also is caused by increased muscle tone in the laryngeal muscles. Normal loudness variations are achieved by varying the tension of the vocal folds. By increasing and decreasing vocal-fold tension, the larynx can precisely regulate the amount of subglottic air that passes through the glottis. Whenever the ability to vary vocal-fold tension is reduced, such as in spastic dysarthria, the ability to vary speech loudness will be reduced as well.

Another characteristic of spastic dysarthria is speaking in short phrases. This is a deficit that is most evident in conversational speech. Darley et al. (1975) suggested that short phrasing is probably a natural consequence of speaking through an abnormally tight larynx. The energy expended on forcing subglottic air through hyperadducted vocal folds makes it difficult for individuals with spastic dysarthria to produce utterances of a longer, more normal length. Short phrasing is considered to be a problem of prosody because the frequent inhalations of air interrupt the normal rhythm of an individual's speech.

Slow rate of speech is yet another prosodic characteristic of spastic dysarthria. It is probably caused by reduced speed and range of movement in the articulators. Weakness in the articulators also can contribute to a slower than normal speaking rate. In addition, Darley et al. (1975) suggested that slow rate might be the result of speaking against tight adduction of the vocal folds, secondary to spasticity in the laryngeal muscles.

Respiration

Problems of respiration do not appear to play as much of a role in spastic dysarthria as they do, for example, in flaccid dysarthria. Much remains unknown about how upper motor neuron damage affects the respiratory system. Darley et al. (1975) suggested that there might be some abnormal respiratory movements in individuals with spastic dysarthria. These deviant movements can cause reduced inhalation and exhalation, uncoordinated breathing patterns, and reduced vital capacity. However, Darley et al. also indicated that the phonation and prosody problems in spastic dysarthria are probably more the result of hyperadduction of the vocal folds than any respiratory problems. It would appear then that, if abnormal respiration is present in spastic dysarthria, it is probably "masked" by the more obvious problems of airflow management at the larynx.

Additional Characteristics of Spastic Dysarthria

Several nonspeech characteristics of spastic dysarthria can help in the diagnosis of this disorder. The first of these is **pseudobulbar affect**—uncontrollable crying or laughing that can accompany damage to the upper motor neurons of the brainstem. It appears to be caused by damage to the areas of the brain that are important in inhibiting emotions. In cases of spastic dysarthria or mixed dysarthria with a spastic component, crying is more common than laughing. The display of pseudobulbar affect may be quite independent of the emotions actually felt by the patient. For example, crying could occur during a normally unemotional situation, such as when the name of a spouse or other family member is mentioned in casual conversation. These unexpected displays of emotion can be embarrassing for the patient and distressing for the family. Treatment options are limited. Sedatives and antipsychotic drugs have been shown to be ineffective in reducing the emotional outbursts. In some instances, however, pseudobulbar affect lessens in severity as a patient's recovery progresses. Not all patients with spastic dysarthria demonstrate pseudobulbar affect, but it is observed more often in this dysarthria than in the other types.

Although drooling can occur in several other dysarthrias, it appears most prominently in spastic dysarthria (Duffy, 2020). It is probably due to impaired oral control of saliva or perhaps to less frequent swallowing. It is not uncommon for affected individuals to claim that their neurologic injury has resulted in the production of too much saliva. Although this is unlikely, there are several treatments for this embarrassing and perhaps unhygienic problem. A behavioral approach to treatment works on cueing the individual to consciously swallow more frequently than normal. Pharmaceutical treatments that reduce saliva production are also available.

Spastic Dysarthria Versus Flaccid Dysarthria

To the untrained ear (and occasionally to the trained ear), the speech characteristics of spastic dysarthria can often sound similar to those of flaccid dysarthria, possibly because these two disorders share many of the same speech characteristics. For example, there can be hypernasality, imprecise consonants, and slow movements of the speech structures in both spastic and flaccid dysarthria. The perceptual similarities between these two dysarthrias are reflected in some of the terms used to describe their symptoms. For example, *bulbar palsy* is a general term meaning atrophy and weakness in the muscles innervated through the medulla (the bulb). This includes the muscles of the tongue, velum, larynx, and pharynx. In fact, bulbar dysarthria was once a common name for flaccid dysarthria. The term *pseudobulbar palsy* (a false bulbar palsy) means weakness and slowness in the same muscles; this term was sometimes used to describe spastic dysarthria. The distinction between bulbar and pseudobulbar palsy is in their different causes. Bulbar palsy is caused by damage to lower motor neurons; pseudobulbar palsy is caused by damage to upper motor neurons.

In several ways, however, the symptoms of spastic and flaccid dysarthria can be clearly distinguished from one another. The following is a summary of the more obvious features of the two. This list might help in making a differential diagnosis between these two types of dysarthria.

- Spastic dysarthria is caused by bilateral damage to the upper motor neurons of the pyramidal and extrapyramidal systems. Flaccid dysarthria is caused by damage to lower motor neurons. Be sure to check the medical reports for any information on the site and type of lesion.
- The hypernasality that could be present in spastic dysarthria is usually not as severe as that heard in flaccid dysarthria. In addition, nasal emission is not common in spastic dysarthria but might be quite evident in flaccid dysarthria. Some writers also have described the hypernasality of spastic dysarthria as being more variable and intermittent than that heard in flaccid dysarthria.
- A very helpful distinction between spastic dysarthria and flaccid dysarthria is that phonation can have a tight, strained-strangled vocal quality in the former and a breathy quality in the latter. Remember, however, in spastic dysarthria, a harsh vocal quality may be heard more frequently than a strained-strangled vocal quality. Do not depend on hearing the strained-strangled quality in all individuals with spastic dysarthria.
- Patients with flaccid dysarthria might demonstrate reduced or absent oral reflexes, such as the gag reflex. In contrast, patients with spastic dysarthria might demonstrate hyperreflexes.
- A slow speech rate combined with harsh or strained-strangled voice quality occurs only in spastic dysarthria.
- Pseudobulbar affect and drooling are associated more with spastic dysarthria than with any other dysarthria.

Key Evaluation Tasks for Spastic Dysarthria

Duffy (2020) identified three evaluation tasks that are particularly helpful in evoking the speech characteristics most associated with spastic dysarthria. In a comprehensive motor speech evaluation, these tasks should be completed especially carefully if spastic dysarthria is suspected.

1. Conversational speech and reading are useful for assessing the resonance (hypernasality), articulation (imprecise consonants), and prosody (monopitch, monoloudness, reduced stress, short phrases) impairments heard in spastic dysarthria.
2. The AMR task will best demonstrate the slow rate of phoneme production associated with this dysarthria.
3. Vowel prolongation will evoke the phonatory deficits (harsh voice quality, strained-strangled voice quality, low pitch) that are so common in spastic dysarthria.

Treatment of Spastic Dysarthria

Depending on the requirements of specific patients, the primary treatment goals for spastic dysarthria might need to target four of the five components of speech production. For example, with some patients it might be necessary to concentrate on decreasing the hyperadduction of the vocal folds (phonation), increasing articulatory precision (articulation), developing more natural intonation in speech (prosody), and decreasing hypernasality (resonance). Respiration is usually not affected significantly in this dysarthria, so the breathing exercises and compensatory strategies mentioned in Chapter 4 will probably not be necessary. In fact, Duffy (2020) and other writers have cautioned against using the pushing and pulling type of phonation and respiratory exercises for spastic dysarthria because these exercises tend to increase the force of muscular contractions in the vocal folds. When a patient has hyperadduction of the vocal folds, one of the last things a clinician should do is increase the adduction.

Treatment of Phonation Deficits

The harsh or strained-strangled vocal quality in spastic dysarthria is caused by hyperadduction of the vocal folds. Because of the increased muscle tone in the laryngeal muscles, the vocal folds are involuntarily adducted too tightly during phonation. Relaxation and easy-onset types of exercises are recommended for this phonatory problem, although there is little research demonstrating the effectiveness of such tasks in spastic dysarthria. Indeed, Dworkin (1991) reported little success in treating vocal-fold hyperadduction with these procedures, a finding echoed by Spencer et al. (2003).

However, anecdotal reports from other clinicians sometimes have been more positive. As suggested by Dworkin, the following exercises might be most successful with patients who have mild hyperadduction, but a trial period of treatment could be given to other patients with this condition.

- Head and neck relaxation—There are various relaxation procedures for this area of the body. Most of them are based on some type of head-rolling motion. One approach is for the clinician to stand behind the seated patient. The clinician tells the patient to relax the neck as much as possible and then takes the patient's head between his or her hands and slowly, gently tilts it back, then forward, and finally to the left and right. At the extreme of each position, the clinician holds the head still for about 10 s before moving to the next position. A modification of this exercise omits the clinician's hands-on role and has the patient making the motion independently, with the clinician talking the patient through the movements. Gentle massage of the sides and back of the patient's neck might also reduce the increased muscle tone in the larynx. Clinicians should consider combining relaxation with the following two phonation exercises. The most logical sequence would be to begin with the relaxation and then move on to easy-onset or yawn-sigh exercises.
- Easy-onset of phonation—Darley et al. (1975) suggested that vocal quality can be improved by instructing the patient to make softer glottal closures during phonation. The first step is to have the patient exhale while producing a smooth, quiet sigh. Once these soft sighs are produced consistently, the patient is asked to gently initiate a prolonged phonation of an open vowel such as /a/. These prolonged phonations are then shaped into words that begin with vowels or breathy consonants such as /w/. The ultimate goal is to build toward easy phonations of sentences during conversational speech.
- Yawn-sigh exercises—This procedure is similar to the easy-onset exercise. The patient is asked to inhale slowly while fully opening the mouth, as if yawning. When the inhalation is complete, the patient begins to exhale while producing a gentle, prolonged sigh. The yawning motion facilitates the relaxation of the neck muscles and should reduce some of the hypertension in the larynx. As with easy onset, the sighing phonations are gradually shaped into open vowels, words beginning with vowels or breathy consonants, and finally into sentences and spontaneous speech.

Treatment of Articulation Deficits

The articulation deficits of spastic dysarthria are usually the result of three conditions affecting the articulators: weakness, reduced speed of movement, and reduced range of movement. The primary articulation error in spastic dysarthria is imprecise consonant production. Stretching exercises and traditional articulation tasks are two types of treatments that have been recommended to enhance a patient's ability to more accurately produce consonant phonemes.

Stretching

It may be beneficial to begin treating the articulation deficits in this dysarthria with gentle, passive stretching exercises. Reducing hypertonicity in the tongue and lips through stretching might result in increased speed and range of tongue and lip movements during speech. Active stretching of the articulators could increase strength as well. As with the relaxation exercises mentioned previously, there is little research on the effectiveness of stretching as a treatment for spastic dysarthria; most evidence is anecdotal. For example, the author had a patient with moderate spastic dysarthria who complained of difficulty making the articulatory contact for /l/ in conversational speech because his tongue felt "so stiff." Shortly after beginning an active tongue-stretching program, the patient gradually began to demonstrate more rapid and accurate lingual movements for /l/ in spontaneous speech. Of course, such reports are not from controlled studies and no causal effect can be assumed, but they might encourage a clinician to try stretching exercises when appropriate.

- Tongue-stretching tasks—Dworkin (1991) described a series of passive tongue-stretching tasks in which the clinician gently grasps the patient's tongue with a gauze pad and carefully pulls it straight forward until resistance is felt. This protruded position is held for 10 s. Then the clinician gently pulls the protruded tongue to the left or right side of the mouth and again holds the position for 10 s. Dworkin cautioned against pulling the tongue too forcefully and encouraged the clinician and patient to have patience during these tasks. Active tongue-stretching movements by the patient also can be used to increase strength, speed, and accuracy of tongue movements (Swigert, 2010). Examples of these tasks include having the patient protrude the tongue fully, elevate the tongue tip toward the nose, lower the tongue tip toward the chin, and hold the tongue at the corners of the mouth. Other active tongue-stretching tasks include elevating the back of the tongue to the soft palate and pressing the tongue tip into the cheek. Although these active tongue-stretching movements have the benefit of promoting increased flexibility, they also might increase hypertonicity in some patients. The clinician should carefully monitor changes in muscle tone. If the active stretching tasks prove to be counterproductive, the passive stretching tasks should be used exclusively.

- Lip-stretching exercises—In passive lip-stretching tasks, the clinician grasps one of the lips gently with a gauze pad and carefully pulls it out and away from the face, holding the position for about 10 s. Active lip-stretching tasks have the patient making the movements, including holding a smile, pursing the lips, and puffing out the cheeks. Again, the clinician should monitor any changes in lip muscle tone when active stretching tasks have been recommended. If increased muscle tone is noted, passive stretching tasks should be used exclusively.

Traditional Articulation Treatments

Traditional articulation treatments also are recommended for imprecise consonant productions in patients with spastic dysarthria. These tasks concentrate on increasing the patient's awareness of articulation errors and practicing the best phoneme productions the patient is capable of achieving.

- Intelligibility drills—Intelligibility drills are tasks in which the patient is given a list of words or sentences to read (Yorkston et al., 1988). The clinician turns away from the patient so that he or she will only be able to understand the patient's speech if it is articulated clearly. By not looking at the target word list or at the patient's mouth, the clinician will depend entirely on the patient's articulation to understand the target word. If the clinician does not understand the target word, the patient needs to determine why the word was unclear and then try saying it again. If this second attempt fails, then the clinician can look at the target word and give the patient specific feedback on why he or she could not understand the utterance (e.g., "I didn't know it was 'sleep' because I couldn't hear the 'p.' Try it again, and let me really hear the 'p' this time.").
- Phonetic placement—This procedure treats articulation errors by instructing patients on the correct position of the articula-

tors before they attempt to produce a target sound. Phonetic placement can be especially valuable in that it educates patients on how certain speech sounds are produced. Many individuals with dysarthria realize they are producing speech sounds incorrectly, but they have little understanding of why their productions are in error. For example, phonetic placement can educate speakers with dysarthria about why their production of a /d/ actually sounds closer to a /z/ or a /p/ sounds more like a /b/ and so forth.

- Exaggerating consonants—Also known as **overarticulation**, exaggerating consonants is a treatment procedure that teaches the patient to fully articulate all consonant phonemes. Darley et al. (1975) suggested that most patients need to concentrate especially on medial and final consonants because these are the sounds most likely to be poorly articulated in connected speech. The improvements in intelligibility can be dramatic when individuals with spastic dysarthria fully articulate the medial and final consonants in words.

Park et al. (2016) used exaggerating consonants as the basis of an intensive treatment program for dysarthria. Their patients had a variety of different types of dysarthria, caused by either traumatic head injury or stroke. The study used a small group repeated measures design to determine the effects of overarticulation (in combination with slower and slightly louder speech) on dysarthric patients' single word and sentence intelligibility. There were 16 treatment sessions (1-hr sessions, four times a week, for 4 weeks). The patients were first oriented to the treatment tasks so that they knew what was expected. The treatment sessions started with 10 min of prepractice where patients reviewed a random selection of the tasks that were to be used later in the session. The following 10 min required the patients to repeat 10 functional phrases five times each (e.g., "What are we doing tomorrow?"). The next 10 min had the patients repeating 10 service requests five times each (e.g., "Where is the _____?"). During the final 30 min, the patients read aloud, described pictures, and engaged in conversation. Feedback during most the sessions consisted of whether the patients' utterances were clear or unclear. Homework also was a part of the treatment procedure. The results showed that naive listeners noted improved conversational intelligibility in all patients compared to pretreatment samples. Many of the other outcome measures also were positive.

- Minimal contrast drills—These drills have the patient concentrate on producing pairs of words that vary by only one phoneme. The distinction between the words can be in the voicing (park–bark), manner of production (pine–mine), or place of production (sea–she) of consonants. The distinction also can be between vowels (man–men), but usually working on consonants does more to enhance intelligibility in most patients. These word pairs can be used alone, in phrases, or in sentences, depending on the needs of the specific patient.

Treatment of Prosody Deficits

The monopitch, monoloudness, and reduced stress problems in spastic dysarthria might respond to exercises that help the patient regain the vocal-tract flexibility that is needed to appropriately vary pitch and loudness. As in nearly all treatment tasks in dysarthria, the general sequence of these tasks is from highly structured activities to more spontaneous procedures that encourage the patient to use the skills learned earlier.

- Pitch range exercises—Exercises of this type can be a useful starting place for work on intonation. Dworkin (1991) recommended that these exercises begin with an assessment of the patient's ability to perceive obvious pitch changes in the clinician's voice. If the patient is unable to make these distinctions, the prognosis is poor for improving the patient's pitch control. However, if the patient can tell the difference between the pitch changes, the next set of exercises have the patient prolong an /a/ at the lowest pitch and then at the highest pitch possible. Once the highs and lows have been established, the patient is asked to sing up and down this pitch range by dividing the range into about eight individual notes. In the final exercises, the patient reads printed sentences that have arrows written above and below key words indicating the normal pitch changes for those words. For example, an upward arrow at the end of a question would indicate that the patient should raise pitch on the final word.
- Intonation profiles—This task uses lines to show intonation changes in written sentences. Lines drawn immediately below words indicate a flat intonation. Lines farther below words indicate a drop in pitch. Lines above words indicate a rise in pitch. These lines can be added easily to any written sentence, whether it is a statement or a question. For most patients, it is usually best to start with short, simple sentences and then progress to longer sentences. The ultimate goal is to have the

patient take the pitch changes produced in this structured activity and begin to use them in conversational speech.

- Contrastive stress drills—These tasks are usually designed so that the clinician asks a question, and the patient answers it by adding stress on key words to convey the intended meaning of the answer (McHenry, 1998). For example, the clinician might ask the following question about a picture of a man playing football: "Is the man playing basketball?" The patient will answer, "No. The man is playing football." The clinician's next question might be, "Is the woman playing football?" The patient's answer to this question would be, "No, the man is playing football." A third question might be, "Is the man watching football?" The patient would answer, "No, the man is playing football." The length of the questions and the complexity of the pictures for this task can easily be varied according the abilities of the patient.

- Chunking utterances into syntactic units—Duffy (2020) mentioned that some individuals with dysarthria need to learn to divide their utterances according to normal pauses within and between sentences. This is necessary because their dysarthria has limited the number of words they can produce on a single exhalation. To compensate for this limitation, the following task teaches the patient to inhale at those points in an utterance at which natural syntactic pauses occur. Examples of these natural pauses include after introductory clauses or phrases ("In the morning, [inhale] I went shopping at the store."), between clauses or phrases ("She went there, [inhale] but I missed her."), and between short sentences ("I saw the movie. [inhale] It was pretty good."). By inserting their inhalations at points at which normal pauses occur in an utterance, individuals with spastic dysarthria are often able to maintain a more natural rhythm in their speech. This rhythm is lost when the patient haphazardly places the inhalations within an utterance (Britton et al., 2017).

Treatment of Resonance Deficits

The hypernasality in spastic dysarthria is the result of increased muscle tone in the velum, which results in slowness and reduced range of movement. Although the hypernasality in this dysarthria is often less severe than that of flaccid dysarthria, it can still be quite evident. As in cases of flaccid dysarthria, treatment can be surgical, prosthetic, or behavioral.

Surgical and Prosthetic Treatments

As mentioned in Chapter 4, the surgical treatments for hypernasality include a pharyngeal flap procedure and Teflon paste (or hyaluronic acid) injections into the pharyngeal wall. Although these are possibilities, the palatal lift remains the more common choice for treating severe cases of hypernasality secondary to spastic dysarthria. However, any hyperactive gag reflex or increased muscle tone of the soft palate can make the use of a palatal lift difficult, if not impossible. Consequently, it might be necessary to decrease velar hypertonicity before fitting a patient with spastic dysarthria with a palatal lift.

- Decreasing velar hypertonicity—Dworkin (1991) described a detailed sequence of steps to reduce velar hypertonicity and to simulate the placement of a palatal lift in the mouth. Although the many steps of this procedure are beyond the scope of this book, the initial tasks involve slowly desensitizing the tongue and velum to a foreign object in the mouth. A reduction in velar hypertonicity is achieved by massaging the velum with a tongue blade that is covered by a finger cot. The final step of the treatment sequence is to use the tongue blade to press upward on the velum as if a palatal lift were in place.

Behavioral Treatments for Hypernasality

The following treatment procedures for hypernasality are only recommended for cases of mild severity. They also might be appropriate for fine-tuning velopharyngeal closure after surgical treatment or after a palatal lift has been fitted (Ono et al., 2005).

- Visual feedback—Although nasal air escape in spastic dysarthria is not as common as in flaccid dysarthria, it could be noted in some patients. A mirror can provide visual feedback to the patient regarding small amounts of nasal escape of air during the production of nonnasal phonemes (Rosenbek & LaPointe, 1985). The mirror is held under the nostrils while the patient looks at himself or herself in another larger mirror. The larger mirror provides the patient with a direct view of any fogging of the smaller mirror held under the nose. By trying to minimize nasal escape of air while repeating sentences that contain no nasal consonants, the patient with mild hypernasality might be able to maximize velar closure (Strand & Sullivan, 2001). Such simple devices as the See-Scape or a soft feather held under the nose also can provide this visual feedback (Ono et al., 2005).

- Reduce rate of speech—Reducing the rate of speech can increase intelligibility and lessen the perception of hypernasality in some individuals with flaccid dysarthria (Strand & Sullivan, 2001; Yorkston et al., 2010). Numerous activities can help reduce the rate of speech (see Chapter 8). One that might be appropriate in cases of spastic dysarthria is the use of finger or hand tapping to set the appropriate speaking rate. In this procedure, the patient speaks one word or syllable for every tap of the clinician's finger or hand. In general, slowing the speech rate increases intelligibility because it allows extra time for the articulators to reach their targets, thus resulting in more precise articulation of phonemes. The slower rate could decrease hypernasality because it can give a slow-moving velum extra time to fully and accurately close the velopharyngeal port during connected speech, which also promotes improved production of the pressure consonants.

- Increase loudness—The perception of hypernasality can sometimes be minimized by having the patient speak more loudly. Louder speech tends to mask the hypernasal resonance in individuals with spastic dysarthria. Equally important, the louder speech can often increase intelligibility by simply making it easier for a listener to hear what is being said. Modeling appropriate loudness levels is a key component of this treatment. Visual feedback on loudness is also helpful for most patients. A sound pressure level meter (either as a stand-alone instrument or an app on a smartphone) can give patients a visual cue as to what the desired loudness should be.

Summary of Spastic Dysarthria

- Spastic dysarthria can be caused by any process that results in bilateral damage to the pyramidal and extrapyramidal systems.
- In general, the bilateral damage to the pyramidal system results in muscle weakness and slowness in the articulators during speech. The bilateral damage to the extrapyramidal system results in increased muscle tone (spasticity) in the articulators, which could be most evident in the hyperadduction of the vocal folds during phonation.
- The speech characteristics of spastic dysarthria include imprecise consonants, monopitch, reduced stress, and harsh vocal quality.

■ Treatment of spastic dysarthria can concentrate on reducing the increased muscle tone by relaxation and stretching exercises. Traditional articulation tasks can target the imprecise consonant productions that are so common in this dysarthria.

Study Questions

1. Define spastic dysarthria in your own words.
2. Which nervous system tracts must be damaged before spastic dysarthria can occur?
3. What role does damage to the pyramidal and extrapyramidal tracts play in the symptoms of spastic dysarthria?
4. What is the most common cause of spastic dysarthria?
5. Why is it impossible for a single-hemisphere stroke to cause spastic dysarthria?
6. What was the most common articulation deficit in Darley et al.'s subjects with spastic dysarthria?
7. What is pseudobulbar affect?
8. What do the terms bulbar palsy and pseudobulbar palsy mean?
9. What is a treatment for hyperadduction of the vocal folds?
10. Describe a tongue-stretching exercise.

Chapter 6

Unilateral Upper Motor Neuron Dysarthria

- **Definitions of Unilateral Upper Motor Neuron Dysarthria**
- **Neurologic Basis of Unilateral Upper Motor Neuron Dysarthria**
- **Causes of Unilateral Upper Motor Neuron Dysarthria**
  - Stroke
  - Tumors
  - Traumatic Brain Injury
- **Speech Characteristics of Unilateral Upper Motor Neuron Dysarthria**
  - Articulation
  - Phonation
  - Resonance
  - Prosody and Respiration
- **Key Evaluation Tasks for Unilateral Upper Motor Neuron Dysarthria**
- **Treatment of Unilateral Upper Motor Neuron Dysarthria**
- **Summary of Unilateral Upper Motor Neuron Dysarthria**
- **Study Questions**

Definitions of Unilateral Upper Motor Neuron Dysarthria

There are fewer published definitions of unilateral upper motor neuron dysarthria than of any other type of dysarthria. One reason for this is the relatively recent recognition of this dysarthria as a motor speech disorder. Darley et al. (1969a, 1969b, 1975) did not classify it as one of the separate dysarthrias, and there were few clinical studies of this disorder before the 1980s. Most of the research on unilateral upper motor dysarthria has been done since the mid-1980s. This is curious because the effects of unilateral upper motor neuron damage on speech production have been recognized for many years (see the 1897 description by Marie and Kattwinkel in Chapter 1). The available definitions all mention that articulation deficits are the primary characteristic of this dysarthria. Many also mention that these articulation deficits are almost always mild. The following two quotes are typical descriptions of unilateral upper motor neuron dysarthria:

[A] motor speech disorder caused by damage to the upper motor neurons that supply cranial and spinal nerves involved in speech production, the dominant speech problem is imprecise productions of consonants, but slow diadochokinesis and voice disorder also commonly occur. (Singh & Kent, 2000, p. 248)

This is a recently documented form of dysarthria involving damage on a single side of the brain, presumably in the corticobulbar tract. At one time it was thought that dysarthria associated with upper motor neuron disease had to involve bilateral lesions. Stated otherwise, unilateral lesions of the corticobulbar tract were not expected to produce dysarthria because of the extensive bilateral innervation of speech mechanism musculature. Based on reviews of a fair number of cases, however, it now seems clear that unilateral upper motor neuron damage can produce dysarthria, albeit of a mild and often temporary kind. (Weismer, 2007, pp. 68–69)

Although Weismer's quote mentions the temporary nature of this dysarthria in many patients, readers should not assume that all individuals with unilateral upper motor neuron dysarthria will spontaneously recover from the speech deficits associated with it. The effects of this dysarthria can be persistent, and many patients with it will be appropriate candidates for speech treatment.

Neurologic Basis of Unilateral Upper Motor Neuron Dysarthria

Chapter 2 explained how upper motor neurons transmit motor impulses from the higher centers of the brain to the brainstem and spinal cord and how these neurons eventually synapse with the lower motor neurons in the cranial and spinal nerves. That chapter also discussed how upper motor neurons are divided into the pyramidal and extrapyramidal tracts. Chapter 5 showed that a key to understanding spastic dysarthria is knowing that both the left and right pyramidal and extrapyramidal tracts must be damaged for spastic dysarthria to result. That is, spastic dysarthria is present only when there is bilateral damage to both of these tracts (Figure 6–1). The damage to the pyramidal system will result in weakness and loss of fine motor control in the muscles of speech production, and the damage to the extrapyramidal system will cause increased muscle tone (spasticity) and abnormal reflexes in many of these same muscles. The combination of these symptoms results in the speech characteristics of spastic dysarthria.

What happens, however, when the damage to upper motor neurons occurs on only one side of the brain (Figure 6–2)? In other words, how is speech production affected by unilateral damage to upper motor neurons? Because most of the cranial nerves serving the speech muscles (except the lower face and tongue) receive bilateral innervation from the upper motor neurons, the speech deficits seen after unilateral upper motor neuron damage almost always are less severe than those occurring after bilateral damage. Nevertheless, unilateral damage to the upper motor neurons can cause obvious speech production deficits, despite this bilateral innervation of most cranial nerves.

The most apparent consequences of unilateral upper motor neuron damage are to the muscles of the lower face and tongue. Because the cranial nerves serving these structures are innervated primarily by the upper motor neurons on only one side of the brain, unilateral damage can affect the muscles of the lower face and tongue on the side opposite the damage (Figure 6–3). For example, if upper motor neuron damage occurred on the left side of the brain, the lower right side of the face and tongue might show signs of weakness. In cases of severe unilateral damage, these two structures could be nearly paralyzed on the affected side. More typically, however, this unilateral weakness of the tongue and lower face will usually result in movements that are slow and have reduced range of motion. The tongue might deviate to the affected side when protruded, and lower facial droop might be evident.

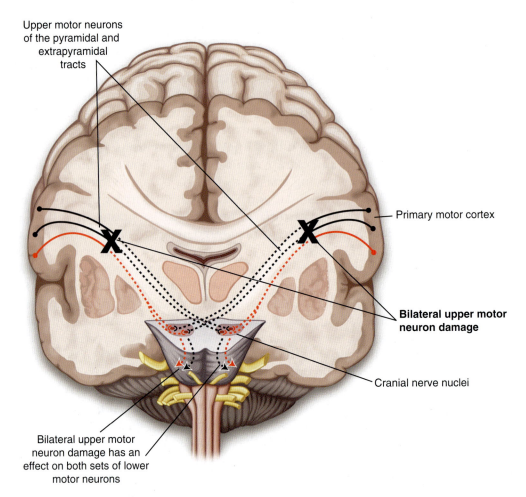

FIGURE 6–1. As discussed in Chapter 5, spastic dysarthria is caused by bilateral upper motor neuron damage to the pyramidal and extrapyramidal systems.

Patients with these problems often report that their tongue movements are slow and clumsy.

Although the effects of unilateral upper motor neuron damage on the lower face and tongue are recognized widely, the effects of this damage on the other structures of speech production are less clearly defined and less well understood. The traditional view is that because the upper motor neurons bilaterally innervate the velum, pharynx, and larynx, these speech structures should not be affected significantly by unilateral upper motor neuron damage. This is because the upper motor neurons on the unaffected side will provide sufficient innervation to the cranial nerves serving the two sides of these structures.

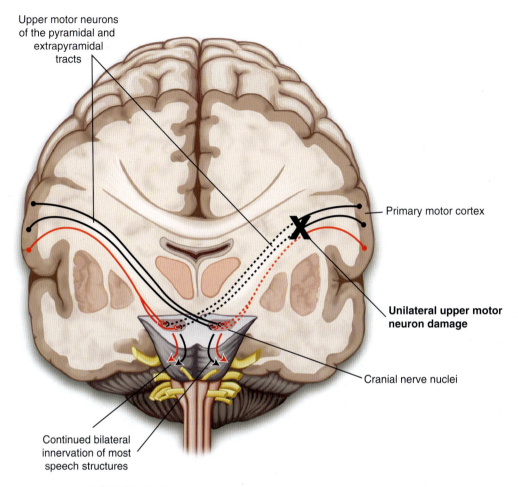

FIGURE 6–2. Unilateral upper motor neuron damage usually will have only a mild effect on speech production because most speech structures will still receive innervation from the opposite, undamaged hemisphere. The lower face and the tongue will demonstrate the most significant effects of unilateral damage because these speech structures primarily receive only unilateral upper motor neuron innervation.

In reality, however, the clinical picture is not that definite. It appears that unilateral upper motor neuron damage can affect the function of these bilaterally innervated speech structures. For example, some patients with unilateral upper motor neuron dysarthria have a harsh vocal quality. Ideally, this disorder of phonation should not occur in cases of unilateral upper motor neuron damage, because the vagus nerve, which innervates the larynx, receives bilateral innervation; the upper motor neurons on the unaffected side should provide innervation to both sides of the larynx, and vocal-fold adduction should be relatively unaffected.

However, because the harsh vocal quality strongly suggests some type of laryngeal dysfunction, it would appear that the innervation from the unaffected hemisphere is not a perfect replacement for the innervation from the damaged upper motor neurons in the opposite hemisphere. The question of why some bilaterally innervated speech structures show impaired function after unilateral upper motor neuron damage is discussed again later in this chapter.

Causes of Unilateral Upper Motor Neuron Dysarthria

Any condition that damages the upper motor neurons on one side of the brain can cause unilateral upper motor neuron dysarthria. Moreover, this dysarthria can occur after damage in either the left or right hemisphere. When the damage is in the left hemisphere, unilateral upper motor neuron dysarthria often co-occurs with aphasia or apraxia of speech. When the damage happens in the right hemisphere, this dysarthria can co-occur with the cognitive and visual deficits associated with injury to that side of the brain. Typically, pathologies that cause focal lesions are the most common cause of unilateral upper motor neuron dysarthria. It is not often associated with degenerative diseases, infections, or metabolic disorders, all of which usually result in widespread neurologic damage.

Stroke

Without doubt, the most frequent cause of unilateral upper motor neuron dysarthria is stroke. In a study of 56 subjects with this dysarthria, Duffy and Folger (1986) found that 91% of the cases had been caused by a stroke. Strokes that result in this dysarthria can occur almost anywhere in the brain that contains upper motor neurons. This would include many cortical and subcortical areas, as well as the brainstem. Strokes affecting the internal capsule and nearby areas are frequent causes of unilateral upper motor neuron dysarthria. The internal capsule is the point where many descending upper motor neurons are compacted closely as they course downward between the thalamus and the basal ganglia (Figure 6–4). Several arteries supply blood to the internal capsule, and even small strokes can have major consequences because of the close proximity of so many upper motor neurons in this area.

Strokes involving the frontal lobe also are leading causes of unilateral upper motor neuron dysarthria. Given the importance of

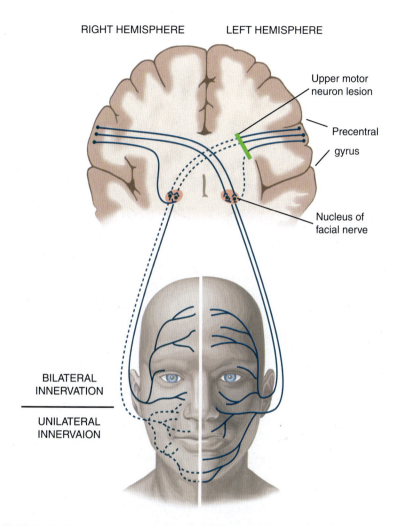

FIGURE 6–3. Unilateral upper motor neuron damage will affect only the muscles of the lower face and tongue because most other speech structures are innervated by upper motor neurons on both sides of the brain.

the frontal lobes in formulating and initiating movement, it should not be surprising that unilateral damage to one of them can result in dysarthric speech.

Tumors

Although not a common cause of unilateral upper motor neuron dysarthria, brain tumors can certainly lead to this disorder. Several ways in which a brain tumor can cause the focal, unilateral upper motor neuron damage that results in this dysarthria are listed here.

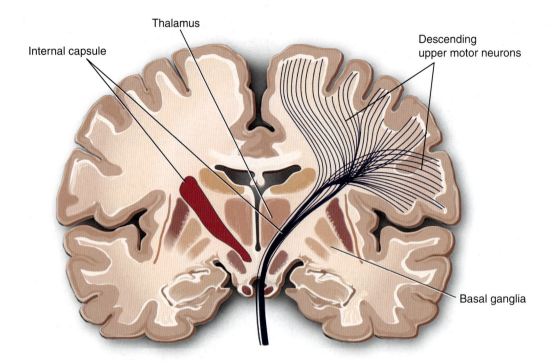

FIGURE 6–4. The internal capsule is the point where descending upper motor neurons are squeezed together as they pass between the basal ganglia and the thalamus. Damage to the internal capsule could have a significant effect on motor function because even a small lesion can damage many upper motor neurons.

- A brain tumor may directly cause the destruction of nearby upper motor neurons as it grows. This loss of neurons will degrade the transmission of motor impulses from the higher brain centers to the cranial and spinal nerves.
- A growing tumor can displace and "squeeze" upper motor neurons as it becomes larger. This direct pressure from the tumor can compromise the function of the neurons.
- The growing tumor could compress the arteries or veins serving upper motor neurons and interfere with the normal blood flow to or from these cells. The resulting reduction in blood flow would have a negative effect on the function of the neurons.

Tumors such as these could cause unilateral upper motor neuron dysarthria if their effects were restricted to only one side of the brain. However, many brain tumors can have bilateral effects on brain function, even if they are located in only one hemisphere. For example, a tumor in the left hemisphere that caused a generalized increase in intracranial pressure would actually affect the functioning of both hemispheres. Such a tumor probably would not cause unilateral upper motor neuron dysarthria because it would have a bilateral influence on brain function.

Traumatic Brain Injury

As with brain tumors, TBIs are not a common cause of unilateral upper motor neuron dysarthria. Most TBIs result in diffuse damage that affects both hemispheres because the whole brain is usually stretched and distorted at the moment of impact. As a result, lesions typically occur in both hemispheres following a TBI. Nevertheless, it is possible to have head injury in which a lesion is restricted primarily to one side of the brain. In such cases, the damage can affect upper motor neurons unilaterally, either at the cortical, subcortical, or brainstem levels. When this happens, it is possible that unilateral upper motor neuron dysarthria could result.

Speech Characteristics of Unilateral Upper Motor Neuron Dysarthria

In most cases of unilateral upper motor neuron dysarthria, the effects of the disorder on motor speech production usually are judged to be mild or moderate. This dysarthria is often a short-term disorder for mildly impaired patients, with recovery occurring over a period of days or weeks. In these milder cases, dysarthria might be the most obvious or perhaps the only indicator that some type of neurologic event has taken place (Duffy, 2020). In the more serious cases, unilateral upper motor neuron dysarthria will probably co-occur with other disorders, such as aphasia, apraxia, limb hemiparesis, visual deficits, or cognitive impairments. When there are co-occurring speech and language disorders, it might be difficult to clearly diagnose this dysarthria because the patient's verbal output could be limited. As a result, the dysarthria might "take a back seat" to these other deficits. Nevertheless, the speech characteristics of unilateral upper motor neuron dysarthria are distinguishable from other dysarthrias and need to be identified accurately during a diagnostic evaluation (Table 6–1).

Articulation

As indicated in the definition at the beginning of this chapter, unilateral upper motor neuron dysarthria is principally a disorder

TABLE 6–1	Percentage of 56 Individuals With Unilateral Upper Motor Neuron Dysarthria Who Demonstrated the Following Speech Production Errors
Percentage of Individuals	**Speech Production Errors**
95	Imprecise consonants
72	Slow AMRs
39	Harsh voice quality
33	Imprecise AMRs
33	Irregular AMRs
18	Slow rate
14	Irregular articulatory breakdowns
11	Mild hypernasality
9	Reduced loudness
5	Strained-harsh voice quality
4	Increased rate of speech in segments
4	Excess and equal stress

Note: From *Motor Speech Disorders: Substrates, Differential Diagnosis, and Management* (p. 228), by J. Duffy, 1995, St. Louis: Mosby. Copyright 1995 by W. B. Saunders Company. Reprinted with permission.

of articulation. This should not be surprising, given that unilateral upper motor neuron damage typically affects the tongue and lower face much more than it does other speech production structures. The most likely causes of the articulation deficits associated with this dysarthria are weakness, reduced range of motion, and decreased fine motor control of the tongue and lips.

Few studies have examined the speech characteristics of unilateral upper motor neuron dysarthria. One of the most comprehensive was conducted by Duffy and Folger (1986), who found that 98% of their subjects with this dysarthria had articulation deficits. The primary difficulty for nearly all of these subjects was imprecise consonant production. Most of the subjects' articulation deficits had severity ratings in the mild to moderate range. Irregular articulatory breakdowns also were present in some of the subjects but were significantly less common than the problem with consonants. In addition, nearly all subjects had slow AMRs, and 33% had irregular AMRs. The slow AMRs were often so mild that they seldom resulted in slower than normal connected speech rates.

In another study of unilateral upper motor neuron dysarthria, Hartman and Abbs (1992) also found that imprecise consonant productions were a common feature of their subjects' speech. However, the irregular articulatory breakdowns noted by Duffy and Folger (1986) were not evident in this study. The authors attributed this finding to differences between the subjects in the two studies, suggesting that their subjects had lesions that were more focal than Duffy and Folger's subjects.

Ropper (1987) examined the speech of 10 subjects with unilateral upper motor neuron dysarthria secondary to right hemisphere strokes. As with the two studies described earlier, articulatory deficits were the subjects' primary speech disorder, with most subjects showing signs of oropharyngeal weakness. As in the study by Hartman and Abbs (1992), the subjects in Ropper's study did not demonstrate the irregular articulatory breakdowns that were noted by Duffy and Folger (1986).

Phonation

Several studies have indicated that a mild to moderate harsh vocal quality can be present in some cases of unilateral upper motor neuron dysarthria (Duffy & Folger, 1986; Ropper, 1987). For example, Duffy and Folger (1986) reported that 39% of their subjects had this harsh quality in their speech. As mentioned earlier, this is a curious phenomenon because it suggests that the larynx can be affected by unilateral upper motor neuron damage. Conventional thinking has always suggested that most of the cranial nerves are bilaterally innervated by upper motor neurons. Consequently, both the left and right branches of a cranial nerve would still receive full or nearly full upper motor neuron innervation when one upper motor neuron pathway is damaged. In the case of the vagus (X) cranial nerve, which serves the larynx, unilateral upper motor neuron damage should not affect phonation because both sides of the laryngeal muscles are thought to receive adequate upper motor neuron innervation from the undamaged side of the brain.

However, the presence of a harsh vocal quality after unilateral upper motor neuron damage indicates that the function of the larynx is somehow being compromised by the unilateral lesion. Duffy (2020) suggested several reasons for the harshness sometimes noted in unilateral upper motor neuron dysarthria, as listed here.

- It could be the result of mild vocal-fold weakness or spasticity following unilateral upper motor neuron damage.
- A previously unknown lesion could be present, and this combined with a new upper motor neuron lesion on the opposite side of the brain now causes vocal-fold spasticity.

- The harsh vocal quality could be a dysphonia that appears normally in many elderly individuals.
- It might be caused by a general medical condition such as illness or inactivity and, therefore, cannot be attributed directly to the upper motor neuron damage.

Any of these are possible explanations for the harsh vocal quality noted in some patients with this dysarthria. One of the most interesting aspects of this question is the implication that there is still plenty to be learned about how the nervous system controls the speech mechanism. Watch the PluralPlus UUMN Dysarthria Case 1 video for an example of a patient with harsh vocal quality.

Resonance

Duffy and Folger (1986) found that 11% of their subjects with unilateral upper motor neuron dysarthria had hypernasality. As with the harsh vocal quality noted in their study, it is surprising to find that velopharyngeal function is affected by unilateral upper motor neuron damage because the vagus nerve, which serves the velar and pharyngeal muscles, is bilaterally innervated by the upper motor neurons. It is likely that the causes of this hypernasality could be related to several of those outlined in the section on phonation: general weakness or illness, prior lesions to upper motor neurons in the opposite hemisphere, and so forth. In particular, it could be that the unilateral damage to the upper motor neurons causes a mild muscular weakness in the velum and results in the noted hypernasality.

Prosody and Respiration

Prosody and respiration are rarely impaired in cases of unilateral upper motor neuron dysarthria. Given that this dysarthria is generally a mild to moderate articulation disorder, this should not be surprising. Duffy (2020) reported that when prosody is affected, the most likely cause is a slightly slow rate of speech. The respiration of patients with unilateral upper motor neuron dysarthria is seldom impaired significantly, especially in the long term. This is probably the result of the widely distributed innervation of the intercostal muscles and the bilateral innervation of the diaphragm. Although some abnormal intercostal muscle movement has been noted in patients with single-hemisphere strokes (Przedborski et al., 1988), respiration deficits usually are not a problem in cases of unilateral upper motor neuron dysarthria.

Key Evaluation Tasks for Unilateral Upper Motor Neuron Dysarthria

1. As with any dysarthria, the medical records can provide valuable diagnostic information about the cause and the site of lesions. Facts about the site of lesions can be especially helpful in diagnosing unilateral upper motor neuron dysarthria. As stated earlier in this chapter, it is important to remember that sometimes this dysarthria is the only evidence that a stroke or other neurologic event has occurred. The lesion might be too small for neurologic imaging procedures to detect, especially early after the onset of symptoms.

2. Conversational speech or reading a paragraph are useful tasks for evoking the imprecise consonant productions that are so common in this dysarthria. These tasks also can be useful in detecting the irregular articulatory breakdowns that sometimes are present.

3. The AMR task is helpful in highlighting a slowed rate of phoneme production. Remember that in many individuals with unilateral upper motor neuron dysarthria, a slightly slow AMR might not reflect slow connected speech.

4. A prolonged vowel will be useful in detecting the harsh voice quality heard in some patients with this dysarthria.

Treatment of Unilateral Upper Motor Neuron Dysarthria

Unilateral upper motor neuron dysarthria presents a few unique situations for the clinician. When it accompanies the language and apraxia deficits of a left hemisphere lesion or the visual and cognitive deficits of a right hemisphere lesion, the relatively mild articulation problems of this dysarthria are often a low treatment priority. The other coexisting deficits almost always are allotted the bulk of treatment time, which usually is appropriate. The result, however, is that this dysarthria is frequently not treated. On the other hand, when this dysarthria is the only evidence of a neurologic pathology (usually a stroke) and there are no obvious language or cognitive deficits, the resulting articulation problems could be so minor that a clinician might decide not to treat them. These two circumstances could partially explain the scarcity of treatment studies on unilateral upper motor neuron dysarthria.

Although it is understandable that this dysarthria receives little treatment in cases of aphasia and other serious disorders, unilateral upper motor neuron dysarthria should be treated in many cases, and probably in a majority of them. Duffy (2020) and Swigert (2010) recommended traditional articulation tasks for individuals with this dysarthria. The following activities might be appropriate for individuals with unilateral upper motor neuron dysarthria.

- Intelligibility drills—Intelligibility drills are tasks in which the patient is given a list of words or sentences to read (Yorkston et al., 1988). Then the clinician turns away from the patient so that he or she will only be able to understand the patient's speech if it is articulated clearly. By not looking at the target word list or at the patient's mouth, the clinician will depend entirely on the patient's articulation to understand the target word. If the clinician does not understand the target word, the patient needs to determine why the word was unclear and then try saying it again. If this second attempt fails, then the clinician can look at the target word and give the patient specific feedback on why he or she could not understand the utterance (e.g., "I didn't know it was 'sleep' because I couldn't hear the 'l.' Try it again, and let me really hear the 'l' this time.").

- Phonetic placement—This procedure treats articulation errors by instructing patients on the correct position of the articulators before they attempt to produce a target sound. Phonetic placement can be especially valuable in that it educates patients on how certain speech sounds are produced. Many individuals with dysarthria realize they are producing speech sounds incorrectly, but they have little understanding of why their productions are in error. For example, phonetic placement can educate speakers with dysarthria about why their production of a /d/ actually sounds closer to a /z/ or a /p/ sounds closer to a /b/ and so forth.

- Exaggerating consonants—Also known as overarticulation, exaggerating consonants is a treatment procedure that teaches the patient to fully articulate all consonant phonemes. Darley et al. (1975) suggested that most patients need to concentrate especially on medial and final consonants, because these are the sounds most likely to be poorly articulated in connected speech. The improvements in intelligibility can be dramatic when individuals with unilateral upper motor neuron dysarthria fully articulate the medial and final consonants in words.

Park et al. (2016) used exaggerating consonants as the basis of an intensive treatment program for dysarthria. Their patients had a variety of different types of dysarthria, caused by either traumatic head injury or stroke. The study used a small group repeated measures design to determine the effects of overarticulation (in combination with slower and slightly louder speech) on dysarthric patients' single-word and sentence intelligibility. There were 16 treatment sessions (1-hr sessions, four times a week, for 4 weeks). The patients were first oriented to the treatment tasks so that they knew what was expected. The treatment sessions started with 10 min of prepractice where patients reviewed a random selection of the tasks that were to be used later in the session. The following 10 min required the patients to repeat 10 functional phrases five times each (e.g., "What are we doing tomorrow?"). The next 10 min had the patients repeating 10 service requests five times each (e.g., "Where is the _____?"). During the final 30 min, the patients read aloud, described pictures, and engaged in conversation. Feedback during most of the sessions consisted of whether the patients' utterances were clear or unclear. Homework also was a part of the treatment procedure. The results showed that naive listeners noted improved conversational intelligibility in all patients compared to pretreatment samples. Many of the other outcome measures also were positive.

- Minimal contrast drills—These drills have the patient concentrate on producing pairs of words that vary by only one phoneme. The distinction between the words can be in the voicing (park–bark), manner of production (dime–mime), or place of production (sea–she) of consonants. The distinction also can be between vowels (man–men), but working on consonants does more to enhance intelligibility in most patients. These word pairs can be used alone, in phrases, or in sentences, depending on the needs of the specific patient.

Summary of Unilateral Upper Motor Neuron Dysarthria

- As its name implies, unilateral upper motor neuron dysarthria is caused by damage to the upper motor neurons on only one side of the brain. This contrasts with spastic dysarthria, which is caused by damage to the upper motor neurons on both sides of the brain.
- Unilateral upper motor neuron dysarthria is almost exclusively a disorder of articulation. This dysarthria is often present with aphasia and apraxia of speech when the damage occurs in

the left hemisphere of the brain. When the right hemisphere is damaged, this dysarthria often co-occurs with the visual and cognitive deficits associated with injury to that side of the brain.

- Treatment of unilateral upper motor neuron dysarthria includes such traditional articulation tasks as intelligibility drills and phonetic placement.

Study Questions

1. Define unilateral upper motor neuron dysarthria in your own words.
2. Why does unilateral damage to the upper motor neurons result in less severe symptoms as compared with bilateral damage to these neurons?
3. Unilateral upper motor neuron dysarthria is primarily a disorder of what?
4. What is the most common cause of unilateral upper motor neuron dysarthria?
5. Why are traumatic head injuries not a common cause of unilateral upper motor neuron dysarthria?
6. What is the most common articulation disorder in cases of unilateral upper motor neuron dysarthria?
7. What did Duffy suggest as the cause of harsh vocal quality in unilateral upper motor neuron dysarthria?
8. Why are there so few treatment studies for unilateral upper motor neuron dysarthria?
9. Describe intelligibility drills.
10. What are minimal contrast drills?

Chapter 7

Ataxic Dysarthria

Definitions of Ataxic Dysarthria

Neurologic Basis of Ataxic Dysarthria

   Neural Pathways to and From the Cerebellum

The Cerebellum and Speech

Causes of Ataxic Dysarthria

   Degenerative Diseases

   Stroke

   Toxic Conditions

   Traumatic Head Injury

   Tumors

   Other Possible Causes

Speech Characteristics of Ataxic Dysarthria

   Articulation

   Prosody

   Phonation

   Resonance

   Respiration

Key Evaluation Tasks for Ataxic Dysarthria

Treatment of Ataxic Dysarthria

   Respiration

   Prosody

      Rate Control

      Stress and Intonation

   Articulation

Summary of Ataxic Dysarthria

Study Questions

Definitions of Ataxic Dysarthria

Damage to the cerebellum is the most common feature in the published definitions of ataxic dysarthria (sometimes called cerebellar dysarthria). It is mentioned in nearly all instances. This cerebellar damage results in speech errors that are primarily articulatory and prosodic. These two types of errors often combine to give the speech of individuals with ataxic dysarthria an unsteady, slurred quality. All three of the following definitions are good introductions to ataxic dysarthria.

[A] dysarthria associated with damage to the cerebellar system and characterized by speech errors relating primarily to timing, giving equal stress to each syllable; articulation problems are typically characterized by intermittent errors ranging from mild to severe; vocal quality [can be] harsh, with monotonous pitch and volume; prosody may range from reduced to unnatural stress. (Nicolosi et al., 1983, p. 79)

Ataxic dysarthria is a disorder of sensorimotor control for speech production that results from damage to the cerebellum or to its input and output pathways. The dragging and blurred quality of ataxic dysarthria speech has sometimes been likened to "drunken speech." (Cannito & Marquardt, 1997, p. 217)

Acute and chronic, hereditary or acquired cerebellar disorders are often accompanied by [ataxic dysarthria], especially in patients with lesions in the left paravermian region [of the cerebellum]. The disorders typically result in slow speech with difficulty pronouncing words and scanning syllables. (Rampello et al., 2016, p. 357)

Neurologic Basis of Ataxic Dysarthria

Up to now, this textbook has discussed dysarthrias that are caused by damage to motor neurons. Flaccid dysarthria (Chapter 4) is caused by damage to the lower motor neurons; spastic dysarthria (Chapter 5) is caused by bilateral damage to the upper motor neurons; and unilateral upper motor neuron dysarthria (Chapter 6) is caused by unilateral damage to the upper motor neurons. This chapter examines ataxic dysarthria, which is caused by damage to the cerebellum or to the neural pathways that connect the cerebellum to other parts of the CNS. Incidentally, the term *ataxia* means widespread incoordination and comes from the Greek word for "lack of order."

Although the cerebellum was discussed in Chapter 2, it would be beneficial to review some of the information about it. The cerebellum is located below the occipital lobe and is attached to the back of the brainstem (Figure 7–1). It is shaped somewhat like a "small brain" in that it has two hemispheres, a deep fissure between the hemispheres, and a cortical surface of gray matter that has many convolutions. The cerebellum is more complex and fully developed in humans than in any other animal species. This complexity reflects a human's need for very precise muscular control over certain movements, such as those for speech.

The cerebellum is a very important part of the motor system. Its primary function is to coordinate the timing and force of muscular contractions so that skilled, voluntary movements appropriate for an intended task are created. It accomplishes this by processing sensory information from all over the body and integrating that information into the execution of a movement. The processing and integration function of the cerebellum is obvious because there are about 40 neural fibers conveying information into the cerebellum for every neural fiber conveying information out (Brodal, 2010). Although it is not clearly understood how it performs these functions, the general cellular layout of the cerebellum and its neural pathways has been documented in detail.

Neural Pathways to and From the Cerebellum

The cerebellum is attached to the brainstem and communicates with the rest of the CNS through three bundles of neural tracts called the **cerebellar peduncles** (Figure 7–2 and Figure 7–3). By exchanging information through these neural tracts, the cerebellum is able to monitor ongoing movements and communicate with the cortex concerning planned upcoming movements. Through the first of these tracts, the **inferior peduncle**, the cerebellum receives sensory information from the entire body about the position of body parts—including the eyes, the vestibular system of the inner ear, the joints of the limbs, the skin, tendons, and muscles—before, during, and after a movement. With this information, the cerebellum is able to recognize what the body is doing during a movement and whether a motor impulse to the muscles is accomplishing the intended result. Overall, this access to sensory information allows the cerebellum to monitor the timing and force of movements while they are being performed. For example, if a body part encounters some unexpected resistance during a movement, the cerebellum detects that resistance immediately through its access to sensory information from the affected body part. The cerebellum can then

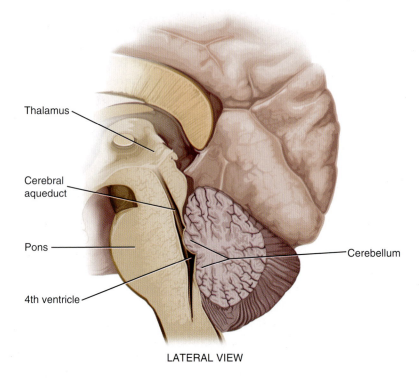
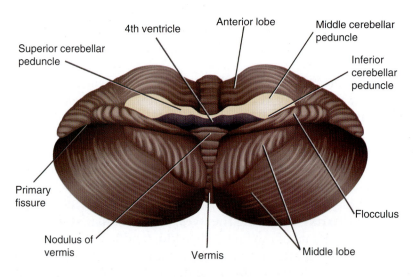

FIGURE 7-1. A lateral view of the cerebellum showing how it is attached to the brainstem and an inferior view of the cerebellum.

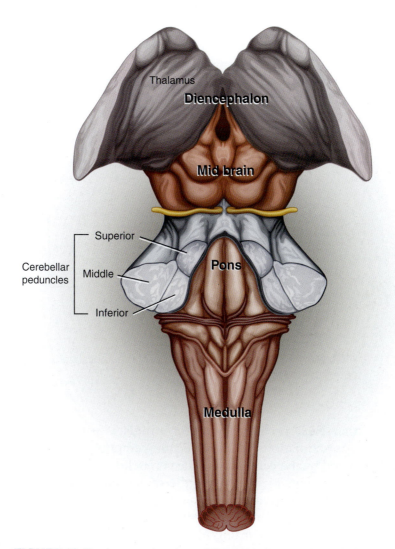

FIGURE 7–2. A posterior view of the brainstem and cerebellar peduncles. In this illustration, the cerebellum has been removed.

send adjusting motor impulses to that body part via the superior peduncle (discussed later) to compensate for the resistance, thereby keeping the timing and force of the movement appropriate for the task.

The second pathway, the **middle peduncle**, is the largest of the cerebellar peduncles. The neural tracts that travel through the middle peduncle connect the cortex with the cerebellum. These tracts are especially important to the motor system, because it is through them that the cerebellum receives preliminary information from the cortex regarding planned movements. It is thought

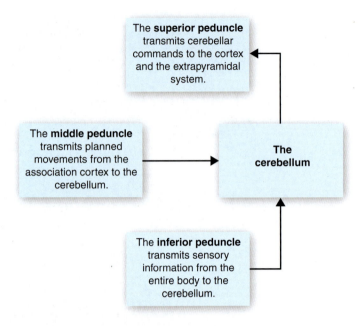

FIGURE 7–3. A schematic diagram of the neural pathways leading into and out of the cerebellum.

that these preliminary motor impulses from the cortex are rough approximations of intended movements and need to be coordinated by the cerebellum. The cerebellum coordinates these planned movements by integrating the sensory information it receives from the body with an individual's experience of what the appropriate movement should be. The intended movements are then smoothed and refined according to the current conditions of the body and sent back to the cortex via the thalamus. These processed motor commands are then sent to the motor areas of the cortex, where they are transmitted to the appropriate muscles.

The third pathway, the **superior peduncle**, is the cerebellum's main output channel to the rest of the CNS, providing several destinations for the neurons coursing through it. One of these destinations is the cerebral cortex. It is through the neural fibers in the superior peduncle that the cerebellum sends its processed motor impulses to the motor areas of the cortex, thereby completing the corticocerebellar control circuit. The entire corticocerebellar control circuit, therefore, starts in the cortex and courses down into the cerebellum through the middle peduncle. The fibers of this neural circuit exit the cerebellum through the superior peduncle and travel back up to the cortex after passing through the thalamus.

Along with the neural tracts coursing out of the superior peduncles to the cortex, additional tracts travel out of the superior peduncle and connect the cerebellum directly to neurons of the extrapyramidal tract. By way of these connections to the extrapyramidal system, the cerebellum can stimulate or inhibit the actions of voluntary muscles. Unlike the neural impulses traveling through the corticocerebellar control circuit, these cerebellar commands to the extrapyramidal system do not travel to the cortex before being sent to the muscles. Instead, these commands take a complex course through the extrapyramidal system as they make their way to the appropriate lower motor neurons. Once these cerebellar motor impulses reach the lower motor neurons, they are then able to coordinate and quickly adjust the movements of the voluntary muscles according to the changing positions and circumstances of the body.

Incidentally, the neurons that course through these three cerebellar pathways are called **cerebellar control circuits**, not upper motor neurons. Although they do transmit motor impulses, these neurons do not actually synapse with lower motor neurons, which, by definition is what upper motor neurons do. Most neurons coursing out of the cerebellar peduncles synapse with either true upper motor neurons (primarily those of the extrapyramidal system) or interneurons in the brainstem and spinal cord.

The Cerebellum and Speech

Without doubt, the cerebellum plays an important role in coordinating the many intricate muscular contractions needed to produce intelligible speech. However, the precise nature of the cerebellum's influence on speech is unclear. There are probably at least two ways in which the cerebellum influences speech movements. One of these is through the corticocerebellar control circuit discussed previously. The planned motor impulses of a planned speech act are sent from the cortex to the cerebellum. The cerebellum coordinates and refines these preliminary speech movements according to (a) sensory information about the positions and conditions of the articulators, and (b) prior practice with regard to what the skilled target movement should be. These coordinated motor impulses are then sent to the thalamus for additional refinement and then forwarded to the motor cortex. From there, the motor impulses are transmitted to the appropriate muscles for speech production.

Another way in which the cerebellum might influence speech movements is through its connections to the extrapyramidal system.

As described in the preceding section of this chapter, the cerebellum can make rapid adjustments in the timing and force of movements to compensate for unexpected changes in the circumstances of a movement. For example, if someone is attempting to talk with food in his or her mouth, the cerebellum will detect that tongue movements are being slowed by the presence of the food. To maintain intelligible articulation of speech sounds, the cerebellum will adjust the firing of the appropriate motor neurons to the tongue so that intelligible articulation can be maintained despite this resistance to tongue movement during speech. Because of this remarkable dual ability to coordinate and modify both planned and ongoing speech movements, the cerebellum is a key player in the motor speech system. However, because it is so important, damage to the cerebellum or to its control circuits can significantly harm an individual's ability to produce normal speech.

Causes of Ataxic Dysarthria

Damage to different parts of the cerebellum or its control circuits can result in a variety of movement disorders. In general, individuals with cerebellar damage have problems coordinating their voluntary movements. It seems as if they have trouble controlling the timing and force of their movements, especially at the beginning and ending of an action. For example, their movements might be wavering and jerky when reaching to pick up an object. This unsteadiness indicates that the range and direction of movements also can be affected by cerebellar damage. Altogether, these movement deficits of timing, force, range, and direction are known as **cerebellar ataxia**.

Impairment of equilibrium during walking can be one of the more obvious symptoms of cerebellar damage. In these cases, individuals walk with a wide-based, staggering gait, frequently giving the impression that they are just about to fall. Cerebellar damage also can cause deficits in voluntary eye movements, intention tremors, hypotonia of the muscles, and problems with motor learning.

Because so much about the operation of the cerebellum is unknown, neuroscientists are unclear about how different types of cerebellar damage affect speech production. Darley et al. (1975) stated that ataxic dysarthria often occurs when there is generalized or bilateral damage to the cerebellum. They also reported that speech coordination might be especially dependent on a part of the cerebellum at the midpoint between the cerebellar hemispheres, called the **vermis** (see Figure 7–1). Some research has suggested that focal lesions also can cause ataxic dysarthria. Duffy (2020) cited several studies suggesting that ataxic dysarthria can be caused by focal damage to the superior peduncle, the lateral portions of the cerebellar hemispheres, or areas near the vermis.

Degenerative Diseases

A number of degenerative disorders result in progressive cerebellar dysfunction and are frequent causes of ataxic dysarthria. **Autosomal dominant cerebellar ataxia of late onset** is a hereditary disease that usually begins in middle age. Ataxic dysarthria is only one of many features that could be present in this disorder. Progressive cerebellar ataxia, retinal degeneration, muscle rigidity, sensorineural deafness, balance deficits, dementia, and a number of other neurologic features also might be evident. The presence of these symptoms can vary significantly among individuals with this disease, even among affected members of the same family. It is a terminal disease, with death usually occurring within several years of the first appearance of symptoms.

Idiopathic sporadic late-onset cerebellar ataxia is similar to autosomal dominant cerebellar ataxia of late onset, except that it usually does not include as many neurologic symptoms. It often results only in progressive cerebellar ataxia, ataxic dysarthria, and balance deficits. This disorder also tends to begin in middle age, but its survival rate is about 20 years from onset. As its name suggests ("idiopathic" means spontaneous occurrence of a pathologic condition with an unknown or obscure origin), the cause of idiopathic sporadic late-onset cerebellar ataxia is unclear, but it might be the combined result of unrecognized genetic and environmental factors (Lieto et al., 2019).

Friedreich's ataxia is a progressive hereditary disease that can affect the spinal cord as well as the cerebellum and is accordingly classed as a spinocerebellar disease. Although often described as a common cause of cerebellar ataxia, it is actually a rare disorder with a prevalence of only 2 per 100,000 population. The symptoms of Friedreich's ataxia, which usually become evident when individuals are 10 to 15 years of age, include cerebellar ataxia affecting gait and manual dexterity, dysarthria, and visual disorders (Tai et al., 2018). The less common symptoms include dementia and sensorineural deafness. Few people with this disorder survive past their 40s, with death often occurring after coma or heart failure. The dysarthria associated with Friedreich's ataxia is not necessarily purely ataxic in nature because this disorder does not usually affect only the cerebellum and its control circuit. Evidence of lower motor neuron weakness and certain signs of extrapyramidal system involvement might also be present. Because these other areas of the motor system can be affected, the dysarthria associated with Friedreich's ataxia is often of a mixed type, which is examined in Chapter 10.

Olivopontocerebellar degeneration is another progressive cerebellar disorder that tends to run in families. This disorder results in atrophy of the middle cerebellar peduncle, much of the cerebellum, and parts of the pons. One of the primary symptoms of olivopontocerebellar degeneration is cerebellar ataxia. The neuron degeneration associated with this disorder also can involve the basal ganglia and some of the corticospinal tract. Symptoms of a parkinsonian nature, such as muscular rigidity and reduced range of movement, also are often present. As with Friedreich's ataxia, the dysarthria associated with olivopontocerebellar degeneration is usually more mixed in nature rather than a pure ataxic type.

Stroke

As with the other areas of the brain, the cerebellum has a rich arterial blood supply. Several arteries serve the cerebellum, including the superior cerebellar artery and the anterior inferior cerebellar artery. Blockage of blood flow through either of these arteries can cause ataxic dysarthria. Ruptured aneurysms or arteriovenous malformations in these arteries also have been linked to ataxic dysarthria. In fact, about 10% of intracerebral hemorrhages primarily affect the cerebellum or the neurons in the cerebellar control circuits (Heilman et al., 1977). Most cerebellar stokes result in the sudden onset of a number of "cerebellar signs," including limb ataxia, problems with balance, visual deficits, and ataxic dysarthria.

Toxic Conditions

Different toxic and metabolic conditions can affect the functioning of the cerebellum. The toxic conditions that have been associated with cerebellar dysfunction include lead and mercury poisoning, long- and short-term consumption of alcohol, and exposure to chemicals such as acrylamide and cyanide. Most of these conditions are treatable, and any instances of ataxic dysarthria, if present, will usually resolve as the toxic levels of these substances decrease. Toxic levels of phenytoin (Dilantin), an antiseizure drug, also have been associated with ataxic dysarthria. Unlike many of the other toxic conditions, the effects of long-term phenytoin overdosage might be irreversible.

Other conditions that can result in cerebellar dysfunction include prolonged vitamin E or B12 deficiency, severe cases of hypothyroidism, and hereditary disorders such as Wilson's disease. Each of these can cause ataxic dysarthria, although they are not common disorders. Incidentally, Wilson's disease usually results in mixed dysarthria and is discussed in more detail in Chapter 10.

Traumatic Head Injury

Cerebellar tissue can be distorted and stretched by the force of head trauma and can be just as susceptible to the dynamics of an impact as the other parts of the brain. As with most head injuries, traumatic damage to the cerebellum tends to be diffuse. However, the cerebellar peduncles are especially vulnerable to the twisting and rotational forces of such an injury, because the cerebellum is essentially an appendage that is attached to the brainstem. During a rapid, rotational movement of the head, some of the highest amounts of axon stretching could be at these points of attachment. As a result, the axons coursing through the peduncles often are especially susceptible to damage during a head injury.

Tumors

Tumors can affect cerebellar function in several ways. First, a tumor could grow in cerebellar tissue, directly destroying cells and compressing the cerebellum if it grows large enough. Second, a tumor could grow near the cerebellum, for example, on the occipital lobe, which then compresses cerebellar tissue. Third, a brainstem tumor could interfere with the functions of the cerebellar control circuits. The appearance of ataxic dysarthria after the appearance of a cerebellar tumor depends on the location and size of the tumor. Duffy (2013) reported that tumors accounted for about 6% of the cases of ataxic dysarthria at the Mayo Clinic over a 9-year period.

Certain types of tumors tend to appear frequently in the cerebellum. **Metastatic tumors** are among the most common. These tumors are formed when one tumor (the primary tumor) sheds cancerous cells that seed a secondary (metastatic) tumor in another part of the body. Primary metastatic cerebellar tumors are usually located in sites such as the skin (melanomas), lungs, kidneys, or breasts. A slow-growing type of tumor called a **low-grade astrocytoma** can appear frequently in the cerebellum, especially in children. More than 50% of these tumors in children are located in the cerebellum. When it occurs in adults, this type of tumor usually appears between the ages of 30 and 60. **Hemangioblastomas** are benign tumors of proliferated blood vessels found occasionally in the cerebellum. The symptoms of a hemangioblastoma usually appear late in childhood, but sometimes they are not evident until the affected individual is an adult. Progressive cerebellar ataxia and ataxic dysarthria can be among the symptoms of a cerebellar hemangioblastoma.

Other Possible Causes

Although the following are not the most common causes of cerebellar dysfunction, ataxic dysarthria also can result from:

- Viral infections that invade the cerebellum.
- Other infections, such as trichinosis, typhus, and syphilis, that could affect cerebellar functions.
- A bacterial abscess (a localized collection of pus) near the cerebellum that could compress the surrounding brain tissue. Such an abscess will probably present symptoms similar to those of a cerebellar tumor.

Speech Characteristics of Ataxic Dysarthria

In general, individuals with ataxic dysarthria give the impression that the movements of their speech mechanism are poorly coordinated. As in other cerebellar-based movement problems, patients with ataxic dysarthria seem to have problems controlling the timing and force of the many muscular contractions that are needed to produce clearly articulated speech. It is often reported that individuals with ataxic dysarthria have a drunken quality to their speech. Patients frequently report that articulation is slurred and prosody is monotonous. Such symptoms reflect the fact that ataxic dysarthria is primarily a disorder of articulation and prosody (Duffy, 2020). Some medical professionals use the term **scanning speech** when talking about ataxic dysarthria. In that usage, it describes how individuals with this dysarthria often demonstrate a slow, deliberate production of syllables, with each syllable in a word receiving equal stress.

Articulation

Articulation deficits are a significant problem in ataxic dysarthria. Darley et al. (1969a, 1969b) found that imprecise consonant production was the most prevalent speech error in this type of dysarthria (Table 7–1). Another common characteristic is distorted vowels. It is the imperfect articulation of phonemes that gives ataxic dysarthria its characteristic slurred quality. These distortions are caused by cerebellar damage that disrupts the timing, force, range, and direction of movements needed to maintain normal articulation. Such deficits in the performance of complex movements requiring more than one body part are sometimes called **decomposition of movement**.

The articulation errors in ataxic dysarthria, however, might not always be consistent. Some individuals with ataxic dysarthria also might demonstrate **irregular articulatory breakdowns**, meaning that their imprecise consonant and vowel productions can vary from utterance to utterance. These intermittent breakdowns will usually occur most frequently in sentences that contain several multisyllabic words, but the errors might not appear on every production of such a sentence. The breakdowns often give the appearance that the syllables are being compressed during the production of a word. Incidentally, hyperkinetic dysarthria (Chapter 9) is the only

TABLE 7–1 The Most Common Speech Production Errors in 30 Individuals With Ataxic Dysarthria

Rank	Speech Production Errors
1	Imprecise consonants
2	Excess and equal stress
3	Irregular articulatory breakdown
4	Distorted vowels
5	Harsh voice quality
6	Prolonged phonemes
7	Prolonged intervals
8	Monopitch
9	Monoloudness
10	Slow rate

Source: From "Clusters of Diagnostic Patterns of Dysarthria," by F. L. Darley, A. E. Aronson, and J. R. Brown, 1969, *Journal of Speech and Hearing Research, 12,* p. 256. Copyright 1969 by American Speech-Language-Hearing Association. Reprinted with permission.

other dysarthria in which irregular articulatory breakdowns could be present, although Duffy and Folger (1986) did find it in a few of their subjects with unilateral upper motor neuron dysarthria. In general, the articulation errors in most of the other dysarthrias tend to be quite consistent during speech (Darley et al., 1975). Watch the PluralPlus Ataxia Dysarthria Case 1 and 2 videos for examples of the articulation and prosody difficulties in this disorder.

Prosody

Prosodic errors also are prominent in ataxic dysarthria. At least six prosodic deficits can be present in the speech of individuals with this type of dysarthria:

- Equal and excess stress
- Prolonged phonemes
- Prolonged intervals between phonemes
- Monopitch
- Monoloudness
- Slow rate

Darley et al. (1969a, 1969b) ranked each of these within the top 10 most deviant speech characteristics of their subjects with cerebellar lesions.

Equal and excess stress is the tendency of many speakers with ataxic dysarthria to put equal stress on syllables or words that would normally have varied stress patterns. Some speakers with ataxic dysarthria tend to put excessive stress on syllables or words that are not normally stressed to that degree. This stress pattern can be a distinguishing characteristic of ataxic dysarthria. When listening to an individual speaking in this manner, the syllable stress on such words as record (the noun) and record (the verb) might appear to be quite similar, with the listener needing to infer the correct word from the context. This stress pattern gives the impression that each syllable or word is produced separately, without one part of a word or sentence being influenced by the others.

The next two prosodic errors, prolonged phonemes and prolonged intervals between phonemes, are related. One of the hallmarks of cerebellar damage is slow movement on both single and repetitive motion tasks. This slowness includes the movements of the speech musculature, resulting in a slowed production of phonemes and a lengthening of the intervals between phonemes. Netsell and Kent (1976) indicated that these prolongations are probably caused by decreased muscle tone (hypotonia). They suggested that this hypotonia results in a general slowness in the contractions of the speech muscles, resulting in an overall prolongation of speech production. These prolongations of phonemes and intervals contribute to a slow rate of speech, which is another prosodic defect that is very common in ataxic dysarthria.

Darley et al. (1969a, 1969b) noted monopitch in 20 and monoloudness in 18 of their 30 subjects with cerebellar damage. They suggested that these two prosodic errors also are caused by hypotonia of the speech muscles. It is logical to assume that the equalizing of stress also contributes to the perception of these two characteristics in individuals with ataxic dysarthria.

Phonation

Few phonatory deficits are usually noted in ataxia dysarthria. Darley et al. (1969a, 1969b) found that harsh vocal quality is certainly the most prominent phonatory deficit that could be evident in this dysarthria. They identified this phonatory problem in 21 of their 30 subjects. These researchers suggested that this condition is caused by decreased muscle tone in the laryngeal and respiratory structures, which prevents the full contraction of these muscle groups.

Another possible phonatory problem in ataxic dysarthria is voice tremor. Cerebellar damage might cause tremors that affect various body parts, and when the laryngeal or respiratory muscles are involved, the result can be a distinguishable voice tremor. Although not common, it has been observed in some individuals with this dysarthria (Ackermann & Ziegler, 1991; Darley et al., 1969a, 1969b).

Resonance

Hypernasality is seldom a serious problem in ataxic dysarthria. Darley et al. (1969a, 1969b) did not rank it as one of the significant speech errors in their study of subjects with cerebellar lesions, although 10 of their 30 subjects demonstrated some instances of it. These researchers, nevertheless, concluded that it is not a prominent characteristic of this dysarthria. Duffy (2020) also reported that abnormal resonance is infrequent, but he noted that intermittent hyponasality could be evident in some individuals, probably because of timing errors between the muscles of the velum and the other muscles of articulation.

Respiration

Cerebellar damage can cause uncoordinated movements in the respiratory muscles, which can contribute to the speech deficits heard in ataxic dysarthria. Although few studies have examined the respiration of individuals with ataxic dysarthria, several have shown that respiration during speech can contain exaggerated or paradoxical movements (Luchsinger & Arnold, 1965; Murdoch et al., 1991). Paradoxical movements occur when different muscle groups work against each other rather than in coordination. Such abnormal respiratory movements can affect speech production. Exaggerated movements of the respiratory muscles can lead to excessive loudness variations during many speech tasks, including conversation.

Paradoxical movements of the intercostal muscles and the diaphragm can reduce the vital capacity of the lungs and thereby limit the amount of subglottic air available for speech. Insufficient subglottic air pressure during conversational speech often leads the affected individual to speak on residual air. This, in turn, can lead to an increased rate of speech, decreased loudness, and a harsh vocal quality. Ultimately, these abnormal respiratory movements can affect the prosody of individuals with ataxic dysarthria. Incidentally, Darley et al. (1969a, 1969b) did not notice any rapid involuntary inhalations or exhalations of air in their subjects with ataxic dysarthria. Such involuntary respiratory movements are observed much more frequently in cases of hyperkinetic dysarthria (Chapter 9).

Key Evaluation Tasks for Ataxic Dysarthria

1. Speech alternate motion rates can be one of the most valuable evaluation tasks when ataxic dysarthria is suspected. The overall rate will probably be slower than normal. In addition, many individuals with this dysarthria will be unable to maintain a steady rhythm as they repeat the target sounds. In the most severe cases, they might speed up abruptly and then, just as unexpectedly, slow down during this speech production task. Their difficulty in maintaining a regular rhythm highlights how cerebellar damage can affect the timing of movements by different muscle groups.
2. Reading, conversational speech, and repeating sentences containing numerous multisyllabic words also are important evaluation tasks (Duffy, 2020). The complexity of these longer speech activities will reveal any inaccurate speech

movements. As such, they can be especially effective at evoking the irregular articulatory breakdowns that often appear in ataxic dysarthria. Remember that these breakdowns tend to occur more frequently on multisyllabic words than on words of shorter length. Furthermore, these three tasks should reveal any prosodic errors that might be present in connected speech.

Treatment of Ataxic Dysarthria

As stated previously, ataxic dysarthria is the result of damage to the cerebellum or the cerebellar control circuit. This damage often affects the speed, force, and timing of movements by the articulators, which results in movements that are typically described as "uncoordinated." In a majority of instances, the most evident speech errors in this dysarthria are those related to articulation and prosody.

Respiration

Most patients with ataxic dysarthria do not need to work on strengthening their respiration abilities. Rather, they usually should concentrate on controlling their airflow more accurately during speech. The uncoordinated movements of their respiratory muscles can leave them speaking on residual air, which affects prosody and phonation. There are numerous tasks that could be useful in helping these patients gain better breath control during speech.

- Slow and controlled exhalation—In this simple task, the patient is asked to inhale fully and then exhale in a slow, steady stream. Using a stopwatch, the clinician times the length of the exhalation. The goal is to increase the length and steadiness of the airflow over several sessions. Dworkin (1991) described an advanced variation on this task in which the patient is asked to inhale fully, begin a slow exhalation for 3 s, stop the exhalation by holding the breath for about 1 s, then continue with the exhalation. The difficulty of this task can be increased until the patient is holding and releasing the air three times on a single breath.

- Speak immediately on exhalation—Because of poor coordination of the respiratory and laryngeal muscles, many patients with ataxic dysarthria waste a significant amount of their subglottic air by beginning their phonations a second or two after they have started to exhale. The task of speaking immediately on exhalation concentrates on making sure patients initiate phonation the moment they begin an exhalation. Swigert (2010) suggested that the patient place a hand on the abdomen and begin a simple /m/ phonation the moment the hand starts to move inward on the exhalation. The clinician can place his or her hand on the patient's hand to know when to cue the patient to begin the phonation, if necessary.

- Stop phonation early—Because individuals with ataxic dysarthria often have shallow respiration, they might try to speak for a longer period than their limited subglottic air supply allows. This results in speaking on residual air and frequently leads to harsh vocal quality, decreased loudness, and increased rate of speech. Consequently, it is often necessary for the patient to learn to end an utterance before running low on air. This can often be initially accomplished by having the clinician provide verbal and visual cues that tell the patient when to stop phonating and take another breath. Over time, as the patient becomes more independent at stopping phonation before speaking on residual air, the clinician's cues can be withdrawn.

- Optimal breath group—This task is somewhat similar to the stopping phonation early procedure. The optimal breath group task teaches the patient how many syllables or words can be said clearly on one full inhalation (Linebaugh, 1983). Once a baseline has been established, the patient can work on increasing the length of the breath group, perhaps through deeper inhalations, more controlled exhalations, or beginning phonations immediately on exhalation. The optimal breath group task is similar to cued reading materials and chunking utterances into syntactic units activities, which are described later.

Prosody

The prosodic problems experienced by individuals with ataxic dysarthria usually involve rate, stress, and intonation. By slowing their rate, these individuals often can improve their intelligibility. By incorporating more typical stress and intonation into their utterances, their speech could exhibit a more natural quality.

Rate Control

Although a slow or irregular rate of speech is characteristic of ataxic dysarthria, many individuals with this disorder still attempt to speak at a rate that is too rapid for their speech production capabilities. By speaking too rapidly, they do not give their articulators sufficient time to reach target positions, nor do they give a listener enough time to assimilate the spoken message. The amount of slowing needed to improve intelligibility does not always have to be significant. Often minimal decreases in rate can result in noticeably more understandable speech. The following rate control tasks are some of the procedures that might successfully slow the speaking rate of individuals with ataxic dysarthria. These tasks are highly structured and are probably most appropriate for the initial treatment steps in which increasing a patient's awareness of a slower, more intelligible rate is the primary goal.

- Reciting syllables to a metronome—Dworkin (1991) suggested using a metronome to set the pace of syllable production. In this task, the metronome is set to the appropriate rate, and the patient is asked to recite or read familiar passages such as the Pledge of Allegiance, a well-known poem, or something similar. The patient should produce one syllable for every beat of the metronome. Although the resulting speech will sound automated, this is acceptable because the goal in this task is to build the patient's awareness of a more appropriate speech rate. With enough practice, the slower pace set by the metronome could become habituated into the patient's conversational speech.
- Finger or hand tapping—Finger or hand tapping can be substituted for a metronome to set the pace of appropriate syllable production. Initially, the clinician sets the pace by tapping with a finger or hand, with the patient following the tempo while reading a familiar passage. Once the pace is established, the patient can try to do the tapping. Be aware, however, that the typically uncoordinated movements of such a patient might make it very difficult for him or her to maintain a regular pace when trying to tap independently.
- Cued reading material—Various rate cueing techniques can be used with written sentences or paragraphs. One type of cueing is to have the clinician point to a word or syllable at the desired rate and ask the patient to read the material at that pace. Another type of cueing is to have reading material that

has slash marks or spaces to indicate when pauses are necessary while reading aloud. For example, a prepared sentence from a story might look like this: "With a feeling of deep /// yet most singular affection /// I regarded my friend." At the slash marks, the patient should pause for a brief moment before continuing to read. Such reading materials also can be a useful tool in introducing a patient to the optimal breath group duration tasks that were discussed in the section on respiration deficits. They could also be useful for introducing patients to the task of chunking utterances into syntactic units (discussed later).

Stress and Intonation

Stress and intonation exercises for individuals with ataxic dysarthria should concentrate on developing more natural pitch and loudness variations in connected speech. The following tasks might be appropriate for the initial steps of a treatment plan that addresses the stress and intonation problems of patients with ataxic dysarthria.

- Contrastive stress drills—These tasks are usually designed for the clinician to ask a question, with the patient answering it by adding stress on key words to convey the intended meaning of the answer (McHenry, 1998). For example, the clinician might ask the following question about a picture of a man playing football: "Is the man playing basketball?" The patient will answer, "No. The man is playing football." The clinician's next question might be, "Is the woman playing football?" The patient's answer to this question would be, "No, the man is playing football." The length of the questions and the complexity of the pictures for this task can easily be varied according to the abilities of the patient.
- Pitch range exercises—Exercises of this type can be a useful starting place for work on intonation. Dworkin (1991) recommended that these exercises begin with an assessment of the patient's ability to perceive obvious pitch changes in the clinician's voice. If the patient is unable to make these distinctions, the prognosis is poor for improving the patient's pitch control. However, if the patient can tell the difference between the pitch changes, the exercises might help. First, have the patient prolong an /a/ at the lowest pitch and then at the highest pitch possible. Once the highs and lows are established, the patient is asked to sing up and down this pitch

range by dividing the range into about eight individual notes. In the final exercises, the patient reads printed sentences that have arrows written above and below key words indicating the normal pitch changes for those words. For example, an upward arrow at the end of a question would indicate that the patient should raise the pitch on the final word; a downward arrow at the end of a statement would indicate a decrease in pitch.

- Intonation profiles—This task uses lines to show intonation changes in written sentences. Lines immediately below the sentence indicate a flat intonation. Lines above words indicate a rise in pitch. Lines below words indicate a drop in pitch. These lines can be added easily to any written sentence, no matter whether it is a statement or a question. For most patients, it is usually best to start with short, simple sentences and then progress to longer sentences. The ultimate goal is to have the patient generalize the pitch changes learned in this structured activity to conversational speech.

- Chunking utterances into syntactic units—Duffy (2020) mentioned that some individuals with dysarthria need to learn to divide their utterances according to normal pauses within and between sentences. This is necessary because their dysarthria has limited the number of words they can produce on a single exhalation. To compensate for this limitation, this task teaches the patient to inhale at the points in an utterance at which natural syntactic pauses occur. Examples of these natural pauses include after introductory clauses or phrases ("In the morning, [inhale] I went shopping at the store."), between clauses or phrases ("She went there, [inhale] but I missed her."), and between short sentences ("I saw the movie. [inhale] It was pretty good."). By inserting inhalations at points at which normal pauses occur in an utterance, individuals with ataxic dysarthria are often able to maintain a more natural rhythm in their speech. This rhythm is lost if inhalations are placed haphazardly within an utterance.

Articulation

Although articulation might improve with a slowed rate of speech, individuals with ataxic dysarthria also might need to concentrate directly on improving their productions of phonemes.

- Intelligibility drills—Intelligibility drills (Yorkston et al., 1988) are tasks in which the patient is given a list of words or sentences to read. Then the clinician turns away from the patient so that he or she will only be able to understand the patient's speech if it is articulated clearly. By not looking at the target word list or at the patient's mouth, the clinician will depend entirely on the patient's adequate articulation to understand the target word. If the clinician does not understand the target word, the patient needs to determine why the word was unclear and then try saying it again. If this second attempt fails, then the clinician can look at the target word and give the patient specific feedback on why he or she could not understand the utterance (e.g., "I didn't know it was 'sleep' because I couldn't hear the 'p.' Try it again, and let me really hear the 'p' this time.").

- Phonetic placement—This procedure treats articulation errors by instructing patients on the correct position of the articulators before they attempt to produce a target sound. Phonetic placement can be valuable in that it educates patients on how certain speech sounds are produced. Many individuals with dysarthria realize they are producing speech sounds incorrectly, but they have little understanding of why their productions are in error. For example, phonetic placement can help speakers with ataxic dysarthria understand why their production of a /d/ actually sounds closer to a /z/ or their /p/ sounds closer to a /b/ and so forth.

- Exaggerating consonants—Also known as overarticulation, exaggerating consonants is a treatment procedure that teaches the patient to fully articulate all consonant phonemes. Darley et al. (1975) suggested that most patients need to concentrate especially on medial and final consonants because these are the sounds most likely to be poorly articulated in connected speech. The improvements in intelligibility can be dramatic when individuals with ataxic dysarthria fully articulate the medial and final consonants in words.

    Park et al. (2016) used exaggerating consonants as the basis of an intensive treatment program for dysarthria. Their patients had a variety of different types of dysarthria, caused by either traumatic head injury or stroke. The study used a small group repeated measures design to determine the effects of overarticulation (in combination with slower and slightly louder speech) on dysarthric patients' single-word and sentence intelligibility. There were 16 treatment sessions (1-hr sessions, four times a week, for 4 weeks). The patients were first oriented to the treatment tasks so that they knew what was expected. The treatment sessions started with 10 min of prepractice where patients reviewed a random selection of the tasks that were to be used later in the session. The following 10 min required the patients to repeat 10 functional phrases five times each (e.g., "What are we doing tomorrow?"). The next 10 min had the patients repeating 10 service requests five times each (e.g., "Where is the _____?"). During the final 30 min, the patients read aloud, described pictures, and engaged in conversation. Feedback during most of the sessions consisted of whether the patients' utterances were clear or unclear. Homework also was a part of the treatment procedure. The results showed that naive listeners noted improved conversational intelligibility in all patients compared to pretreatment samples. Many of the other outcome measures also were positive.

- Minimal contrast drills—These tasks have the patient concentrate on producing pairs of words that vary by only one phoneme. The distinction between the words can be in the voicing (park–bark), manner of production (pine–mine), or place of production (sea–she) of consonants. The distinction also can be between vowels (man–men) but working on consonants does more to enhance intelligibility in most patients. These word pairs can be used alone, in phrases, or in sentences, depending on the needs of the specific patient.

Summary of Ataxic Dysarthria

- Ataxic dysarthria can be caused by any process that results in damage to the cerebellum or the cerebellar control circuits. Degenerative disease and stroke are common causes of ataxic dysarthria.
- Usually, articulation and prosody are affected most significantly in cases of ataxic dysarthria.
- The speech characteristics of ataxic dysarthria include imprecise consonant production and irregular articulatory breakdowns.
- Treatment for ataxic dysarthria often concentrates on controlling respiration for speech, increasing articulatory accuracy, and developing optimal rate and intonation in connected speech.

Study Questions

1. Define ataxic dysarthria in your own words.
2. What is the primary function of the cerebellum?
3. Describe the neural pathways leading to and from the cerebellum.
4. What are the two ways that the cerebellum probably influences speech production?
5. What is autosomal dominant cerebellar ataxia of late onset?
6. Describe the three ways in which a tumor can affect cerebellar function.
7. Which two components of speech production are usually affected most in cases of ataxic dysarthria?
8. What is decomposition of movement?
9. Is hypernasality a significant problem in most cases of ataxic dysarthria?
10. Describe an exercise that can help individuals with ataxic dysarthria more accurately control their airflow during speech production.

Chapter 8

Hypokinetic Dysarthria

Definitions of Hypokinetic Dysarthria

Neurologic Basis of Hypokinetic Dysarthria

   Characteristics of Parkinsonism

   Causes of Parkinsonism

Causes of Hypokinetic Dysarthria

   Idiopathic Parkinson's Disease

   Neuroleptic-Induced Parkinsonism

   Postencephalitic Parkinsonism

   Traumatic Head Injury

   Toxic Metal Poisoning

   Stroke

Speech Characteristics of Hypokinetic Dysarthria

   Prosody

   Articulation

   Phonation

   Respiration

   Resonance

Key Evaluation Tasks for Hypokinetic Dysarthria

Treatment of Hypokinetic Dysarthria

   Pharmacologic Treatments for Parkinsonism

   Surgical Treatments for Parkinsonism

   Stem-Cell Implantation

   Behavioral Treatments for Parkinsonism

     Articulation

     Phonation

     Respiration

     Prosody

Summary of Hypokinetic Dysarthria

Study Questions

Definitions of Hypokinetic Dysarthria

Most definitions of hypokinetic dysarthria mention that individuals with this disorder have reduced vocal loudness, a harsh or breathy vocal quality, and abnormal speaking rates. Although these are not all of the characteristics of hypokinetic dysarthria, they are among the most common ones. It is interesting to note that many individuals with this dysarthria have slow speaking rates, but in some there can be an abnormally increased rate of speech. The following two definitions encompass many of the most important aspects of hypokinetic dysarthria.

> [Hypokinetic dysarthria (HD)] is manifested in all dimensions of human speech and voice production, specifically in the areas of articulation, phonation, prosody, speech fluency, and faciokinesis. HD is characterized by rigidity and bradykinesia, together with reduced muscular control of the larynx, articulatory organs, and other physiological support mechanisms of human speech production. Since self-monitoring of speech is abnormal in [Parkinson's disease (PD)], HD has a serious impact on the quality of life of PD patients. (Chen et al., 2020, p. 712)

> [Hypokinetic dysarthria is] a distinctive perceptual motor speech disorder associated with basal ganglia control circuit pathology. . . . This may appear in all of the respiratory, phonatory, resonatory, articulatory and prosody levels of speech, but its characteristics are most evident in voice, articulation and prosody. This specific speech disorder is characterized by reduced loudness, imprecise consonants, vowel centralization, and rate changes accompanied by involuntary facial movements. [Its] deleterious effects on patient's communication and social participation may lead to social isolation, reducing the quality of life. (Muñoz-Vigueras et al., 2021, p. 640)

Neurologic Basis of Hypokinetic Dysarthria

In several ways, hypokinetic dysarthria is unique. It is the only dysarthria in which increased rate of speech can be one of the symptoms. It also is the only dysarthria in which the vast majority of cases share the same causative factor (**parkinsonism**). Because it accounts for so much of the hypokinetic dysarthria seen in clinical caseloads, parkinsonism is considered the de facto cause of this dysarthria throughout most of this chapter. Keep in mind, however, that parkinsonism is not the only cause of hypokinetic dysarthria.

A few other disorders can lead to this dysarthria, and they are discussed in the section on causes in this chapter.

Hypokinetic dysarthria occurs when the symptoms of parkinsonism affect the muscles of speech production. The parkinsonian symptoms that have the greatest effect on speech are muscle rigidity, reduced range of motion, and slowed movement. In nearly every instance, these symptoms are caused by dysfunction in the basal ganglia or by damage to the basal ganglia's neural connections to other parts of the CNS. The term **hypokinetic** might be misleading to readers encountering it for the first time. Initially, it might be confused with hypotonia, which is decreased muscle tone. A beginning clinician might consequently assume that an individual with parkinsonism will have weak and floppy muscles. This assumption would be quite wrong, however. Literally, hypokinetic means "less motion," not decreased muscle tone. In fact, individuals with parkinsonism usually demonstrate increased muscle tone. When applied to individuals with parkinsonism, "hypokinetic" describes their decreased range and frequency of movement. For example, individuals with parkinsonism usually demonstrate a shuffling, "baby step" type of walking known as festinating gait, and their ability to express emotion through their facial expressions will be greatly diminished, a phenomenon known as *masked facies*. In addition, they might blink their eyes infrequently and have difficulty starting or stopping movements. The reasons for these behaviors are discussed in the following sections.

Characteristics of Parkinsonism

Parkinsonism has a distinctive collection of symptoms. One of the most prevalent symptoms is **resting tremor**, present in about 80% of patients. Parkinsonian tremors are seen most commonly in the fingers and hands, but they also can involve the limbs and face. These tremors have a frequency of about four to six oscillations per second. They are called resting tremors because they are most noticeable while the body is not moving. Interestingly, the tremors might become less pronounced or disappear completely when the body is completely relaxed or when an affected body part is being moved voluntarily. During moments of agitation or nervousness, however, the tremors tend to become significantly worse.

A very common symptom of parkinsonism is **bradykinesia**, which causes slow and reduced range of movement. The shuffling walk and the lack of facial expression mentioned previously are good examples of bradykinesia. Limb, trunk, and neck movements also are frequently affected by bradykinesia. Typically, the movements of affected body parts are slow, labored, and very limited in their range. In addition to the difficulties of walking and facial expression, bradykinesia also can affect speech, finger movements, writing, and many other voluntary movements. It is important to note, however, that the slowness and reduced range of movement of bradykinesia is not the result of muscle weakness. Individuals with parkinsonism usually demonstrate nearly normal muscle strength. As with all the symptoms of parkinsonism, bradykinesia is caused by dysfunction in the basal ganglia.

Muscular rigidity is the result of increased muscle tone. The muscles of individuals with this condition are always in a greater than normal state of contraction, both at rest and during movement. Rigidity most typically affects the neck, trunk, and limbs. The effects of rigidity can usually be observed easily. For instance, constant resistance is present when an affected body part is pulled to an extended position. This is sometimes described as "lead pipe resistance," because it feels to the person who is doing the pulling that a piece of soft metal is being bent. In some joints, however, there might be a subtle, rhythmic alteration in the rigidity as a body part is being moved. This intermittent change in rigidity is described as "cogwheel resistance" because of its step-by-step, ratchet-like motion. Although rigidity and bradykinesia are separate symptoms of parkinsonism, rigidity can exacerbate the slowed and restricted movements of bradykinesia.

It should be noted that there are differences between rigidity and spasticity, although they are both the result of increased muscle tone. One of the clearest distinctions between them is how they react to passive movement. In spasticity, increasing resistance to the passive movement is followed by an abrupt relaxation of the muscle being tested. The increase in resistance is especially evident when the passive movement is rapid. In contrast, rigidity demonstrates a more or less constant resistance to the passive movement, no matter how quickly the examiner moves the affected body part (Wiederholt, 2000).

Akinesia is a delay in the initiation of movements and is yet another common characteristic of parkinsonism. Examples of akinesia can be seen in many of the movements of individuals with parkinsonism. For instance, when an individual with parkinsonism is asked to verbally answer a question, there might be a noticeable pause before any words are spoken. This delayed initiation of speech could last only a few seconds, but sometimes it is much longer. Although it is rare, someone with severe akinesia might become stuck in a certain posture and be completely unable to move. Strangely, when an individual is stuck in one of these frozen positions, a brief touch from another person is sometimes all that is needed to initiate or continue a movement. In addition to this difficulty in initiating movements, many individuals with parkinsonism can have trouble stopping a movement once it is started. For instance, while reaching for a glass of water, they might knock it over because they were unable to stop reaching once the movement was initiated. Not surprisingly, it is often reported that individuals with akinesia are reluctant to actively move about their home or other surroundings because they are afraid of being injured when they do so.

Disturbances of **postural reflexes** also are seen in individuals with parkinsonism. Such disturbances are especially evident when these individuals are doing relatively automatic tasks. For example, they might have difficulty maintaining their balance while walking. In addition, the normal walking arm swing will be absent; their arms will hang stiffly at their sides. If pushed lightly while standing, they are likely to fall because they cannot quickly shift their center of balance. They might be unable to rise from a chair because they do not naturally shift their trunk forward as they attempt to stand. Normally, the basal ganglia help regulate these postural reflexes through neural connections with the extrapyramidal system. However, when the basal ganglia are not functioning properly, these postural problems of balance and movement can become obvious. These impaired reflexes contribute greatly to the 62% to 68% of people with Parkinson's disease who have falls and related injuries.

Although tremor, bradykinesia, rigidity, akinesia, and disturbed postural reflexes are the primary symptoms of parkinsonism, there are numerous other symptoms that could appear in individuals with this disorder, including depression, swallowing difficulties, dementia, and hypokinetic dysarthria. These additional symptoms do not appear in all individuals with parkinsonism; nevertheless, they can be common features of this disorder.

Causes of Parkinsonism

As already mentioned, parkinsonism is caused by dysfunction in the basal ganglia, which are a collection of subcortical, gray matter structures that play an important role in controlling movement (Figure 8–1). The individual members of the basal ganglia are the caudate nucleus, the globus pallidus, and the putamen (Andreatta, 2023; Seikel et al., 2020). Because the caudate nucleus and the putamen are made of many of the same type of neurons and are functionally related, they are known together as the striatum. The basal ganglia are located deep in the brain and are quite complex in their interconnections with each other and with other parts of the CNS. One of the most important neural pathways of the basal ganglia is the looped control circuit that connects it to the cerebral cortex (Figure 8–2). The first part of this control circuit is composed

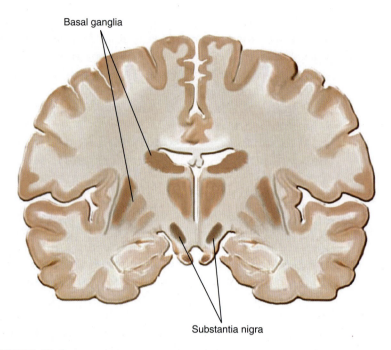

FIGURE 8–1. The substantia nigra produces dopamine for the basal ganglia. In cases of Parkinson's disease, neurons in the substantia nigra gradually die, causing a progressive reduction of dopamine to the basal ganglia.

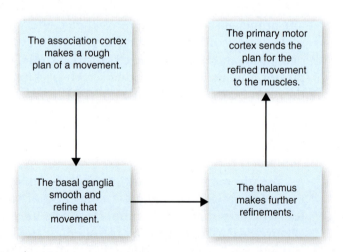

FIGURE 8–2. A schematic diagram of the basal ganglia control circuit.

of neural fibers that descend from the cortex. Through these fibers, the cortex transmits information about planned upcoming movements to the basal ganglia. The basal ganglia, in turn, smooth and refine these planned movements, especially movements that are going to be slow and continuous. Once this refinement is completed, the basal ganglia send the refined neural impulses for the planned movements up to the motor cortex, where they are then transmitted through the pyramidal system to the lower motor neurons and out to the muscles.

To function properly, the basal ganglia depend on the balanced interaction of several neurotransmitters. Two of the most important are dopamine and acetylcholine. Dopamine is largely an inhibitory neurotransmitter and tends to slow neural activity within the striatum. The dopamine used by the striatum is produced by special neurons in the substantia nigra—a collection of gray matter cells located near the basal ganglia. Acetylcholine also affects the function of the basal ganglia, but unlike dopamine, it has an excitatory effect on these areas of the brain. It tends to facilitate neural firing.

In general, parkinsonism is caused by a reduction of dopamine in the striatum. The loss of dopamine has a profound effect on the workings of the striatum because it is placed in a state of neurochemical imbalance. When this imbalance occurs, there is too much excitatory neurotransmitter (acetylcholine) acting on the neurons of the striatum as compared with the amount of inhibitory neurotransmitter (dopamine) available. The higher levels of this excitatory neurotransmitter in the striatum are thereby thought to be the primary cause of the rigidity, bradykinesia, and other symptoms of parkinsonism.

The causes of reduced dopamine in the striatum are varied. In most cases, such as **idiopathic** Parkinson's disease, the cause is not well understood. In this disease, the dopamine-producing neurons in the substantia nigra slowly begin to degenerate for unclear reasons. As these neurons degenerate, they produce less and less dopamine for use in the striatum, which then is unable to function properly. These dopamine-producing neurons can be damaged in numerous other ways, including by the effects of drugs and toxic poisoning, damage from infections, tumors, head injury, cerebral anoxia, and cerebrovascular disease.

Causes of Hypokinetic Dysarthria

Parkinsonism is a collective term for a group of different disorders that share many of the same symptoms. It is sometimes used interchangeably with the term *Parkinson's syndrome.* In general, the shared symptoms of parkinsonism are those discussed previously: tremor, bradykinesia, muscle rigidity, akinesia, and disturbed postural reflexes. In this section, the major causes of hypokinetic dysarthria are examined, starting with three disorders that are classed as parkinsonism.

Idiopathic Parkinson's Disease

Idiopathic Parkinson's disease is the most common form of parkinsonism and is the single most frequent cause of hypokinetic dysarthria. This disease is the result of the progressive degeneration of dopamine-producing neurons in the substantia nigra. As mentioned previously, the reason why these neurons degenerate is unknown, hence the label "idiopathic." (Note: Some professionals have stopped using "idiopathic" in reference to this disease because of the recent significant progress in understanding its cause. For example, Bloem et al. (2021) reported that genetic predisposition, exposure to certain pesticides, and repeated head injuries are definite risk factors for developing this disorder.) Parkinson's disease affects about 20 individuals per 100,000 population each year, with men and women being affected equally. It usually occurs between the ages of 40 and 70 years and typically follows a slowly progressive course that lasts for years. The first signs of Parkinson's disease often include restlessness, rapid fatigue, and sensory signs such as coldness, numbness, or tingling. Duffy (2020) noted that hypokinetic dysarthria also can be one of the first symptoms of this disease. As the disease progresses, these early signs are joined by the major symptoms of tremor, rigidity, and so forth. In about 50% to 75% of cases, **L-dopa** treatments are successful in treating most of the major symptoms. These treatments can reduce the severity of the symptoms, but they do not stop the progression of the disease.

Additional symptoms of this disorder include dementia, which is present in 8% to 30% of cases. It usually is difficult to determine whether this dementia is caused by Parkinson's disease or if is an accompanying occurrence of Alzheimer's disease. Significant depression also has been reported in as many as 50% of patients. Warlow (1991) reported that most individuals with Parkinson's disease are ultimately confined to bed and die of pneumonia, urinary tract infections, or septicemia (the persistent presence of toxic microorganisms in the blood, commonly called blood poisoning).

Neuroleptic-Induced Parkinsonism

Neuroleptic-induced parkinsonism, a negative side effect of using antipsychotic (**neuroleptic**) drugs, is the second most common form of parkinsonism. These neuroleptic drugs can be very successful in treating the confusion and agitation in psychotic patients, but their long-term use can result in this form of parkinsonism. The neuroleptic drugs that have this side effect include chlorpromazine, trifluoperazine, and prochlorperazine. The appearance of parkinsonian symptoms depends on the drug and the dosage levels. For example, about 90% of patients taking trifluoperazine could show subtle, variable signs of tremor, rigidity, and, in particular, bradykinesia. It usually takes about 2 to 4 weeks of taking the drug before these parkinsonian symptoms appear. It is not clearly understood how neuroleptic drugs cause the symptoms of parkinsonism, but it is known that some of these drugs increase the amount of acetylcholine in the basal ganglia. Consequently, it is supposed that this increase in acetylcholine results in relatively lower levels of dopamine in the basal ganglia and thereby causes the parkinsonian symptoms.

The signs of neuroleptic-induced parkinsonism usually disappear within weeks of discontinuing use of the drugs. However, stopping the drug treatment is often not an option for many of these individuals because their psychosis will return. In these cases, the individual will continue to take the neuroleptic medication, but they also will take additional medications to treat their parkinsonian symptoms. Interestingly, L-dopa cannot be used to treat the hypokinetic movement disorders in these individuals because it tends to increase their psychotic symptoms.

Postencephalitic Parkinsonism

Postencephalitic parkinsonism is caused by viral encephalitis. It is a relatively uncommon disorder, and, unlike idiopathic Parkinson's disease, it can affect children. In postencephalitic parkinsonism, the effects of the infection are concentrated in the substantia nigra; this results in decreased amounts of dopamine in the basal ganglia. The parkinsonian symptoms appear several weeks or months after the acute stage of the infection. In the majority of cases, these symptoms are identical to those in idiopathic Parkinson's disease. In some instances, the initial symptoms of the infection are so mild that they are unrecognized. Nevertheless, the basal ganglia are not receiving enough dopamine, and the result can be parkinsonism. Certain cognitive deficits are associated with children in whom postencephalitic parkinsonism develops, including increased distractibility and impaired abstract reasoning. Pharmacologic treatment of this disorder is the same as for idiopathic Parkinson's disease, usually L-dopa therapy.

Traumatic Head Injury

Head trauma can selectively damage the substantia nigra or basal ganglia. The trauma can be either a single event or repeated injuries over time. Duffy (2020) noted that the cumulative effects of repeated blows to the head, such as what occurs in boxing, can damage the substantia nigra and might result in **punch drunk encephalopathy**, a disorder characterized by memory deficits, slowed movements, and dysarthria.

Cerebral anoxia also has been known to selectively affect the basal ganglia to a greater degree than other areas of the brain, although the exact reason for this is unknown. In such cases, bradykinesia and rigidity could appear days or weeks after the patient returns to consciousness. Co-occurring cognitive and pyramidal system deficits probably will be present as well.

Toxic Metal Poisoning

An often-cited cause of parkinsonian symptoms is long-term exposure to manganese, a metal used in the manufacturing of iron, aluminum, and copper alloys. The early signs of manganese poisoning, which occurs most often in miners, include irritability, insomnia, and emotional outbursts. Dementia usually co-occurs with the parkinsonian signs in the later stages of long-term exposure to this metal.

Stroke

Although references are sometimes made to "arteriosclerotic parkinsonism" or "vascular parkinsonism," Wiederholt (2000) stated that there is no credible evidence for such a diagnostic classification. Nevertheless, it has been documented that a single stroke can affect the basal ganglia and cause the sudden onset of parkinsonian symptoms, although it certainly is rare. Warlow (1991) indicated that such a stroke results in parkinsonian symptoms on the side of the body opposite to the lesion, with a majority of cases showing spontaneous improvement over time. Compared to a single stroke resulting in parkinsonism, it is more likely that parkinsonian symptoms will appear in an individual who has suffered multiple strokes. In such instances, numerous associated disorders probably exist, including other motor system deficits, visuospatial impairments, and speech and language problems.

Speech Characteristics of Hypokinetic Dysarthria

The speech of individuals with hypokinetic dysarthria is usually quite distinctive, with errors of prosody and articulation being the most noticeable speech characteristics. Overall, individuals with hypokinetic dysarthria give the impression that the sequencing and placement of their articulatory movements are fairly accurate, but the range of these movements is greatly restricted. It is as if their speech movements are compressed and abbreviated. As is discussed in the following sections, most of the speech characteristics of hypokinetic dysarthria are a result of bradykinesia (reduced range and speed of movement), akinesia (delays in the initiation of movement), and muscle rigidity. In the most severe cases, the tremors so commonly associated with parkinsonism also can affect the speech musculature, resulting in tremulous phonations.

Prosody

Darley et al. (1969a, 1969b) found that monopitch, reduced stress, and monoloudness were the three most prominent speech characteristics of hypokinetic dysarthria (Table 8–1). They attributed these prosodic errors to a limited range of motion in the laryngeal musculature and to a lack of "vigor" in the contractions of these muscles. These prosodic errors are most evident in verbal tasks that normally include variations in pitch and loudness, such as conversational speech, reading sentences or paragraphs, and trying to verbally convey emotions.

Darley et al. also noted inappropriate silences in the speech of their subjects. These silent pauses are probably the result of

TABLE 8–1 The Most Common Speech Production Errors in 32 Individuals With Hypokinetic Dysarthria

Rank	Speech Production Errors
1	Monopitch
2	Reduced stress
3	Monoloudness
4	Imprecise consonants
5	Inappropriate silences
6	Short rushes
7	Harsh voice quality
8	Breathy voice (continuous)
9	Pitch level
10	Variable rate

Source: From "Clusters of Diagnostic Patterns of Dysarthria," by F. L. Darley, A. E. Aronson, and J. R. Brown, 1969, *Journal of Speech and Hearing Research, 12*, p. 258. Copyright 1969 by American Speech-Language-Hearing Association. Reprinted with permission.

the akinesia, which makes it difficult for affected individuals to initiate a motor response. Clinical observations suggest that these moments of silence appear most frequently at the beginning of a spoken sentence or between sentences. They often last for only 2 or 3 s, but longer lapses can occur. When combined with the condition's typical expressionless facial movements, these silent moments sometimes mislead beginning clinicians into assuming the patient did not hear a question or perhaps has lost his or her train of thought.

Several speech-rate abnormalities also can be present in hypokinetic dysarthria. An overall increased rate of speech is the most notable of these. Although most individuals with hypokinetic dysarthria do not have a consistently increased speech rate, it has been seen in some cases. It has been suggested that increased speech rate is related to the difficulties some individuals with parkinsonism have in stopping a voluntary movement once it is started (Hirose, 1986). If severe enough, this increased rate of speech can result in the blurred articulation of phonemes. This can contribute to the imprecise production of consonants, which is discussed later. Short rushes of speech are probably more common in hypokinetic dysarthria than a constant increase in speech rate. When these short rushes occur, they might have a stop-and-go quality, with a brief pause being followed by the quick production of several words. Darley et al. (1969a, 1969b) found these short rushes of speech to be the sixth most common characteristic of hypokinetic dysarthria, appearing in 19 of their 32 subjects. Finally, it must be noted that some studies have found cases of decreased rate of speech in individuals with this dysarthria (Ludlow et al., 1987). It would appear, therefore, that there can be significant individual differences in speech rate abnormalities in cases of hypokinetic dysarthria, ranging from slow to fast. Watch the PluralPlus Hypokinetic Dysarthria Case 1 video for an example of this disorder.

Articulation

There can be numerous types of articulation errors in hypokinetic dysarthria. According to Darley et al. (1969a, 1969b), one of the most common is imprecise consonants. In many cases, the imprecise production of consonants is caused by reduced range of movement by the articulators, which consequently results in distorted and incorrect productions of phonemes. For instance, stop consonants can sound very much like fricatives because the articulators are unable to completely block the airflow. Fricative consonants can have a distorted "mushy" quality because the point of airflow constriction is slightly larger than what is needed for normal articulation. Affricate consonants can reflect a combination of these errors because they contain both a stop phase and a fricative-like release phase. These types of errors in the production of consonants are sometimes described as "articulatory undershoot" (Duffy, 2020).

Two unusual dysfluencies also have been noted in the speech of individuals with hypokinetic dysarthria. The first of these is repeated phonemes. Duffy (2020) indicated that these repetitions usually take place at the beginning of an utterance or after a pause. They are often very quick and can be produced with very limited movement of the articulators. In fact, they can sound like a prolonged vowel because of how rapidly they are produced. The other type of dysfluency is **palilalia**, the compulsive, increasingly rapid repetition of a word or phrase. Although it was not noted in any of the subjects studied by Darley et al. (1969a, 1969b), palilalia could be present in some individuals with parkinsonism. This phenomenon might be most clearly evident to a listener when the affected individual makes a single-word utterance, perhaps in answer to a yes-or-no question. The response, for example, will be the repetition of "yes, yes, yes, yes, yes, yes" with a quickly increasing rate of speech until the utterance fades into a soft, blurred mumble. Both of these dysfluencies could be neurologically related to the festinating gait of individuals with parkinsonism, in which they sometimes cannot stop themselves from walking past their destination. In a very similar manner, some hypokinetic speakers might not be able to stop saying a syllable or word once they have started an utterance. Watch the PluralPlus Hypokinetic Dysarthria Case 2 video for an example of palilalia in a patient with Parkinson's disease.

Phonation

A harsh or breathy voice quality is common in most individuals with hypokinetic dysarthria, although these might not be the most noticeable speech errors in this disorder. Logemann et al. (1978) found that 89% of their 200 subjects with Parkinson's disease had vocal qualities that were breathy, hoarse, rough, or tremulous. This finding indicates how widespread these errors of phonation can be in this dysarthria. Darley et al. (1969a, 1969b) also noted phonatory deficits in their subjects but ranked them in the bottom half of the most prominent speech errors in hypokinetic dysarthria. They described these errors as either a harsh or breathy voice quality and ranked them, respectively, as the seventh and eighth most prominent speech characteristics of their 32 subjects with parkinsonism.

Several studies provide evidence that the harsh or breathy vocal quality of hypokinetic dysarthria is caused by incomplete vocal-fold closure during phonation (Garratt et al., 1987; Uziel et al., 1975). When the vocal folds fail to completely close during phonation, air leaks through the partly open glottis and causes an audibly turbulent noise. In more severe cases, vocal quality could become so breathy as to be more of a whisper. When combined with decreased loudness (discussed later), this whispering vocal quality often makes the individual's speech unintelligible. Duffy (2020) stated that it can be the most obvious and troublesome aspect of hypokinetic speech. In addition to this whispered dysphonia, moments of **aphonia** (complete loss of phonation) also can occur in connected speech, even in patients with moderate severity.

Low pitch can be another phonatory characteristic of hypokinetic dysarthria. Darley et al. (1969a, 1969b) rated it as the ninth most prominent speech error in their subjects with hypokinetic dysarthria. However, other studies have found increased pitch in hypokinetic speakers (Canter, 1963; Ludlow & Bassich, 1984). Taken as a whole, these studies suggest that patients with hypokinetic dysarthria can have significant individual-to-individual differences in pitch.

Respiration

Respiratory difficulties have been noted in some individuals with hypokinetic dysarthria. For example, it has been observed that these individuals could have breathing rates that are faster than normal. It also has been noted that these individuals frequently have paradoxical movements of the muscles of exhalation and inhalation, which means that the respiratory muscles of the chest and the diaphragm are not coordinated during breathing. Also, many individuals with hypokinetic dysarthria have reduced range of movement in their respiratory muscles. These respiratory problems result in shallow breath support, poorly controlled exhalations of air for speech, and short breathing cycles. Each of these factors can contribute to many of the speech errors in hypokinetic dysarthria. The rapid, short breathing cycles, for instance, might be a partial cause of the short rushes of speech discussed previously. The shallow breath support could contribute significantly to the breathy, soft phonations of this dysarthria.

Resonance

Although hypernasality can be present in some cases of hypokinetic dysarthria, it is usually mild. Most individuals with this dysarthria do not have significant deficits of resonance. For instance, Logemann et al. (1978) found mild hypernasality in only 10% of their subjects with Parkinson's disease.

Key Evaluation Tasks for Hypokinetic Dysarthria

Duffy (2020) recommended the following four key evaluation tasks to help highlight the speech errors commonly heard in hypokinetic dysarthria.

1. Conversational speech and reading are useful for evoking the many errors of prosody that could be present in this dysarthria. These errors include monopitch, reduced stress, monoloudness, and inappropriate silences. Connected speech samples also can be useful in detecting whether short rushes of speech are present. This is heard when several words of a longer utterance are said hurriedly, with a brief pause before and after it.
2. Speech AMRs can highlight articulation errors, including imprecise consonant productions, variable rates of articulation, and the blurring of syllables.
3. Vowel prolongations can be helpful in assessing vocal quality.
4. Conversational speech, AMRs, and vowel prolongation also can be used to detect other characteristics of hypokinetic dysarthria, such as decreased loudness, low pitch, and repeated phonemes.

Treatment of Hypokinetic Dysarthria

Treatments for hypokinetic dysarthria can be divided into three categories: pharmacologic, surgical, and behavioral. Of these three, pharmacologic intervention is the most widely used, usually in the form of drugs based on L-dopa. Surgical treatments include ablation procedures (purposefully making lesions in parts of the basal ganglia) and deep brain stimulation. The behavioral treatments for hypokinetic dysarthria include many of the same techniques described in prior chapters of this book, but there are several treatment procedures for hypokinetic dysarthria that have not been discussed yet, such as the Lee Silverman Voice Treatment.

Pharmacologic Treatments for Parkinsonism

A number of drug-based treatments are available for hypokinetic movement disorders. One treatment approach is to replace dopamine in the striatum. Direct dosages of dopamine will not work, however, because they cannot pass the blood–brain barrier and, consequently, will not reach the striatum. (The blood–brain barrier is the body's mechanism that controls the flow of matter from the bloodstream to the extracellular fluid in the brain. Part of this barrier's effectiveness is the tight arrangement of the cells in the walls of the cerebral capillaries.) Because of the blood–brain barrier, dopamine replacement treatments use a precursor of dopamine known as L-dopa, a chemical that can reach the striatum and then is converted into dopamine by the brain. Once in the striatum, this drug compensates for the dopamine that is not being produced by the substantia nigra.

Another treatment approach attempts to correct the neurotransmitter imbalance in the basal ganglia by decreasing the amount of acetylcholine activity in the striatum. Anticholinergic drugs act to either deplete acetylcholine in the basal ganglia or to interfere with its effect on these brain structures. In some individuals with parkinsonism, the best treatment results occur when L-dopa is combined with certain anticholinergic drugs.

The effectiveness of these treatments is well established. L-dopa can significantly reduce tremor, bradykinesia, akinesia, and rigidity in many hypokinetic movement disorders. In addition, L-dopa treatment can prolong life if it is started early enough in the course of some disorders. Although L-dopa is effective for many symptoms of hypokinetic disorders, Wiederholt (2000) reported that this drug has the least effect on the speech disturbances associated with these disorders. In addition, the side effects of L-dopa can range from minor to quite serious. The minor problems include gastrointestinal disturbance, poor control of blood pressure, insomnia, and agitation. The more serious side effects usually appear after a prolonged course of treatment and include such significant psychiatric symptoms as hallucinations, severe agitation, decreased social inhibitions, and paranoid delusions. Prolonged treatments with L-dopa also can cause abnormal involuntary movements (choreiform movements) of the limbs, head and neck, and orofacial muscles.

Anticholinergic drugs also can reduce the major symptoms of many hypokinetic movement disorders, but their negative effects can be just as significant as those caused by L-dopa treatment. The minor side effects include dry mouth, dizziness, dilated pupils, and clumsiness. The more serious side effects include inappropriate emotional outbursts, delusions, hallucinations, and confusion.

Unfortunately, the pharmacologic treatments for hypokinetic movement disorders are not cures. They can reduce many of the symptoms and can slow the progression of some degenerative disorders, but they do not stop the disease, and they do not return an affected individual to completely normal motor functions. In fact, these drugs eventually become ineffective in treating progressive hypokinetic disorders.

Surgical Treatments for Parkinsonism

Because they are complicated and invasive procedures, the surgical treatments for parkinsonism are usually performed only when a patient is truly incapacitated and medications have lost their effectiveness. The two general types of surgical treatment for parkinsonism are ablative surgery (thalamotomy and pallidotomy) and deep brain stimulation. In the **ablative procedures**, lesions are purposefully produced in small amounts of brain tissue to reduce neuron activity in a specific area of the brain. In a pallidotomy, a hole is drilled into the skull, and a small electrical probe is inserted into the globus pallidus of the basal ganglia. The tip of the probe then is heated for a short time to destroy nearby neurons. The loss of these neurons reduces brain activity in that part of the basal ganglia, and, consequently, a patient's muscle rigidity, tremor, and bradykinesia can be reduced to some degree. Although they were the surgical treatment of choice years ago, thalamotomies and pallidotomies are rarely performed today, primarily because they cause permanent lesions and their results have not been consistent. Both have been supplanted by the more recently developed procedure known as deep brain stimulation.

Deep brain stimulation is a more effective means of reducing many of the symptoms of parkinsonism, and unlike the ablative procedures, it does not result in permanent lesions. Moreover, it can be reversed if desired. In this treatment, a small electrode is inserted into either the globus pallidus or subthalamic nucleus (a gray-matter structure connected to the globus pallidus, sometimes considered to be part of the basal ganglia). When turned on, the electrode sends a low-level electrical current to the surrounding neurons, which interrupts neural activity in that part of the brain. The electrode is controlled and powered by a small pulse generator that usually is placed under the skin near the collarbone. Exactly how the current interferes with neural activity is not clearly understood, but its effects on the symptoms of parkinsonism can be immediate. In many cases, tremor, bradykinesia, rigidity, muscle tone, and postural reflexes can all be improved. In fact, some patients are able to reduce their medications after the surgery and still have noticeable increases in their physical abilities. Unfortunately, the effects of deep brain stimulation are not permanent. Although improved motor function for 1 to 2 years after implantation is well documented, Limousin and Foltynie (2019) found that long-term data are limited. Current evidence shows positive effects for about 10 years, but this varies significantly patient to patient. Factors affecting long-term effectiveness include where the electrodes are implanted, age of the patient, and the severity of symptoms at the time of surgery.

Stem-Cell Implantation

Stem cells are unique in that they can transform themselves into different types of cells. They are found naturally in embryos and in adult tissues, and they can be grown in the laboratory. Because of stem cells' ability to change into other cells, recent research has concentrated on transplanting them into areas of the nervous system in which lesions have been found in the hope that they can assume the functions of the damaged cells. A significant amount of this research has concentrated on using stem cells to treat parkinsonism. Currently, most of this research has been on mice with laboratory-induced parkinsonism. Although the results are preliminary, they have been encouraging, showing that stem cells implanted into the striata of mice with parkinsonism can eventually produce dopamine. In 2018, human trials were first conducted using (adult) induced pluripotent stem cells, which are uniquely able to give researchers insight into what has gone wrong in diseased neurons, as well as provide potential methods of reestablishing normal function (Kim et al., 2022). These cells are not derived from fetal tissue, and because they are patient specific, the problem of immune rejection is greatly reduced (Stoddard-Bennett & Reijo Pera, 2019). Although this progress in stem-cell therapy is promising, much more research is needed before it can be approved as a treatment for parkinsonism.

Behavioral Treatments for Parkinsonism

Although the medical treatments can have positive effects on the speech deficits in parkinsonism, behavior- and instrumentation-based tasks are still an important part of the clinical treatment plan. There are numerous procedures that speech-language pathologists can use to help these patients communicate more effectively, many of which have research showing that they can be effective (Moya-Galé & Levy, 2019).

Articulation

The most common articulation deficit in hypokinetic dysarthria is imprecise consonant production, which is sometimes described as giving the patient's speech a "mushy" quality. As previously mentioned, this problem is often the result of reduced range of motion in the articulators. This deficit can be compounded by the increased rate of speech that occurs in some patients with parkinsonism. The articulation errors in hypokinetic dysarthria can be treated in several ways. In general, the treatments are divided into rate reduction, stretching, and traditional articulation tasks.

Rate Reduction. In many individuals with hypokinetic dysarthria, slowing the rate of speech can improve articulation because it allows the articulators more time to reach the target positions needed to accurately produce phonemes. The slower rate also gives the listener more time to process what is being spoken. Prosody also might appear more natural when the rate of speech is slowed. A number of different rate control procedures have been used to slow the speech of individuals with hypokinetic dysarthria, as listed here.

- **Pacing boards**—These are devices with finger-width slots along their length (Figure 8–3). Using pacing boards is simple.

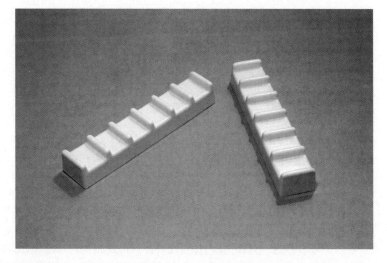

FIGURE 8–3. Inexpensive plastic pacing boards can be useful in slowing the rate of speech in some individuals with hypokinetic dysarthria.

The patient is instructed to place a finger in the first slot and begin reading or repeating a short sentence; each time a word is spoken the patient moves the finger to the next slot. That is, the patient should only say one word every time the finger is moved to the next slot on the board. By slowing their rate of speech, this procedure can produce noticeable improvements in intelligibility in many individuals with hypokinetic dysarthria. One of the drawbacks of a pacing board can be the patient's reluctance to use it in public when speaking to strangers. As a consequence, pacing boards are often used only in the home, although they are very portable and are used successfully in public by some individuals with this dysarthria.

- Hand or finger tapping—In the beginning of this task, the clinician sets the pace for repeating or reading sentences by tapping his or her hand or finger. The patient attempts to speak one syllable for each of the clinician's taps. Once this rate is established, the patient does the tapping to control the rate of speech production. One problem with this procedure is that many individuals with parkinsonism have difficulty maintaining a slow, steady rate as they tap. As a result, their tapping will increase along with their rate of speech. Pacing boards seem to be a good option for patients who have this problem. The requirement of having to move their finger up and over to the next slot tends to keep their rate of speech steadier than only using hand or finger tapping to set the rate.

- Alphabet boards—Another way to slow the rate of someone with this dysarthria is the use of an alphabet board (Figure 8–4). This is simply a piece of paper with all of the letters of the alphabet printed in large, dark print. The numbers 1 to 10 also could be printed on it. The patient is told to use the board by pointing to the first letter of every word as it is being spoken. This procedure can increase intelligibility in two ways. It slows the patient's speech and allows for better articulatory contact. It also gives the listener a visual cue as to what word is being spoken. As with pacing boards, the use of an alphabet board can have an immediate effect on intelligibility. There are drawbacks, however. Many patients will be reluctant to use this procedure in public, which could limit its use to the home. In addition, individuals with hypokinetic dysarthria with even mild dementia might find this procedure beyond their cognitive capabilities.

- **Delayed auditory feedback** (DAF)—This electronic device "feeds" patients their own voice after a short delay, usually of approximately 50 to 150 ms. To maintain fluent speech while listening to their own delayed speech, most patients must slow their rate of speaking. Although used frequently to slow the

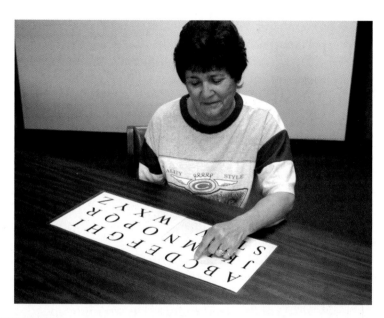

FIGURE 8–4. By pointing on an alphabet board to the first letter of every word they speak, individuals with hypokinetic dysarthria are forced to slow their rate of speech. The listener also receives a first-letter visual cue of the target word, which often facilitates comprehension.

speaking rate of people who stutter, DAF also has been used to slow the rate of speech in individuals with hypokinetic dysarthria. The effectiveness of this procedure to slow the rate of speech and increase intelligibility has been demonstrated in some studies (Yorkston et al., 1988) but not in others (Dagenais et al., 1998). Downie et al. (1981) found that DAF was effective in 2 of their 11 subjects with parkinsonism. Because of these mixed results, it might be useful to attempt a short trial period of DAF treatment to determine whether it is effective in reducing a given patient's rate of speech.

- Reciting syllables to a metronome—Dworkin (1991) suggested using a metronome to set the pace of syllable production. In this task, the metronome is set to the appropriate rate, and the patient is asked to recite or read familiar passages such as the Pledge of Allegiance, a well-known poem, or something similar. The patient should produce one syllable for every beat of the metronome. Although the resulting speech will sound automated, this is acceptable because the goal in this task is to build the patient's awareness of a more appropriate speech rate. With enough practice, the slower pace set by the metronome could become habituated into the patient's conversational speech. Free downloadable metronomes are available as smartphone apps. Small, electrical metronomes can be easily purchased as well.

Stretching Tasks. The stretching tasks discussed in the following paragraphs are very similar to those used in treating spastic dysarthria. They are designed to reduce the increased muscle tone of the articulators and increase the range of motion in these same structures.

- Tongue-stretching tasks—Dworkin (1991) described a series of passive tongue-stretching exercises in which the clinician gently grasps the patient's tongue with a gauze pad and carefully pulls it straight forward until resistance is felt. This protruded position is held for 10 s. Then the clinician gently pulls the protruded tongue to the left or right side of the mouth and again holds the position for 10 s. Dworkin cautioned against pulling the tongue too forcefully and encouraged the clinician and patient to have patience during these tasks. Active tongue-stretching movements by the patient also can be used to increase strength, speed, and accuracy of tongue movements (Swigert, 2010). Examples of these tasks include having the patient protrude the tongue fully, elevate the tongue tip toward the nose, lower the tongue tip toward the chin, and hold the tongue at the corners of the mouth. Other active tongue-stretching tasks include elevating the back of the tongue to the soft palate and pressing the tongue tip into the cheek. Although these active tongue-stretching movements have the benefit of promoting increased flexibility, they also might increase hypertonicity in some patients. The clinician should carefully monitor changes in muscle tone. If the active stretching tasks prove to be counterproductive, the passive stretching tasks should be used exclusively.
- Lip-stretching tasks—In passive lip-stretching tasks, the clinician grasps one of the lips gently with a gauze pad and carefully pulls it out and away from the face, holding the position for about 10 s. Active lip-stretching tasks have the patient making the movements, including holding a smile, pursing the lips, and puffing out the cheeks. Again, the clinician should monitor any changes in lip muscle tone when active stretching tasks have been recommended. If increased muscle tone is noted, passive tasks should be used exclusively.
- Jaw-stretching tasks—Swigert (2010) recommended two stretching tasks to lessen rigidity in the jaw muscles. First, the patient attempts to hold a maximum opening of the jaw, both with and without physical assistance from the clinician. Then the patient attempts to hold the jaw lateralized first to the right and then to the left, both with and without physical assistance from the clinician. The clinician determines the length of time

the patient is required to hold the position and the number of repetitions that should be completed during this task.

Traditional Articulation Treatments. Traditional articulation treatments also are recommended for the imprecise consonant productions in patients with hypokinetic dysarthria. These tasks concentrate on increasing the patient's awareness of articulation errors and practicing optimal phoneme productions.

- Intelligibility drills—Intelligibility drills are tasks in which the patient is given a list of words or sentences to read aloud (Yorkston et al., 1988). Then the clinician turns away from the patient so that he or she will only be able to understand the patient's speech if it is articulated clearly. By not looking at the target word list or at the patient's mouth, the clinician will depend entirely on the patient's articulation to understand the target word. If the clinician does not understand the target word, the patient needs to determine why the word or words were unclear and then try saying it again. If this second attempt fails, the clinician can look at the target word and give the patient specific feedback on why the utterance was not understood (e.g., "I didn't know it was 'sleep' because I couldn't hear the 'p.' Try it again, and let me really hear the 'p' this time.").

- Phonetic placement—This procedure treats articulation errors by instructing patients on the correct position of the articulators before they attempt to produce a target sound. Phonetic placement can be especially valuable in that it educates patients on how certain speech sounds are produced. Many individuals with dysarthria realize they are producing speech sounds incorrectly, but they have little understanding of why their productions are in error. For example, phonetic placement can educate speakers with hypokinetic dysarthria why their production of /d/ actually sounds closer to a /z/ or a /p/ sounds closer to a /b/ and so forth.

- Exaggerating consonants—Also known as overarticulation, exaggerating consonants is a treatment procedure that teaches the patient to fully articulate all consonant phonemes. Darley et al. (1975) suggested that most patients need to concentrate especially on medial and final consonants because these are the sounds most likely to be poorly articulated in connected speech. The improvements in intelligibility can be dramatic when individuals with hypokinetic dysarthria fully articulate the medial and final consonants in words.

    Park et al. (2016) used exaggerating consonants as the basis of an intensive treatment program for dysarthria. Their patients had a variety of different types of dysarthria, caused by either traumatic head injury or stroke. The study used a small group repeated measures design to determine the effects of overarticulation (in combination with slower and slightly louder speech) on dysarthric patients' single-word and sentence intelligibility. There were 16 treatment sessions (1-hr sessions, four times a week, for 4 weeks). The patients were first oriented to the treatment tasks so that they knew what was expected. The treatment sessions started with 10 min of prepractice where patients reviewed a random selection of the tasks that were to be used later in the session. The following 10 min required the patients to repeat 10 functional phrases five times each (e.g., "What are we doing tomorrow?"). The next 10 min had the patients repeating 10 service requests five times each (e.g., "Where is the _____?"). During the final 30 min, the patients read aloud, described pictures, and engaged in conversation. Feedback during most the sessions consisted of whether the patients' utterances were clear or unclear. Homework also was a part of the treatment procedure. The results showed that naive listeners noted improved conversational intelligibility in all patients compared to pretreatment samples. Many of the other outcome measures also were positive. This technique was adapted for telehealth applications in a small study with 15 participants receiving Be Clear treatment 4 days a week for 4 weeks. The results were modest yet promising (Whelan et al., 2022).

- Minimal contrast drills—These drills have the patient concentrate on producing pairs of words that vary by only one phoneme. The distinction between the words can be in the voicing (park–bark), manner of production (pine–mine), or place of production (sea–she) of consonants. The distinction also can be between vowels (man–men), but working on consonants does more to enhance intelligibility in most patients. These word pairs can be used alone, in phrases, or in sentences, depending on the needs of the specific patient.

Phonation

Because many individuals with hypokinetic dysarthria adduct their vocal folds only partially, they might have a harsh or breathy vocal quality when speaking. When this abnormal vocal quality is combined with poor respiratory support, their speech also could have significantly reduced loudness. Most of the following treatment tasks are the same as those used for flaccid dysarthria. These activities are designed to increase phonatory effort to bring the vocal folds together in a more fully adducted position.

- Pushing and pulling procedures—Sometimes described as "effortful closure techniques," pushing and pulling procedures help the vocal folds adduct by providing an overall increase in muscle contractions in the torso and neck (Ramig, 1995). In contrast to cases of flaccid dysarthria, in which these procedures are used to enhance muscle contraction in the laryngeal muscles, they are used in hypokinetic dysarthria to overcome reduced range of motion in the laryngeal muscles. Examples of these techniques include having a sitting patient push up on the arms of a chair while phonating an open vowel or having the patient pulling up on the edge of a heavy table while prolonging a vowel.
- Hard glottal attack—Some patients can demonstrate a better quality phonation when they begin an utterance with a hard glottal attack (Dworkin & Meleca, 1997). Dworkin (1991) described a complete exercise for this procedure. The basic steps are to have the patient hold a deep breath, bear down, and attempt to phonate a tight /a/. This tight phonation should be modified into a more normal vocal quality as soon as possible to avoid the adverse side effects of consistent hard glottal attacks during speech.
- Voice amplifiers—A small, portable voice amplifier can be a useful tool for individuals whose voice quality is breathy and soft. These devices have a detachable microphone that the patient speaks into and a speaker that amplifies the voice. A volume knob controls the output from the amplifier. Although these devices are simple to use, some training usually is needed to help the patient determine how far to hold the microphone from the mouth and how to adjust the volume knob. These devices can be quite helpful for some patients. As a trial, the author once recommended a voice amplifier for a patient with Parkinson's disease whose voice was very soft. Ironically, his wife was very hard of hearing. Once they learned how to use the device, the two of them were so pleased with its performance that they were no longer interested in continuing the regular treatment sessions. I wish all dismissals from treatment were so satisfactory.
- Instrumental biofeedback—A number of electronic devices or computer programs can provide visual or auditory feedback on pitch, loudness, or rate of speech. For example, a sound pressure level meter (or the smartphone app) can be an effective

tool to help patients reach and maintain higher levels of vocal loudness. The clinician often will increase the required loudness levels incrementally—perhaps first requiring the patient to reach 40 dB readings on the meter while prolonging a vowel, then with words or phrases, then sentences, and finally in conversation. The clinician subsequently requires the patient maintain 45 or 50 dB readings for the same tasks. Ultimately, the treatment goal should be at about 60dB, which is the average loudness of normal conversational speech. Numerous computer programs also can provide a visual display of loudness. By speaking into a microphone connected to the computer, the patient is able to see the intensity level of his or her speech on the monitor. By watching the screen while they speak, patients are able to adjust their loudness to reach the desired levels.

Several studies have documented the effectiveness of instrumental biofeedback devices to enhance the speech of individuals with hypokinetic dysarthria (Johnson & Pring, 1990; Rubow & Swift, 1985; Scott & Caird, 1983). Although initial treatment gains can be achieved with these devices, it should not be assumed that using them ensures the successful transfer of these gains to outside settings. Rubow and Swift (1985) found that their subject's in-clinic improvements in speech loudness did not carry over to locations outside the clinic. Such difficulties with carryover are not a problem only in the treatment of hypokinetic dysarthria with instrumental biofeedback. They are common to the treatment of all speech and language deficits.

- Lee Silverman Voice Treatment-LOUD (LSVT LOUD)—This is an effortful phonation program that was created by Ramig et al. (1995). Its positive effects on the speech of individuals with Parkinson's disease have been noted in a number of studies (Bryans et al., 2021; Liotti et al., 2003; Muñoz-Vigueras et al., 2021; Sapir et al., 2007; Yuan et al., 2020). LSVT LOUD is an intensive program in which patients with parkinsonism are guided through a daily schedule of maximum effort in their phonations and in which they are constantly reminded to "THINK LOUD." There are five guiding principles to the procedure:
    1. LSVT LOUD concentrates strictly on increasing vocal loudness. Articulation errors and other speech deficits are not directly addressed in the treatment sessions. The authors stated that bringing additional treatment tasks into the procedure only complicates the treatment and that

the increased effort to produce a louder voice usually promotes increased articulatory accuracy as a positive side effect.

2. It requires multiple repetitions of high-effort phonations from the patient. The emphasis is on producing phonations that have normal loudness, quality, and duration. The treatment procedure starts with prolonging a vowel with maximal effort and then moves on to words, sentences, and connected speech.

3. The treatment sessions must be completed daily. The clinician-led sessions need to be 50 to 60 min in length for a total of 16 individual sessions in a month. (Group sessions also have been incorporated into the treatment process.) For the days away from the clinician, the patient is given specific instructions on what needs to be done at home.

4. Patients must be "calibrated" for what is normal loudness. Many patients with parkinsonism seem to have problems with their sensory perception of what is loud. When speaking with normal loudness during an effortful phonation activity, they often will say that it seems as though they are shouting. To overcome this misperception, patients are given much feedback on how their louder phonations actually sound to listeners, and they are encouraged to be aware of how their louder phonations feel while they are producing them.

5. The progress must be quantified, meaning that objective measures must be obtained of the patient's performance throughout treatment. In general, this is accomplished by using a sound pressure level meter to document the loudness of phonations, a tape recorder to document the quality of phonations, and a stopwatch to measure the duration of phonations.

The actual treatment procedures used in this program are not unique. They include traditional tasks such as pushing and pulling procedures, a more open-mouth posture, modeling, and plenty of repetition. It is the intensity of the program and the hierarchy of treatment tasks that makes it distinctive. Because all components of the program should be used as designed by the authors, clinicians must attend a workshop to become certified administrators of the LSVT LOUD program.

SPEAK OUT! and The LOUD Crowd is another effortful phonation treatment for hypokinetic dysarthria (Boutsen et al., 2018;

Levitt et al., 2015). This treatment is divided into two parts. The first is SPEAK OUT!, where patients work in individual treatment sessions with a certified speech-language pathologist. The second part is The LOUD Crowd, consisting of group therapy maintenance sessions. Patients in SPEAK OUT! practice speaking with intent, which means consciously attending to each word spoken, so that speech becomes more deliberate and less automatic. There are similarities between SPEAK OUT! and LSVT LOUD. For example, both procedures require patients to concentrate on producing loud, controlled speech. Both procedures also are structured to raise the patient's awareness of how his or her speech sounds to listeners. One noted difference is that LSVT LOUD requires 16 hr of treatment, whereas SPEAK OUT! requires 8 hr, with patients eventually transitioning to the group maintenance sessions. As with LSVT LOUD, research into SPEAK OUT! suggests that it can be an effective treatment for hypokinetic dysarthria (Behrman et al., 2020).

Incidentally, a number of studies have examined the effects of LSVT LOUD on other types of dysarthria (Sapir et al., 2003; Wenke et al., 2010; Wenke et al., 2008, 2011). The basis of these studies is the finding that when patients with hypokinetic dysarthria effortfully increase their vocal loudness, articulation and phonation improve as well. Wenke et al. (2010) compared LSVT LOUD to traditional treatment with 26 patients with a variety of different dysarthrias (flaccid, spastic, ataxic, hypokinetic, and mixed). The LSVT LOUD treatments followed the standard procedures. The traditional treatments were individualized to each patient's needs and consisted of such familiar procedures as phonetic placement, rate reduction, contrastive stress drills, easy onset of phonation, and optimal breath group. The results showed no significant differences between the two procedures on any of the measured variables, including for the 6-month posttreatment reassessment. The importance of this finding is that LSVT LOUD is a relatively simple therapy task. Patients need only to concentrate on being loud. In contrast, traditional treatments usually require patients to attend to multiple elements of their speech, often simultaneously. Youssef et al. (2015) conducted a similar comparison of LSVT LOUD and traditional dysarthria treatment. They also found no significant differences between the two. It could be that with more research, LSVT LOUD will prove to be an effective treatment for more than just hypokinetic dysarthria.

Respiration

The shallow breath support that can occur in hypokinetic dysarthria could cause shortened phrases and decreased loudness in the speech of affected individuals. In addition, it can contribute to the breathy quality of their phonation. The respiratory treatments for hypokinetic dysarthria are many of the same used in the treatment of flaccid dysarthria.

- Speaking immediately on exhalation—Because of their shallow breath support, many patients with hypokinetic dysarthria have very limited amounts of subglottic air. By cueing the patients to begin phonating immediately on exhalation, they can use more of their available subglottic air pressure. Swigert (2010) suggested that the first step in this exercise is to have the patient place a hand on the abdomen and begin a simple /m/ phonation the moment the hand starts to move inward on exhalation. If necessary, the clinician can place his or her hand on the patient's hand to know when to cue the patient to begin the phonation.
- Cueing for complete inhalation—Sometimes breath support for speech can be increased just by reminding the patient to inhale fully before speaking. The clinician will probably need to give frequent reminders about this early in treatment. The ultimate goal is to have these deeper inhalations become a habitual part of the patient's conversational speech. To maximize the efficient use of subglottic air, it is often effective to combine the cues to inhale completely with reminders to speak immediately on exhalation.
- Slow and controlled exhalation—In this simple task, the patient is asked to inhale fully and then exhale in a slow, steady stream. Using a stopwatch, the clinician times the length of the exhalation. The goal is to increase the length and steadiness of the airflow over several sessions. Dworkin (1991) described an advanced variation on this task in which the patient is asked to inhale fully, begin a slow exhalation for 3 s, stop the exhalation by holding the breath for about 1 s, then continue with the exhalation. The difficulty can be increased until the patient is holding and releasing the air three times on a single breath.
- Stop phonation early—Because of paradoxical respiratory muscle movements, individuals with hypokinetic dysarthria often have shallow respiration. Typically, these patients might try to phonate for a longer period than their limited subglottic air supply allows. This results in speaking on residual air, which can cause a harsh vocal quality, decreased loudness, and an increased rate of speech. Consequently, it is often necessary for a patient to learn to stop an utterance before running low on air, which can be accomplished initially by

the clinician providing verbal and visual cues that tell the patient when to stop phonating and take another breath. Over time the cues can be discontinued as the patient becomes more independent at stopping phonation before speaking on residual air.

- Optimal breath group—This task is similar to the stopping phonation early procedure. The optimal breath group task teaches the patient how many syllables or words can be said clearly on one full inhalation (Linebaugh, 1983). Once a baseline has been established, the patient can work on increasing the length of the breath group, perhaps through deeper inhalations, more controlled exhalations, or beginning phonations immediately on exhalation.

Prosody

As already mentioned, prosody often can be improved by slowing the rate of speech in individuals with hypokinetic dysarthria. The following paragraphs describe some of the other procedures recommended for making the prosody of these speakers appear more natural.

- Intonation profiles—This task uses lines to show intonation changes in written sentences. Lines immediately below words indicate a flat intonation. Lines farther below words indicate a drop in pitch. Lines above words indicate a rise in pitch. These lines can be added easily to any written sentence, whether it is a statement or a question. For most patients, it is usually best to start with short, simple sentences and progress to longer sentences. The ultimate goal is to have the patient take the pitch changes produced in this structured activity and begin to use them in conversational speech.
- Contrastive stress drills—These tasks are usually designed for the clinician to ask a question, with the patient answering it by adding stress on key words to convey the intended meaning of the answer (McHenry, 1998). For example, the clinician could ask the following question about a picture of a man playing football: "Is the man playing basketball?" The patient will answer, "No. The man is playing football." The clinician's next question might be, "Is the woman playing football?" The patient's answer to this question would be, "No, the man is playing football." A third question might be, "Is the man watching football?" The patient would answer, "No, the

man is playing football." The length of the questions and the complexity of the pictures for this task can easily be varied to match the abilities of the patient.

- Chunking utterances into syntactic units—Duffy (2020) mentioned that some individuals with dysarthria need to learn to divide their utterances according to normal pauses within and between sentences. This is necessary because their disorder has limited the number of words they can produce on a single exhalation. To compensate for this limitation, the following task teaches the patient to inhale at the points in an utterance at which natural syntactic pauses occur. Examples of these natural pauses include after introductory clauses or phrases ("In the morning, [inhale] I went shopping at the store."), between clauses or phrases ("She went there, [inhale] but I missed her."), and between short sentences ("I saw the movie. [inhale] It was pretty good."). By inserting inhalations at points at which normal pauses occur in an utterance, individuals with hypokinetic dysarthria are often able to maintain a more natural rhythm in their speech. This rhythm is lost when the patient haphazardly places inhalations within an utterance.

Summary of Hypokinetic Dysarthria

- Any process that damages the basal ganglia can cause hypokinetic dysarthria. This dysarthria is closely associated with parkinsonism, which includes such disorders as idiopathic Parkinson's disease and drug-induced parkinsonism.
- The symptoms of parkinsonism are tremor, bradykinesia, muscular rigidity, akinesia, and disturbances of postural reflexes.
- The most common cause of hypokinetic dysarthria is idiopathic Parkinson's disease. This disease is caused by decreased amounts of the neurotransmitter dopamine in the portion of the basal ganglia called the striatum.
- The speech characteristics of hypokinetic dysarthria include harsh vocal quality, reduced stress, monoloudness, and imprecise consonants.
- Treatment of hypokinetic dysarthria should concentrate on improving articulatory precision, increasing phonatory effort, and promoting more natural prosody. Individuals with increased rate of speech can often benefit from rate control tasks.

Study Questions

1. Define hypokinetic dysarthria in your own words.
2. What are the five primary symptoms of parkinsonism?
3. Describe how the substantia nigra and the striatum are involved in the cause of parkinsonism.
4. What is L-dopa?
5. What can be the adverse side effects of L-dopa treatment?
6. What is postencephalitic parkinsonism?
7. About what percentage of individuals with idiopathic Parkinson's disease eventually have dementia?
8. What is the most common phonation deficit in individuals with hypokinetic dysarthria?
9. Describe two rate control treatment tasks for individuals with increased rate of speech.
10. Describe two treatment tasks for reducing the harsh or breathy vocal quality that is so common in hypokinetic dysarthria.

Chapter 9

Hyperkinetic Dysarthria

Definitions of Hyperkinetic Dysarthria

Neurologic Basis of Hyperkinetic Dysarthria

   What Causes Hyperkinetic Movement?

Causes of Hyperkinetic Dysarthria

   Chorea

      Sydenham's Chorea

      Huntington's Disease

      Stroke

      Tardive Dyskinesia

      Other Causes of Chorea

   Speech Characteristics of Hyperkinetic Dysarthria of Chorea

      Prosody

      Articulation

      Phonation

      Respiration

      Resonance

      Summary of Distinctive Speech Errors in Chorea

   Myoclonus

   Tic Disorders

   Essential (or Organic) Tremor

   Dystonia

      Causes of Dystonia

   Speech Characteristics of Hyperkinetic Dysarthria of Dystonia

      Articulation

      Prosody

      Phonation

      Respiration

      Resonance

Key Evaluation Tasks for Hyperkinetic Dysarthria

Treatment of Hyperkinetic Dysarthria

   Medical Treatments

   Behavioral Treatment for Huntington's Disease

   Behavioral Treatment for Dystonia

   Behavioral Treatment for Tic Disorders

Summary of Hyperkinetic Dysarthria

Study Questions

Definitions of Hyperkinetic Dysarthria

Hyperkinetic dysarthria is difficult to define because it can be caused by so many disorders. Unlike hypokinetic dysarthria, which is so often caused by parkinsonism, hyperkinetic dysarthria can be caused by a long list of disorders. These hyperkinetic disorders do have a few factors in common, however. For example, most of them seem to be caused by dysfunction in the basal ganglia, and they all produce involuntary movements that interfere with normal speech production. Both of the following definitions of hyperkinetic dysarthria mention the origin of these disorders and their effects on speech production.

> Speakers with hyperkinetic dysarthria present with dysphonia that is most often characterized by an alteration in voice quality and excessive variation in pitch and loudness. These characteristics are associated with atypical involuntary movements that may be rhythmic or irregular and rapid or slow, and are caused by disorders of the basal ganglia or cerebellar control circuits. Although hyperkinetic dysarthria encompasses a variety of different motor symptoms like tremor, dystonia, chorea, dyskinesia, myoclonus, and tics, 70% of patients with hyperkinetic dysarthria present with tremor or dystonia. (Lester-Smith et al., 2021, p. 2)

> Hyperkinetic dysarthria is characterized by variable articulatory imprecision, vocal harshness, and prosodic abnormalities. It is associated with damage to the extrapyramidal system, more specifically, lesions in the basal ganglia and their major pathways, which are important in the planning and programming of learned movements. (Zraick & LaPointe, 1997, p. 251)

In contrast to hypokinetic, which literally means "too little movement," hyperkinetic means "too much movement." Hyperkinetic movement disorders are characterized by excessive involuntary movements of various body parts. Chorea, myoclonus, tics, dystonia, and essential tremor are all examples of hyperkinetic movement disorders. The involuntary movements associated with these disorders frequently interfere with an affected individual's voluntary movements. When these involuntary movements interfere with speech production, the result is hyperkinetic dysarthria. Hyperkinetic dysarthria is unique among the other dysarthrias in that a clinician can often make an accurate diagnosis by just observing the individual's uncontrolled movements (Duffy, 2020).

Hyperkinetic movement disorders include many different involuntary motions, ranging from subtle movements of the lips, hands, or vocal folds to very large movements that involve many parts of the body. Every hyperkinetic disorder has its own characteristic movement pattern, with each resulting in distinctive patterns of speech errors. For example, the rapid and jerky muscle contractions of myoclonus cause different speech errors from those caused by the slow, sustained muscle contractions of dystonia. Consequently, hyperkinetic dysarthria is actually a group of various motor speech disorders; each is associated with one of the hyperkinetic movement disorders. For example, when describing the dysarthria of an individual with myoclonus or dystonia, it is more accurate to speak of the hyperkinetic dysarthria of myoclonus or the hyperkinetic dysarthria of dystonia than it is to use only the general term *hyperkinetic dysarthria*.

Neurologic Basis of Hyperkinetic Dysarthria

Many of the disorders that cause hyperkinetic dysarthria are associated with damage to the basal ganglia. As mentioned in previous chapters, the basal ganglia are a group of subcortical, gray-matter structures that help control movements (Figure 9–1). The separate structures that make up the basal ganglia are the caudate nucleus, putamen, and globus pallidus (Andreatta, 2023; Seikel et al., 2020). The caudate nucleus and the putamen are together known as the striatum because they share many of the same types of cells and many of the same functions. All the structures of the basal ganglia have a complex array of interconnections among themselves and with many other parts of the brain. One of these interconnections is a looping neural pathway that starts in the cerebral cortex, travels down to the basal ganglia, and then goes back up to the cortical motor areas of the cerebrum. This pathway is called the basal ganglia control circuit (Figure 9–2).

The exact function of the basal ganglia and this control circuit are not fully understood, but these structures do play an important role in smoothing out the rough and exaggerated movements that are initially planned in the cerebral cortex. As discussed in Chapter 2, it is thought that the motor impulses of a planned movement are sent from the cortex to the basal ganglia (specifically to the striatum), where the movements are processed and refined. Once these planned movements have been processed, they are sent out from the basal ganglia via the globus pallidus to the thalamus and then up to the motor centers of the cortex. From the motor centers of the cortex, these motor impulses are sent out to the upper motor neurons and finally to the lower motor neurons. At the neuromuscular junction, the lower motor neurons transmit the neural

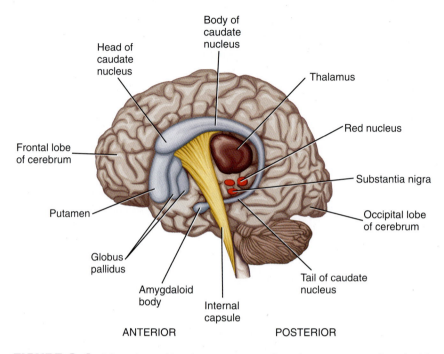

FIGURE 9–1. Many hyperkinetic movement disorders are associated with damage to the basal ganglia. The basal ganglia (putamen, caudate nucleus, and globus pallidus) are shown in relationship to other parts of the brain.

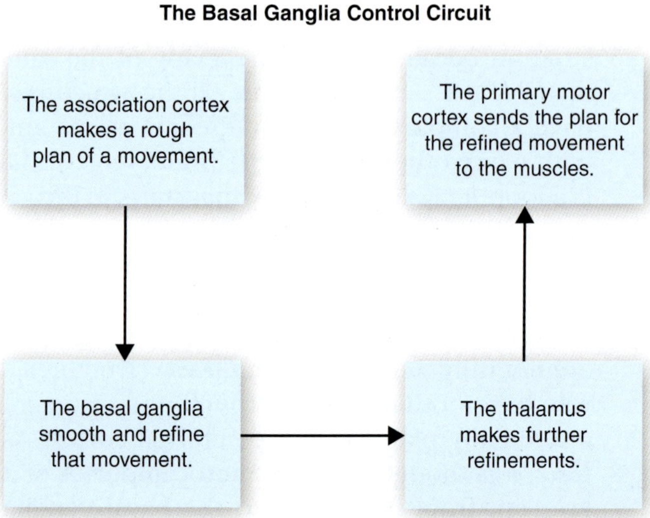

The Basal Ganglia Control Circuit

The association cortex makes a rough plan of a movement.

The primary motor cortex sends the plan for the refined movement to the muscles.

The basal ganglia smooth and refine that movement.

The thalamus makes further refinements.

FIGURE 9–2. A schematic diagram of the basal ganglia control circuit.

244

impulses of the movement to the muscles, which then contract and perform the movement.

What Causes Hyperkinetic Movement?

Even though most hyperkinetic movement disorders seem to be associated with damage to the basal ganglia, neuroscientists have difficulty explaining exactly why the involuntary movements occur. In large part, this is because the researchers are not yet completely sure how the basal ganglia functions. As with all complex mechanisms, it is hard to determine why something is not working properly when its normal function is not well understood.

Although much remains to be learned about hyperkinetic movements, several important observations have been made about the workings of the basal ganglia. One is that different disorders associated with the basal ganglia can have nearly opposite effects on movements. Parkinson's disease and Huntington's disease are two good examples of this. Both disorders are centered in the basal ganglia, yet the motor symptoms of each are very different from one another. Parkinsonism is a hypokinetic disorder and is characterized by rigid and restricted movements. In contrast, Huntington's disease is a hyperkinetic disorder, characterized by rapid, dance-like involuntary movements. How is it that these two disorders of the basal ganglia have such different effects on movement?

Currently, it is the parkinsonism portion of this question that is best understood. As discussed in Chapter 8, parkinsonism is caused by the degeneration of dopamine-producing neurons near the striatum. The loss of these neurons reduces the amount of dopamine in the striatum, which ultimately causes a diminution of movements. As a result, individuals with parkinsonism demonstrate rigidity, akinesia, and other symptoms of the disorder.

Although the dopamine-deficiency explanation of the symptoms of parkinsonism is well understood, the causes of hyperkinetic movement disorders are less clear. One theory suggests that the excessive involuntary movements in some of these disorders are caused by an imbalance of either dopamine or acetylcholine in the basal ganglia—an imbalance that is the inverse of that which causes parkinsonism. For example, any condition that causes too much dopamine to be released into the basal ganglia has an excitatory effect on movement. Similarly, any condition that results in too little acetylcholine in the basal ganglia also has an excitatory effect on movement. In either condition, hyperkinetic movements can be the result. This theory is supported by the experience of individuals with parkinsonism given too much L-dopa (i.e., too much dopamine), in whom hyperkinetic movements develop, a condition known as L-dopa-induced dyskinesia (Fabbrini & Guerra, 2021).

However, research indicates that the true cause of hyperkinetic movements is probably much more complicated than a simple imbalance of one or two neurotransmitters. The complexity of the basal ganglia can be appreciated from the fact that in just the striatum there are more than 100 different neuroactive chemicals (Brodal, 2010). Many of the functions and interactions of these chemicals are unclear, but they undoubtedly play varied roles in the proper functioning of the basal ganglia. Research suggests that the involuntary movements of hyperkinetic disorders are caused in part by disruptions in the functions of these neurochemicals, although the process is far from being fully understood. Until the intricate functions of the basal ganglia are better comprehended, the exact reasons for the involuntary movements of hyperkinetic disorders will remain ill-defined.

Causes of Hyperkinetic Dysarthria

Several hyperkinetic movement disorders can lead to hyperkinetic dysarthria. The disorders examined in this chapter are chorea, myoclonus, tics, essential tremor, and dystonia. As mentioned, most of these hyperkinetic movement disorders are associated with damage to the basal ganglia, the basal ganglia control circuit, or both. Degenerative diseases, traumatic head injury, stroke, infections, and other causes can lead to this damage. However, some of the hyperkinetic disorders, such as essential tremor, seem to have no observable neurologic pathology associated with them.

The involuntary movements linked to hyperkinetic disorders can vary, both in severity and in type of movement. In mild cases, the movements could be small tremors of one muscle. In severe cases, the movements could be so pronounced and affect so much of the body that activities such as walking, eating, and talking are practically impossible. Naturally, there can be definite differences between the dysarthria associated with mild tremor and the dysarthria associated with extreme involuntary movements of large muscle groups.

The overall impression of hyperkinetic dysarthria is that involuntary movements are interfering with an affected individual's efforts to produce speech (Duffy, 2020). A further impression is that speech production might be normal if the involuntary movements would somehow cease. The specific characteristics of the hyperkinetic dysarthria associated with each of the hyperkinetic movement disorders are discussed in the following sections of this chapter. Most of the information will concentrate on the hyperkinetic dysarthria associated with chorea and dystonia because the speech disorders of these two conditions are the most fully documented.

Chorea

Chorea is a movement disorder distinguished by random involuntary movements of the limbs, trunk, head, and neck. Choreic motions are often described as dance-like because they appear to be smooth and coordinated. In fact, the term comes from *choreia,* the Greek word for dance, which incidentally also is the root of the word *choreography*. Although choreic movements might seem to be coordinated, they are actually unpredictable and purposeless. They are sometimes even jerky or abrupt. Other descriptions of chorea have characterized the movements as writhing, highly complex, fleeting, and irregular. In mild cases of chorea, the motions might not be immediately obvious to an observer; instead, they might give the impression that the affected individual is only restless or jittery. When the movements are infrequent, the affected individual might try to hide them by turning them into purposeful gestures, such as scratching the chin or stretching an arm. In severe cases, the motions are constant, stopping only when the individual is asleep. When they are severe, the choreic motions will interfere with nearly all attempts at voluntary movement. As a result, problems with walking, swallowing, speech, and other discrete movements are common in individuals with advanced chorea.

Sydenham's Chorea

Several neurologic disorders share the symptom of chorea. One of these is Sydenham's chorea, a rare condition that usually affects children between 5 and 15 years of age. The familiar name for this condition is Saint Vitus's dance. Its greatest rate of occurrence is in children who have had a streptococcal fever. It appears during the recovery from this infection. Sydenham's chorea is likely an autoimmune disorder where antibodies that fight the infection also react to neurons in the striatum (Feinstein & Walker, 2020). About 40% of the children with this disorder have hyperkinetic dysarthria during the course of their illness. Penicillin and other medications can successfully treat this condition, and many cases clear in 3 to 4 months even without treatment.

Huntington's Disease

Huntington's disease is a progressive disorder that is caused by the gradual degeneration of neurons in the basal ganglia and cerebral cortex. The loss of neurons is especially evident in the caudate nucleus and putamen (the striatum) in the basal ganglia. Huntington's disease is an inherited (autosomal dominant) disorder; it develops in half of the children of a parent carrying the defective huntingtin gene. Normally, this gene produces a protein that seems to be important for neuron function in the brain, among other important duties. When mutated, however, it causes the development of Huntington's disease. It is a rare disorder; prevalence is about 6 per 100,000 population. Although the first symptoms can appear in childhood or adolescence, onset typically occurs during middle age. The average course of the disease is about 15 years, but some individuals survive for 25 or 30 years after the symptoms first appear.

The clinical features and progression of Huntington's disease are very unfortunate. The earliest signs are subtle intellectual deficits that might be evident only in neuropsychological testing. For example, performance scores on cognitive assessments might decline in affected individuals for months or years before other symptoms of the disease are apparent. Inevitably, a significant dementia will develop, in which patients show personality changes, impaired problem-solving abilities, and word-finding difficulties. Individuals with Huntington's disease eventually become inattentive, vague, withdrawn, and depressed. Angry outbursts and suicidal thoughts are not unusual. Along with this cognitive decline, a generalized chorea develops as the loss of basal ganglia neurons progresses. The choreic movements interfere with voluntary actions, resulting in a lurching walk, poorly coordinated fine motor movements, dysphagia, and hyperkinetic dysarthria. In the final stages of the disease, many individuals with Huntington's disease are bedridden, mute, and akinetic (Bachoud-Lévi et al., 2019).

The cause of the neuron degeneration in Huntington's disease is unclear. Several factors seem to play a role, including glutamate excitotoxicity, inflammation responses, and oxidative stress (Kumar et al., 2020). In any case, it is known that the loss of these neurons accompanies significant decreases in neurotransmitter receptors in the basal ganglia, as well as reductions in important enzymes and other neuroactive chemicals in the brain. These complex neurologic changes are thought to be responsible for many of the symptoms of this disease, although researchers are uncertain precisely how the loss of neurons in the striatum causes choreic movements.

Watch the PluralPlus Hyperkinetic Dysarthria Case 1 video for an example of a patient with Huntington's disease.

Stroke

Although it is rare, strokes have been known to cause chorea (Carbayo et al., 2020). Usually these are strokes affecting the basal ganglia or nearby subcortical structures such as the thalamus. The resulting chorea is commonly called *hemichorea* because the involuntary movements occur only on the side of the body that is opposite to the site of the lesion, assuming that the stroke damage is restricted to only one side of the brain.

Sometimes stroke damage to the subthalamic nucleus (a collection of subcortical motor neurons near the substantia nigra) can cause a condition known as **hemiballism.** This disorder is characterized by wild and violent involuntary movements of the limbs that are contralateral to the lesion. Although this disorder is a diagnostic category distinct from chorea, hemiballistic movements are described occasionally as being extreme versions of choreic movements. Self-injury and exhaustion are very possible in cases of hemiballism. In most instances, the movements can be treated successfully with medications, and they usually remit spontaneously after a period of days, weeks, or months.

Tardive Dyskinesia

Tardive dyskinesia is a movement disorder that can cause choreic movements of the face, mouth, and neck. In some instances, the limbs also are affected. Tardive dyskinesia is caused by taking certain medications, usually antipsychotic drugs, over a period of months or years. The term *tardive dyskinesia* is an apt description of this disorder because the choreic movements appear after long-term use of these drugs. (*Tardive* means being late in appearing, as in being tardy; *dyskinesia* means a disorder of voluntary movement.) This condition is more likely to develop in women than in men, and elderly individuals are more susceptible than the young. Unfortunately, stopping the medications will not reverse the condition in most cases. In fact, tardive dyskinesia will sometimes appear only after the medications are withdrawn, a condition known as withdrawal-emergent dyskinesia.

The movements of the face and mouth in tardive dyskinesia include lip smacking, tongue protrusions, chewing motions, and grimacing (Debrey & Goldsmith, 2021). Such movements can cause hyperkinetic dysarthria by interfering with normal voluntary attempts at speech production. The impact on articulation can vary from mild to severe, depending on the intensity of the dyskinetic movements and which muscle groups are affected. It is not exactly clear why these drugs cause hyperkinetic movements. It is possible that these medications make certain neurotransmitter receptors in neurons of the basal ganglia supersensitive to dopamine. As a consequence, the basal ganglia will react as if they were receiving too much dopamine, even if only normal amounts are present, which then causes the involuntary movements of tardive dyskinesia.

Other Causes of Chorea

Quite a few conditions can cause choreic movements. These include cerebral anoxia and carbon monoxide poisoning. Both of these can selectively damage the basal ganglia and other related subcortical structures, although chorea is not a typical symptom of either condition. Pregnancy and the use of oral contraceptives also can cause chorea, but the incidence is very low. Cancerous tumors can release proteins and hormones into the body that affect normal organ function. If these substances reach the basal ganglia, chorea could be the result. Additional causes of chorea can include tick encephalitis, hyperthyroidism, syphilis, vitamin B12 deficiency, and celiac disease (Feinstein & Walker, 2020).

Speech Characteristics of Hyperkinetic Dysarthria of Chorea

Chorea can have a significant effect on speech production. The degree of the chorea influences how severely speech is affected. Individuals with mild chorea typically will have fewer speech errors than someone who has a more significantly impairment. In fact, individuals with very mild cases of chorea might have minimal problems with their speech. In more moderately and severely affected individuals, however, a wide variety of speech errors will be evident. The variety of errors is based primarily on two factors. First, the movements of chorea can affect many different muscle groups, including the muscles of the face, neck, head, and torso. The voluntary movements of all these muscles are susceptible to interference from the involuntary movements of chorea. As a consequence, all the components of speech production (articulation, phonation, respiration, resonance, and prosody) might be more or less equally affected by hyperkinetic movements. This is in contrast to many of the other dysarthrias, in which at least one of the components of speech production is usually less affected than the others are. For example, in spastic dysarthria, respiration is usually far less impaired than phonation and articulation.

Second, the movements of chorea are unpredictable. At a given moment, the choreic movements could affect any number of muscle groups. For instance, during speech, one minute, the muscles of the lips and tongue might be affected, and the next, the muscles of respiration will cause a sudden inhalation of air during phonation. A moment later, yet another muscle group might be affected. It also is possible that all the muscles of speech production will be affected simultaneously by the involuntary movements. On the other hand, there could be short periods during which the interference from the choreic movements is minimal. At those moments, speech production might be fully intelligible, if only briefly.

The following paragraphs examine the effects of chorea on each component of speech production, based mostly on Darley et al.'s (1969a, 1969b) analysis of the speech errors of 30 subjects with chorea. The complete ranking of the speech errors is presented in Table 9–1. Note that a few of the errors appear to be contradictory, such as monoloudness and excess loudness variations. In general, such errors reflect the variability and unpredictable nature of choreic movements, which can cause, for instance, both monoloudness and excessive loudness in the same individual at different times.

Prosody

Darley et al. found that chorea affects prosody more than any other component of speech production. The two prosodic errors that were most evident in their subjects were prolonged intervals between syllables and words and variable rate of speech. Duffy (2020) suggested that these errors are caused by the unpredictable timing of the choreic movements and by an individual's attempts to compensate for the movements. For example, an individual might wait for the completion of an interfering choreic motion before continuing with an utterance. This would cause a prolonged interval between syllables or words. On the other hand, a speaker could hurry through an utterance before the next choreic movement occurs and thus have a variable rate of speech. Some of the other noted prosodic errors are monopitch, inappropriate silences, and monoloudness.

Articulation

Imprecise consonant production, distorted vowels, and prolonged phonemes were common articulation errors in Darley et al.'s (1969a, 1969b) subjects with chorea. The first two of these articulation errors

TABLE 9–1	The Most Common Speech Production Errors in 30 Individuals With Hyperkinetic Dysarthria of Chorea

Rank	Speech Production Errors
1	Imprecise consonants
2	Prolonged intervals
3	Variable pitch
4	Monopitch
5	Harsh voice quality
6	Inappropriate silences
7	Distorted vowels
8	Excess loudness variation
9	Prolonged phonemes
10	Monoloudness
11	Short phrases
12.5	Irregular articulatory breakdown
12.5	Excess and equal stress
14.5	Hypernasality
14.5	Reduced stress
16	Strained-strangled quality

Source: From "Clusters of Diagnostic Patterns of Dysarthria," by F. L Darley, A. E. Aronson, and J. R. Brown, 1969, *Journal of Speech and Hearing Research, 12,* p. 260. Copyright 1969 by American Speech-Language-Hearing Association. Reprinted with permission.

are the result of involuntary choreic movements being imposed on the voluntary movements of normal articulation. For example, involuntary contractions of the pharyngeal muscles might change the shape of the vocal tract during speech and thereby cause any vowel spoken at that moment to be distorted. The third articulation error, prolongation of phonemes, can be caused by choreic movements that involuntarily force the holding of an articulatory position longer than is normally required.

Phonation

Choreic movements also can affect phonation. Darley et al. (1969a, 1969b) found harsh vocal quality, excess loudness variations, and strained-strangled vocal quality in many of their subjects. These errors of phonation are caused by intermittent, involuntary hyperadduction of the vocal folds during speech. On the other hand, involuntary vocal-fold abduction during phonation can cause brief instances of breathy vocal quality. In fact, some individuals with chorea might have a harsh or strained-strangled vocal quality in one utterance and then have a breathy vocal quality in a portion of the next. As mentioned, such variability reflects the unpredictable nature of choreic movements. At one moment, the vocal folds might be adducted too tightly; shortly afterward, they might be unable to adduct fully. Choreic movements also could cause instances of **voice stoppage**, in which phonation ceases intermittently during speech.

Respiration

Darley et al. (1969a, 1969b) reported that six of their subjects with chorea had rapid, unexpected inhalations and exhalations of air. These sudden respiratory actions are caused by involuntary movements of the chest or diaphragm. In severe cases of chorea, these respiratory actions can occur at any moment, either while sitting quietly or in the middle of an utterance. During speech, they can cause distracting extraneous phonations, halting utterances, and short phrases. By causing a sudden increase in subglottic air pressure, involuntary exhalations during phonation can contribute to the excess loudness variations noted in the previous paragraph.

Resonance

Hypernasality was noted in 13 of Darley et al.'s subjects. This problem of resonance is caused by involuntary movements that alter the normal timing of velar elevation. Duffy (2020) indicated that hypernasality in chorea is usually intermittent, which reflects the unpredictable nature of the movements. Brief moments of hyponasality also are possible, caused by involuntary velar movements that close the velopharyngeal port during the production of nasal phonemes.

Summary of Distinctive Speech Errors in Chorea

There are many speech errors that can occur in the hyperkinetic dysarthria of chorea. There are so many, in fact, that beginning clinicians can be overwhelmed and confused by their number. To simplify, the following list summarizes speech errors that are generally most evident in individuals with chorea (Duffy, 2020):

- Prolonged intervals between syllables and words
- Variable rate of speech

- Inappropriate silences
- Excess loudness variations
- Prolonged phonemes
- Rapid, brief inhalations or exhalations of air
- Voice stoppages
- Intermittent breathy voice quality

Myoclonus

Myoclonus is a hyperkinetic movement disorder distinguished by involuntary and brief contractions of part of a muscle, a whole muscle, or a group of muscles in the same area of the body. "Myo" means muscle; "clonus" (from the Greek word for turmoil) means alternating contraction and relaxation. The muscle contractions of myoclonus may occur singly, in a repeating irregular pattern, or rhythmically. Furthermore, these contractions cannot be suppressed consciously. Myoclonus can appear in many medical conditions. It can be found in cases of kidney failure, epilepsy, cerebral anoxia, strokes, traumatic head injury, and some progressive neurologic diseases such as Alzheimer's disease and Creutzfeldt-Jakob's disease. It also can appear for unknown reasons. This disorder is not always disabling. In fact, nearly everyone has experienced benign hypnagogic myoclonus, which is the whole-body jerk that sometimes happens immediately before falling asleep.

A focal myoclonus occurs when specific muscles or body parts are affected by the contractions. **Hemifacial spasm** is a good example of a focal myoclonus. In this condition, the muscles around the eye contract involuntarily. These contractions can eventually spread to other muscles, until nearly all of the muscles on the same side of the face are affected. It is a common disorder and is painless, but the social consequences of embarrassment can be significant.

Another example of a focal myoclonus is **palatopharyngolaryngeal myoclonus**, sometimes less accurately known as just palatal myoclonus. Unlike hemifacial spasm, this condition is rare. As its name implies, palatopharyngolaryngeal myoclonus is marked by muscular contractions of the soft palate, the pharynx, and the larynx. The contractions are fairly rhythmic and occur about one to five times per second, even while sleeping (Nathan et al., 2022). Brainstem or cerebellar strokes are the most likely cause of this condition, but others include encephalitis and tumors. In many cases, the cause is unknown (Fleet et al., 2020).

Soft palate contractions are the most frequently noted movement in palatopharyngolaryngeal myoclonus. They consist of brief and rapid elevating contractions that often can be easily observed. The associated contractions of the pharynx can be seen as rhythmic movements of the pharyngeal walls. Interestingly, these pharyngeal contractions can repeatedly open and close the Eustachian tube, which causes an audible (and to the affected individual, a very annoying) clicking sound. The laryngeal contractions of this disorder can sometimes be visible as a twitching of the neck muscles. The effects of palatopharyngolaryngeal myoclonus on speech production are less obvious than might be surmised by the many involuntary movements associated with it. Speech is affected in only the most severe cases of this disorder because the contractions are typically so quick and of such a low intensity (Duffy, 2020). Darley et al. (1975) reported that when speech is involved, there might be intermittent hypernasality, imprecise consonants, and short interruptions of phonation.

Tic Disorders

A **tic** is a rapid movement that can be controlled voluntarily for a time but nevertheless is performed frequently because of a compulsive desire to do so. Affected individuals report that they can suppress a tic for varying periods, but the urge to perform the movement builds irresistibly until they are compelled to do it. There are both motor tics and vocal tics. The most common motor tics involve the face, such as repetitive eye blinks, brief facial twitches, and grimaces. However, motor tics can be more obvious and complex, revealing themselves as hand gestures, squatting, kicking, hopping, and shoulder shrugging. Vocal tics can appear as throat clearing, grunts, and barking noises. Extreme examples of vocal tics include shouting and the compulsive utterance of obscene words (coprolalia). Stress often increases the frequency of tic behaviors.

Tics normally occur in about 10% to 12% of all young children, usually in the form of excessive eye blinks or other brief facial movements. In most of these children, they might occur for less than a month or up to about a year and then disappear. Sometimes, however, a tic will persist. In fact, it might be joined by other tic behaviors over time. Multiple motor and vocal tics are one of the four clinical features of **Gilles de la Tourette's syndrome**, a rare disorder that was first identified in 1885. The other three features are the development of symptoms before the age of 18, the slow appearance and disappearance of tics for at least a year, and certainty that the movements are not attributable to another medical condition (American Psychiatric Association, 2013).

Most children are diagnosed with Tourette's syndrome between the ages of 12 and 17. The prevalence is about 3 per 100,000 population, with boys being affected far more frequently than girls. A fairly strong familial link has been noted; about 35% of individuals with Tourette's syndrome have a close relative with it as well. The motor and vocal tics found in this disorder can include all of those mentioned previously. In addition, vocal tics such as palilalia (the compulsive repetition of one's own speech) and echolalia (the compulsive repetition of someone else's speech) can appear. Seideman and Seideman (2020) reported that Tourette's syndrome is often accompanied by obsessive–compulsive behaviors (in 50% of cases) and attention-deficit/hyperactivity disorder (in 53.4% of cases).

The precise cause of tics is unclear. Some can be traced to mild brain damage or toxic reactions to medications, but determining the specific cause of tics has proven to be difficult. One line of study suggests that they are caused by supersensitive dopamine receptors in the striatum. Another implicates unbalanced levels of dopamine and serotonin. Recent brain imaging research has identified three specific neural circuits between the cortex and basal ganglia that could be involved in tic behaviors, suggesting that complex interactions among several neurotransmitters and disinhibited areas of the striatum influence both the type and location of tics (Martino & Hedderly, 2019).

Essential (or Organic) Tremor

Essential tremor is a benign hyperkinetic movement disorder that causes tremulous movements in affected body parts. The terms *essential* and *organic* are often used synonymously in labeling this disorder. In this context, both terms mean that a disorder has no apparent external cause (i.e., it is idiopathic). Essential tremor is the most common hyperkinetic movement disorder seen by neurologists, occurring in about 300 per 100,000 population. It usually first appears when individuals are in their 40s or 50s, but it has been first noted at much younger and older ages. About 50% of the individuals with essential tremor have family members who also show signs of this disorder, hence the occasional use of the term *familial tremor*.

Essential tremor most often affects the hands, arms, or head. It is an **action tremor**, which means that it is most evident when an individual is performing a movement, such as lifting a glass to the mouth or reaching for something. When the affected body part is at rest, the tremor disappears or is greatly reduced. Stress and fatigue will increase the tremor. Although most cases of essential tremor have a gradual onset, sudden onset of this condition has been noted. Once the tremor does appear, any progression of severity typically occurs at a slow pace. As its name implies, no specific site of lesion has been identified for this disorder, but it has occasionally been associated with hemifacial spasm and focal dystonia (discussed later). Although essential tremor is occasionally confused with parkinsonian tremor, Shanker (2019) indicated a number of characteristics that help distinguish between them:

- Essential tremor is faster than parkinsonism tremor.
- Essential tremor is an action tremor that disappears at rest; parkinsonian tremor is a resting tremor that decreases during movement.
- Individuals with essential tremor do not have other neurologic symptoms such as bradykinesia or akinesia.
- If limb tremor is present in essential tremor, handwriting is normal in size or larger (macrographic). Handwriting is smaller than normal (micrographic) in parkinsonism.

Essential voice tremor occurs in 20% to 30% of individuals with essential tremor (Lowell et al., 2019). It is characterized by phonation that has a tremulous, quavering vocal quality. This tremulous quality is caused by rhythmic, involuntary contractions of the vocal folds, along with vertical laryngeal movements. These contractions occur at a rate of about six per second. The severity range in essential voice tremor is wide. In mild cases, the tremor will be "hidden" by the vigorous vocal-tract movements of conversational speech and be evident only during a prolonged vowel. In fact, Duffy (2020) indicated that some individuals with mild essential voice tremor are not aware that they have the condition. In the more severe cases, tremor of the lips, tongue, or neck might accompany the rhythmic contractions of the larynx. All attempts at phonation will have a clearly evident tremulous quality. If severe enough, these vocal-tract tremors could slow the rate of speech in affected individuals.

Essential voice tremor is progressive, but it is generally considered to be a benign condition. In a longitudinal study of 335 patients with long-term essential voice tremor, only 10% had severe vocal disability (Louis & McCreary, 2021). Treatment for significant cases usually involves medications (Lowell et al., 2021), injections of Botox into laryngeal muscles (Newland et al., 2022), or deep brain stimulation (Ruckart et al., 2022).

Dystonia

Dystonia is a hyperkinetic movement disorder of muscle tone. "Dys" means disordered or abnormal; "tonia" refers to muscle tone.

Dystonia causes involuntary, prolonged muscle contractions that interfere with normal movement or posture. Dystonic movements typically have a slower, more sustained quality than those seen in chorea. Because the effect of dystonia is not necessarily constant, dystonic muscular contractions might appear and disappear during an ongoing movement. These gradual changes in muscle tone are described often as the "waxing and waning" characteristic of dystonia. In severe cases, however, the contractions can be constant, often resulting in painful, fixed contractions of the affected body part. For example, in a severe case of tongue dystonia, the tongue might protrude fully in a very strong and steady muscular contraction, making all attempts at speech uncomfortable and practically impossible.

Dystonia can appear in many muscles of the body. It might affect only one muscle, a single group of muscles, or multiple groups of muscles. Dystonia is categorized according to the number of affected body parts (di Biase et al., 2022):

- Focal dystonia—The dystonic movement or posture is present in only one part of the body, such as the tongue, jaw, arm, or hand.
- Segmental dystonia—The dystonic movement or posture affects two contiguous parts of the body.
- Multifocal—Two noncontiguous body parts are affected.
- Generalized dystonia—The dystonic movement or posture affects the trunk and at least two or more additional body parts.
- Hemidystonia—The dystonic movement or posture affects two or more body parts on the same side of the body (e.g., right arm and right leg).

Sometimes dystonic muscular contractions can be alleviated temporarily by **sensory tricks**. Sensory tricks, also known as *geste antagoniste,* are simple movements or actions that an affected individual can perform to stop the involuntary contractions—at least for a short period. Sensory tricks are very idiosyncratic. A trick that works for one person could have no effect for someone else. A frequently reported sensory trick is a gentle touch to the affected body part. For example, in a case of mandibular dystonia, the sensory trick of lightly touching the jaw might temporarily stop the involuntary muscular contractions. Usually, individuals with dystonia find effective sensory tricks either by accident or experimentation. In one case study, an individual with dystonia of the tongue found that when he put a breath mint between his cheek and gum, his dystonic tongue movements would stop until the mint dissolved. While the mint was in his mouth, his speech articulation was normal. Unfortunately, some individuals' dystonic muscle contractions do not respond to sensory tricks. Even when they do work, sensory tricks tend to lose their effectiveness after long-term use. The reason why they work at all is a mystery. One theory suggests that touching the affected body part causes a change in peripheral proprioceptive feedback that consequently interrupts the abnormal motor output from the brain (Jahanshahi, 2000). Watch the PluralPlus Hyperkinetic Dysarthria Case 2 video for an example of a sensory trick.

Causes of Dystonia

Dystonia can result from numerous conditions including focal cerebrovascular accidents of the basal ganglia, traumatic head injury, carbon monoxide poisoning, cerebral anoxia, and tumors. In these conditions, dystonia can be just one of several symptoms (i.e., a secondary symptom). In some disorders, known as **primary dystonias**, dystonia is the primary symptom.

Oromandibular Dystonia. This is a primary dystonia that can affect the jaw, lips, or tongue muscles in a variety of ways. Tongue protrusion, tongue retraction, jaw closing, jaw opening, jaw deviation, jaw retraction, and lip deviation are all possible in patients with this disorder, and it is common to find combinations of these symptoms in the same individual (Page & Siegel, 2017). For example, a patient could demonstrate both tongue protrusion and jaw opening simultaneously. The range of severity in oromandibular dystonia can be remarkable. Someone with a mild tongue retraction dystonia only might demonstrate subtle distortions of lingual consonants. Conversely, a patient with a severe tongue protrusion or jaw opening dystonia can have both the jaw and tongue fully and painfully extended throughout the day. Such a condition has a significant negative impact on oral communication and eating. Moreover, there can be obvious social consequences when the face and mouth are so visibly distorted by prolonged muscle contractions. Oromandibular dystonia is a rare condition; reported prevalence ranges from 0.1 to 6.9 per 100,000 (Yoshida, 2022). Its cause as a primary dystonia is unknown, although basal ganglia dysfunction is strongly suspected. Watch the PluralPlus Hyperkinetic Dysarthria Case 3 video for an example of a patient with oromandibular dystonia.

Spasmodic Torticollis. **Spasmodic torticollis** is another example of a primary dystonia. This disorder is characterized by intermittent dystonic contractions of the neck muscles, which result in an involuntary turning of the head. The head also usually tilts upward as a result of the contractions. In some cases, spasmodic torticollis eventually develops into a generalized dystonia. The contractions in this disorder can be intermittent, meaning that for varying amounts of time there will be no evidence of dystonia. In severe cases, the head-turning movements can be nearly constant. Stress and anxiety tend to increase the frequency of the contractions. The sensory trick of gently touching the turned-away side of the face can stop the neck muscle contractions in some individuals and allow normal movement for a time. The cause of spasmodic torticollis is unknown, but neuron degeneration in the basal ganglia has been noted in some individuals with the disorder. The speech of affected individuals has been shown to be slow in rate, mildly reduced in intelligibility, and lower in pitch for many females (Duffy, 2020).

Drug-Induced Dystonia. In addition to causing the choreic movements of tardive dyskinesia, the long-term use of certain antipsychotic drugs also can result in a primary dystonia known as **chronic drug-induced dystonia**. As in tardive dyskinesia, withdrawal of the drug might not stop the dystonia. In fact, in some cases the dystonia might appear only after the drug has been withdrawn. Most of the dystonic contractions in this disorder appear near the mouth and face, resulting in grimacing and sustained tongue protrusions. Occasionally, the dystonic movements will generalize to other body parts. Drug-induced dystonia also is known as **tardive dystonia**.

Meige Syndrome. Meige syndrome is a rare idiopathic disease. One of the most prominent symptoms is repetitive eye blinking and abnormal facial movements that are often dystonic in nature. The first signs of this disorder appear in early middle age and get progressively worse. The eye blinks can become so frequent that functional vision is impossible. The involuntary facial movements of this disease can affect the jaw, tongue, mouth, and neck. When the dystonic facial movements are sufficiently strong, they often cause hyperkinetic dysarthria.

Spasmodic Dysphonia. Although it is not always classified as a primary dystonia, **spasmodic dysphonia** has many of the features of a focal dystonia. This disorder is characterized by involuntary vocal-fold movements during phonation. Unlike a typical dystonia, the muscular contractions of spasmodic dysphonia do not usually have a gradual waxing and waning quality. Rather, the involuntary movements are frequently described as being vigorous and active. In a majority of individuals, the spasmodic movements affect the adductor muscles in the larynx, causing what is known as adductor spasmodic dysphonia. In this condition, the vocal folds are involuntarily closed tightly during phonation. It is the most common type, accounting for 85% to 95% of all spasmodic dysphonia cases (Hyodo et al., 2021). This involuntary adduction of the vocal folds can be either constant or intermittent. When constant, an affected person's phonations typically have a continuously strained and effortful quality. When the adduction is intermittent, phonations have a jerky and tight quality. In mild cases, phonations could have only a modestly shaky quality. In the less common abductor form of spasmodic dysphonia, the vocal folds are involuntarily abducted during phonation, resulting in moments of breathiness or aphonia. In a rare, third form of spasmodic dysphonia (known as mixed spasmodic dysphonia), the involuntary movements affect adduction and abduction simultaneously.

An interesting feature of spasmodic dysphonia is that nonlinguistic vocalizations such as laughing or crying are free of the involuntary laryngeal contractions. Many spontaneous, emotionally charged vocalizations also are clear of the dysphonia. This unusual feature of spasmodic dysphonia led many early investigators to assume that its cause was psychogenic. Currently, it is believed that nearly all cases of this disorder have a neurogenic origin, although the pathologic process causing the involuntary vocal-fold movements is unclear. Spasmodic dysphonia's close relationship to a focal dystonia suggests that the cause might be related to a basal ganglia disorder.

Speech Characteristics of Hyperkinetic Dysarthria of Dystonia

Darley et al. (1969a, 1969b) examined the speech errors of 30 subjects with dystonia (Table 9–2). Numerous errors were noted, many of which also were present in their subjects with chorea. The apparent similarity of speech errors in dystonia and chorea can be confusing to many clinicians. However, a careful comparison of Table 9–1 and Table 9–2 reveals several important distinctions between these two hyperkinetic disorders. First, Darley et al. found more errors of articulation in dystonia than in chorea. Three of the top four errors in dystonia were articulation errors; there was only one articulation error (imprecise consonants) in the top four for chorea. Second, the subjects with chorea tended to display more prosodic errors than those with dystonia. Three of the top four errors in chorea were errors of prosody; no prosodic errors were in the top four errors in the subjects with dystonia. In general, the speech errors in individuals with chorea tend to reflect

TABLE 9–2	The Most Common Speech Production Errors in 30 Individuals With the Hyperkinetic Dysarthria of Dystonia

Rank	Speech Production Errors
1	Imprecise consonants
2	Distorted vowels
3	Harsh voice quality
4	Irregular articulatory breakdown
5.5	Strained-strangled quality
5.5	Monopitch
7	Monoloudness
8.5	Inappropriate silences
8.5	Short phrases
10	Prolonged intervals
11	Prolonged phonemes
12	Excess loudness variation
13	Reduced stress
14	Voice stoppages
15	Rate

Source: From "Clusters of Diagnostic Patterns of Dysarthria," by F. L. Darley, A. E. Aronson, and J. R. Brown, 1969, *Journal of Speech and Hearing Research, 12,* p. 259. Copyright 1969 by American Speech-Language-Hearing Association. Reprinted with permission.

errors of prosody, and those in individuals with dystonia tend to reflect errors of articulation. Although such distinctions might be somewhat helpful in diagnosing these two forms of hyperkinetic dysarthria, remember that there will always be numerous individuals with either disorder who do not precisely match these patterns of speech errors.

Articulation

As mentioned, Darley et al. found that articulation errors were the most prominent in their subjects with dystonia. Imprecise consonant production, distorted vowels, irregular articulatory breakdowns, and prolonged phonemes were evident in their subjects' speech. These errors are the result of sustained dystonic contractions of the oral motor muscles that cause incorrect or imprecise positioning of the articulators during speech. The irregular articulatory breakdowns reflect the intermittent nature of many dystonic contractions. When they are present during speech, dystonic movements will interfere with accurate articulation; when they are absent, articulation will be improved considerably.

Prosody

Although typically less prominent than articulation errors, prosodic errors can occur frequently in dystonia. Darley et al.'s (1969a, 1969b) subjects demonstrated monopitch, monoloudness, inappropriate silences, and shortened phrases. They also tended to reduce stress on normally stressed words and syllables. Many of these prosodic errors could be the result of dystonic muscular contractions in the vocal tract that reduce the range and speed of the laryngeal movements needed to produce normal inflections of pitch and loudness.

Phonation

Darley et al. found a harsh vocal quality in 27 of their 30 subjects with dystonia. Many of them also had strained-strangled quality as well. These phonation problems are probably caused by increased muscle tone in the larynx, which results in a tighter, narrower glottal opening during speech. Excess loudness variation also was noted in some of the subjects. As in chorea, excessive loudness variation is most likely the result of momentary hyperadduction of the vocal folds during speech. The co-occurrence of both monoloudness and excessive loudness variation in some individuals with dystonia is explained by the unpredictable waxing and waning quality of dystonic muscular contractions in the larynx. Respiration deficits also might be a factor in these loudness changes (see next section).

Respiration

Respiratory problems are not common in dystonia. However, Duffy (2020) suggested that the excessive loudness variation might be due to the effects of dystonia on respiration. This increase in loudness could be caused directly by dystonic movements that involuntarily contract the respiratory muscles during phonation. It also could be caused indirectly by an affected individual attempting to compensate for abnormal respiratory movements. In either situation, the result could be excessive changes in loudness during speech.

Resonance

Hypernasality was present in 11 of Darley et al.'s (1969a, 1969b) 30 subjects with dystonia; however, it was not severe enough to be included in their ranking of speech errors. This low rating suggests that although hypernasality might be present in dystonia, it is most often quite mild.

Key Evaluation Tasks for Hyperkinetic Dysarthria

1. Vowel prolongation is useful in detecting the harsh or strained-strangled vocal quality that can be present in several of the hyperkinetic dysarthrias. It also might be helpful in evoking a vocal tremor, especially when the tremor is mild. In addition, vowel prolongation can be useful in determining pitch and loudness variations that might be caused by involuntary contractions of the oral, laryngeal, and respiratory muscles.

2. Duffy (2020) suggested that alternate motion rates can highlight the irregular articulatory breakdowns and speech rate variations that can occur in the hyperkinetic dysarthrias.

3. Conversational speech and having the patient read aloud might provide the most comprehensive picture of the speech in individuals with hyperkinetic dysarthria. These two tasks can evoke articulatory errors (e.g., imprecise consonants, vowel distortions, prolonged phonemes), prosodic errors (e.g., silences, monopitch, monoloudness, short phrases), phonatory errors (e.g., harshness, excessive loudness variations), and respiratory errors (e.g., sudden inhalations or exhalations) that could occur in the speech of these individuals.

4. Careful observation of the associated involuntary movements is a critical part of evaluating hyperkinetic dysarthria. Each hyperkinetic disorder has its own general pattern of involuntary movements. The following list highlights the primary distinctions of the hyperkinetic movement disorders mentioned in this chapter:

    - Chorea—Characterized by relatively quick, unpredictable, coordinated movements of the limbs, head, face, mouth, and neck; sometimes having a dance-like quality.
    - Myoclonus—Distinguished by brief contractions of a single muscle or body part. These contractions could occur singly, in a repeating irregular pattern, or rhythmically. Unlike tics, myoclonic contractions cannot be consciously suppressed.

- Tic disorders—Motor or vocal behaviors that can be controlled voluntarily until the compulsive desire to perform the behavior becomes overwhelming. Motor tics include eye blinks, shoulder shrugs, and head jerks. Vocal tics include grunting, humming, and barking noises.
- Essential tremor—A benign action tremor that usually affects the hands, arms, or head. Essential tremor results in essential voice tremor when it affects the vocal folds.
- Dystonia—Characterized by sustained, involuntary contractions of muscles in one or more body parts; these contractions often come and go in a waxing and waning pattern. Dystonic movements are usually slower and more prolonged than those seen in chorea.

Treatment of Hyperkinetic Dysarthria

Given the variety of disorders associated with hyperkinesia, it should not be surprising to find an equally diverse number of treatment options. These treatments generally are based on medical or behavioral interventions.

Medical Treatments

Most of the medical treatments for hyperkinetic dysarthria are pharmacologic—specifically, drugs that suppress the involuntary movements that cause the speech deficits. For example, choreic movements and tic behaviors can be reduced by haloperidol or tetrabenazine; myoclonic jerks can be treated with clonazepam or valproic acid. Unfortunately, no drug-based treatment for any of the hyperkinetic movement disorders has proven to be consistently effective for all patients with these disorders. In addition, most of these medications have significant adverse side effects. For instance, haloperidol can cause sleepiness and dystonic movements. It also can cause tardive dyskinesia if it is taken for prolonged periods.

Perhaps the most successful medication for a hyperkinetic disorder is botulinum toxin (Botox) injections, which are used to treat oromandibular dystonia, spasmodic torticollis, spasmodic dysphonia, and several of the other dystonic movement disorders. For example, Sanuki (2023) reported that Botox injections provide significantly improved phonation in most cases of spasmodic dysphonia, especially for patients with the adductor form of this disorder.

Similarly, Sulica (2010) found that Botox was helpful in treating essential voice tremor, although the benefits were not consistent for all patients. By interfering with the transmission of acetylcholine across the neuromuscular junction, an injection of Botox into muscle tissue can greatly reduce dystonic contractions in affected muscles. The injections are usually effective for several months. Although they must be repeated on a regular basis, Botox injections can provide some degree of relief for many patients experiencing these dystonic movement disorders.

In addition to being used in cases of parkinsonism, deep brain stimulation is used to treat several hyperkinetic movement disorders. In fact, it was recognized as a treatment for dystonia before being approved for parkinsonism. In addition to dystonia, deep brain stimulation also has been used to treat essential tremor, as well as severe cases of Tourette's syndrome, although only experimentally. The implantation of the electrode for hyperkinetic disorders is the same as that described in Chapter 8 for parkinsonism, only the location of the probe in the brain is different. For instance, it is placed in the thalamus when treating cases of essential tremor (as opposed to in the globus pallidus for parkinsonism).

Behavioral Treatment for Huntington's Disease

Yorkston et al. (2012) provided useful suggestions for the speech-language pathologist working on the communication needs of patients with Huntington's disease. In the early stages, the clinician usually has little to do because the patient's speech is still quite intelligible. A few individuals might need to work on maintaining normal prosody and optimal rate, but these problems are not common early in the disease.

In the middle stages of Huntington's, working on rate of speech, rhythmic breathing, and relaxation might help intelligibility because patients often rush to complete their utterances before a choreic movement interrupts them. By learning to keep a normal rate of speech, breathing regularly, and staying relaxed, patients can enhance their intelligibility. Clinicians also should make sure that the patient is speaking only on exhalation, not on inhalation. Traditional speech treatment procedures can be tried at this stage, but the complexity of the activities should be simplified. For example, if omitted final consonants and distorted blends are both affecting intelligibility, work only on the one that most impairs understanding. Remember, however, that it can be difficult to identify specific speech errors in patients with Huntington's disease because of their variable hyperkinetic movements.

Although these techniques can enhance verbal communication to some degree, carryover and maintenance of treatment effects begin to become difficult because of the patient's progressive dementia. Consequently, it is important to work closely with caregivers. Yorkston et al. (2012) suggested teaching caregivers a simple sequence of cues that can be used each time a patient's message is not understood:

1. Tell the patient that you don't understand.
2. Look for cues to help you understand the message (e.g., Has something changed in the room? Is it time for something to happen, such as a meal or a television program?).
3. Ask the patient to say it again, exactly the same way.
4. Use a different way of saying it (e.g., Can the patient repeat just the main word of the message or perhaps spell the word?).

In the late stages of Huntington's disease, the patient might be restricted to single-word verbal utterances, and legible writing usually is not possible. Alternative and augmentative communication techniques can be appropriate, but they must be low-tech and not require any new learning. Simple yes–no systems, basic eye-gaze procedures, and alphabet boards might be appropriate. Continued work with caregivers is important throughout the late stages. They need to learn to simplify their communication interactions with the patient. For example, they should ask only one question at a time (preferably a yes–no question) and wait patiently for a response. By sharing these types of strategies with caregivers, clinicians can help them feel more comfortable during interactions with the patient and be more effective communication partners.

Behavioral Treatment for Dystonia

■ Sensory tricks—Duffy (2020) recommended that clinicians encourage patients with dystonia to find and use sensory tricks that can suppress their involuntary movements. Given that some of these sensory tricks can be quite subtle and need not draw undue attention, this can be a relatively easy treatment option. The drawback, however, is that sensory tricks seldom have long-term effectiveness, nor do they work for every patient. Nevertheless, patients with dystonia should be told about sensory tricks if they have not discovered them for themselves.

- Bite blocks—These devices commonly are used by dentists to comfortably stabilize the jaw during oral care procedures. Bite blocks also can be used as a prosthetic treatment for oromandibular dystonia. They probably are most helpful in cases of dystonic jaw closure, jaw deviation, or jaw retraction. Bite blocks are made of rigid plastic or rubber and are available in a variety of sizes and shapes. For dystonia, they often are used in pairs, with one placed on the left and right back molars. Patients bite down on the blocks as needed for conversation or for drinking liquids. Because the teeth are not clinched together and the jaw is stable, more accurate articulatory contacts can be made while speaking. For a few patients, the voluntary biting down on the blocks also seems to suppress the dystonic contractions at least to some degree. Some patients wear them throughout the day. An additional benefit is that bite blocks are usually not visible because of their small size and their placement in the back of the mouth (Page & Siegel, 2017).

- Easy onset of phonation—There is some anecdotal evidence that easy-onset procedures can lessen involuntary movements affecting the larynx during speech but only in mild cases. The overall goal of the treatment is to have the patient make softer glottal closures while phonating. In the first step, the patient is asked to exhale while producing a smooth, quiet sigh. Once these soft sighs are produced consistently, the patient is asked to gently initiate a prolonged phonation of an open vowel such as /a/. These prolonged phonations are then shaped into words that begin with vowels or a breathy consonant such as /w/. The ultimate goal is to build toward easy phonations of sentences and during conversational speech.

Behavioral Treatment for Tic Disorders

Pharmacological approaches are used frequently to treat tics, and they have been shown to be successful in reducing the severity of the behaviors. Antipsychotic and noradrenergic medications are often prescribed. However, many of these drugs have negative side effects, such as weight gain, fatigue, and slowed mental processing, and they rarely fully suppress tics (Peterson et al., 2016). To supplement and sometimes even to replace medications, a number of behavioral interventions have been developed to help individuals control their urges to tic. The proponents of behavioral treatments recognize that tics have a neurogenic basis, but they also believe that behavioral factors contribute to the frequency and intensity of the tics. For example, when feeling stressful pre-tic urges, affected individuals know that these uncomfortable tensions will be immediately relieved when the tic is performed. This creates a classic situation of negative reinforcement that rewards performing the tic (i.e., the aversive stimulus is removed as soon as the tic is acted out, thereby increasing the likelihood that the tic behavior will be performed again in response to the next pre-tic urge). In general, behavioral treatments for tics attempt to break this reinforcement cycle. Here are some of these techniques:

- Habit reversal training—This procedure teaches individuals to use competing voluntary behaviors to prevent or interrupt tics. For example, when someone with rapid eye-blink tics feels a pre-tic urge, he or she will voluntarily blink slowly before the tic occurs, perhaps keeping the eyes closed for a second or two. The ultimate goal is for the individual to replace tics with controlled movements that are fully voluntary. In a large group study of children with Tourette's syndrome, Piacentini et al. (2010) compared a habit-reversal procedure (augmented with relaxation) to a control treatment that combined supportive psychotherapy and education about the disorder. The results showed that the behavioral procedures resulted in significant reductions in tics for most of the participants when compared to the controls. Moreover, the reductions still were evident 6 months afterward. Yu et al. (2020) and Viefhaus et al. (2020) reported comparable findings in their studies of habit reversal training.
- Relaxation therapy—In this approach, individuals first learn why relaxation can help reduce tics. They then learn to move through a series of progressive muscle relaxation exercises whenever they feel a pre-tic urge emerging or when they are in settings associated with the appearance of tics. Several studies have examined the effectiveness of relaxation therapy (as well as supportive psychotherapy and mental imagery) as treatment for the tic behaviors in Tourette's syndrome (Bergin et al., 1998; Peterson & Cohen, 1998). Overall, the results were inconclusive. For instance, the relaxation technique used by Bergin et al. (1998) taught the subjects to assume a relaxed bodily posture that included lightly closed eyelids, a relaxed neck and limbs, and no eye movements. Although some of the initial findings were positive, there were no long-term reductions in tic behaviors. Hollis et al. (2016) found no evidence that relaxation therapy by itself is an effective treatment for

tics. However, Peterson et al. (2022) found that this technique could be helpful when used as part of a more comprehensive treatment approach, such as how Piacentini et al. (2010) combined it with habit reversal training.

- Exposure response prevention—These exercises teach individuals to resist and tolerate the pre-tic urges that precede the tic behaviors. By consciously suppressing the pre-tic sensations, the subsequent urge to tic also is reduced. Studies that have examined this technique found that most participants were able to reduce their tic behaviors successfully (Meidinger et al., 2005; Frank & Cavanna, 2013). A recent study reported that exposure response prevention (delivered via the Internet) was effective in reducing tics in 221 children with Tourette's syndrome (Andrén et al., 2022).

- Comprehensive Behavioral Intervention for Tics (CBIT)—This is an expanded version of habit reversal, where competing response training is combined with five other behavioral treatments of tics (e.g., awareness training, contingency management). In their systematic review of the literature, Hollis et al. (2016) found that CBIT reduced tics at clinically significant levels. Similarly, Espil et al. (2022) reported that CBIT produced positive results in a group of 80 adolescents with Tourette's syndrome up to 11 years posttreatment.

Summary of Hyperkinetic Dysarthria

- Hyperkinetic dysarthria is actually a collection of separate dysarthrias, each associated with a hyperkinetic movement disorder. For example, there is the hyperkinetic dysarthria of chorea and the hyperkinetic dysarthria of dystonia. In both cases, the dysarthria is caused by involuntary movements that interfere with voluntary attempts at speech. However, because the involuntary movement patterns of the various hyperkinetic movement disorders are different, the effects of each disorder on speech production are different.
- Many, but not all, of the hyperkinetic movement disorders are associated with damage to the basal ganglia. Some of the disorders have no known cause, such as Tourette's syndrome and organic tremor.
- The speech characteristics of hyperkinetic dysarthria vary according to which movement disorder is disturbing speech production.

- The most common treatment for hyperkinetic dysarthria is drug-based. However, certain behavior-based treatment procedures have been found to help some individuals with hyperkinetic dysarthria.

Study Questions

1. Define hyperkinetic dysarthria in your own words.
2. Why is it appropriate to describe hyperkinetic dysarthria as actually being a collection of separate dysarthrias?
3. What is one reason why the function of the basal ganglia is not well understood?
4. How are the involuntary movements of chorea different from those of dystonia?
5. What are the symptoms of Huntington's disease?
6. Why do individuals with chorea sometimes have voice stoppages, unexpected inhalations, and sudden exhalations?
7. Describe fully the cause of tic disorders.
8. What is the most common hyperkinetic movement disorder?
9. What are sensory tricks, and with which hyperkinetic movement disorder are they most closely associated?
10. How are most hyperkinetic movement disorders treated?

Chapter 10

Mixed Dysarthria

Definitions of Mixed Dysarthria
Neurologic Basis of Mixed Dysarthria
Causes of Mixed Dysarthria
- Multiple Sclerosis
  - *Speech Characteristics of Multiple Sclerosis*
- Multisystems Atrophy
  - *Shy-Drager Syndrome*
  - *Progressive Supranuclear Palsy*
  - *Olivopontocerebellar Atrophy*
- Amyotrophic Lateral Sclerosis
  - *Speech Characteristics of Amyotrophic Lateral Sclerosis*
- Wilson's Disease
  - *Speech Characteristics of Wilson's Disease*
- Friedreich's Ataxia

Treatment of Mixed Dysarthria
- Augmentative Communication for Patients With ALS

Summary of Mixed Dysarthria
Study Questions

Definitions of Mixed Dysarthria

Mixed dysarthria can occur when neurologic damage extends into two or more parts of the motor system. As the following quote from Singh and Kent (2000) shows, the speech characteristics of mixed dysarthria are a combination of the characteristics found in the single (or pure) dysarthrias. The location and extent of the neurologic damage determines which characteristics of the pure dysarthrias appear in a particular diagnosis of mixed dysarthria. Weismer's (2007) quote discusses the rationale for how mixed dysarthrias are labeled.

> [A] type of motor speech disorder that is a combination of two or more pure dysarthrias; the neuropathology is varied, depending on the types of dysarthria that are mixed; causes frequently include multiple strokes or neurological diseases; speech disorders are varied and dependent on the types of pure dysarthria that are mixed. (Singh & Kent, 2000, p. 147)

> "Mixed" is a designation for dysarthrias that result from damage to two or more [areas of the motor system]. For example, both upper and lower motor neuron lesions are typical of ALS in fully developed form. The dysarthria in these cases is referred to as a mixed flaccid-spastic type. Another example is multiple sclerosis (MS) in which lesions are typically found in the cerebellum and upper motor neuron. When a dysarthria exists in these cases, it is said to be a mixed spastic-ataxic type. (Weismer, 2007, p. 68)

Neurologic Basis of Mixed Dysarthria

Prior chapters of this book each examined one of the pure dysarthrias, in which a patient's neurologic damage is restricted to a single anatomical portion of the motor system. For example, pure flaccid dysarthria occurs when the neurologic damage is confined to the lower motor neurons. In other words, the damage does not extend to the upper motor neurons, cerebellum, basal ganglia, or other portions of the nervous system. The damage affects only the lower motor neurons. Similarly, in pure ataxic dysarthria, the neurologic damage is confined to the cerebellum or the cerebellar control circuits. It does not extend to the lower motor neurons, the cerebral hemispheres, or other areas of the nervous system.

Realistically, however, the neurologic damage resulting from strokes, head injuries, degenerative and infectious diseases, and tumors often crosses anatomical boundaries and affects various components of the motor system simultaneously. For instance, it is not unusual for a single brainstem stroke to affect both upper and lower motor neurons because portions of these neurons are located in the brainstem. (Upper motor neurons course down through the brainstem to synapse with the lower motor neurons in the cranial and spinal nerves; the cell bodies of lower motor neurons in the cranial nerves are inside the brainstem.) Consequently, it is very possible that both upper and lower motor neurons can be damaged when a stroke interrupts the flow of blood to a certain part of the brainstem. Assuming that a brainstem stroke causes bilateral damage to the pyramidal and extrapyramidal upper motor neurons and damages the lower motor neurons in the cranial nerves used for speech production, the result will probably be a co-occurrence of flaccid and spastic dysarthria. Such a co-occurrence of two pure dysarthrias is a mixed dysarthria. In this example, it would be described as a flaccid-spastic mixed dysarthria.

An individual with mixed dysarthria will demonstrate at least some of the speech characteristics of two or more of the pure dysarthrias. In the example of flaccid-spastic mixed dysarthria, the individual's speech might simultaneously show evidence of hypernasality and nasal emission (the flaccid dysarthria component), a strained-strangled voice quality from hyperadduction of the vocal folds (the spastic component), and imprecise consonant production (a characteristic that is common to both flaccid and spastic dysarthria). The hypernasality and nasal emission could be the result of damage to the lower motor neurons of the vagus cranial nerve. The strained-strangled voice quality would be caused by bilateral damage to the upper motor neurons of the extrapyramidal system. The imprecise consonant production would most likely be the combined result of lower and upper motor neuron damage. Watch the PluralPlus Mixed Dysarthria Cases 1 and 2 videos of patients with flaccid-spastic mixed dysarthria.

Nearly any combination of the pure dysarthrias can appear in a mixed dysarthria, depending on the severity and extent of the neurologic damage (Darley et al., 1975). As mentioned, a brainstem stroke can cause a flaccid-spastic mixed dysarthria because in this area of the brain the lower and upper motor neurons are in close proximity to each other. Another example of mixed dysarthria might be evident in an individual who experiences a traumatic head injury with damage to both the cerebellum and various cranial nerves. The result could be ataxic-flaccid mixed dysarthria. A further example might be a patient with parkinsonism who has a right hemisphere stroke, causing hypokinetic-unilateral upper motor neuron mixed dysarthria. Finally, Guillain-Barré syndrome might develop in a patient with Huntington's disease, resulting in hyperkinetic-flaccid-mixed dysarthria. Although these examples might seem fanciful, mixed dysarthria is actually quite common. In fact, Duffy (2013) stated that clinicians see more cases of mixed dysarthria than any single pure dysarthria and indicated that mixed dysarthria accounted for 29.9% of all the dysarthrias seen at the Mayo Clinic.

Not only can mixed dysarthria be composed of many different combinations of the pure dysarthrias; the relative prominence of each dysarthria type within a mixed dysarthria can vary significantly from individual to individual. In many instances of mixed dysarthria, one of the dysarthric components will be much more noticeable than the other(s). For example, in a flaccid-spastic mixed dysarthria, the flaccid component (perhaps nasal emission) might be much more evident to a listener than the spastic component (perhaps a strained-strangled voice quality). It also is possible, however, for each component of a mixed dysarthria to be more or less equally prominent. In this instance, using the example of flaccid-spastic mixed dysarthria, the listener would judge the nasal emission and the strained-strangled voice quality to be contributing equally to the dysarthric quality of the speaker's speech.

The relative prominence of one dysarthric characteristic over another is usually the result of the severity and extent of the neurologic damage. When the severity is distributed equally over the affected portions of the motor system, the resulting characteristics of the mixed dysarthria may be equally evident. However, when one part of the motor system is more seriously affected than the other, the dysarthric component associated with the more severely damaged portion usually will be more apparent.

It also is important to note that the relative prominence of one dysarthric component over another can change over time. For example, ALS is a progressive motor neuron disease that often first affects lower motor neurons, resulting in flaccid dysarthria. As the disease progresses, however, it eventually begins to affect upper motor neurons as well, causing a flaccid-spastic mixed dysarthria. Initially, in this mixed dysarthria, the flaccid components are more noticeable than the spastic components. In time, however, the upper motor neuron damage usually becomes equal to that of the lower motor neurons. At this stage, the spastic component of the dysarthria may be as evident as the flaccid component. ALS is discussed in greater detail later in this chapter.

Both beginning and experienced clinicians often find it difficult to make a correct diagnosis for mixed dysarthria. This could be due to the multiple speech deficits that are usually present in mixed dysarthria as compared with a pure dysarthria. Although often challenging, it is important to diagnose mixed dysarthria as accurately as possible. A precise diagnosis can provide helpful information about a patient's disorder. To illustrate this, Duffy (2005) used the example of a patient with a diagnosis of Parkinson's disease who presented with a hypokinetic-ataxic mixed dysarthria. Because ataxic dysarthria is not a symptom of Parkinson's disease, the presence of this mixed dysarthria indicated one of two possibilities about the diagnosis of Parkinson's disease: Either the diagnosis was incorrect or the patient had something in addition to Parkinson's disease. The presence of ataxic dysarthria in the patient's speech indicated that further diagnostic work was needed. Situations such as this can occur frequently and demonstrate the value of having a good understanding of all the dysarthrias.

Causes of Mixed Dysarthria

Mixed dysarthria can be caused by various disorders, including single or multiple strokes, brain tumors, traumatic head injuries, degenerative diseases, and infectious diseases. In fact, any disorder that can damage two or more parts of the motor system has the potential to cause mixed dysarthria. Because so many conditions have this potential, a complete listing of all the disorders and combinations of disorders that can lead to this dysarthria would be very long indeed. Accordingly, the following paragraphs concentrate on several specific diseases that typically have mixed dysarthria as a prominent symptom. Remember, however, that numerous other conditions can cause mixed dysarthria in addition to those discussed here.

Multiple Sclerosis

Multiple sclerosis (MS) is a progressive disease in which the myelin covering of axons in the CNS degenerates (Figure 10–1). MS is the most common of the demyelinating diseases. It occurs in about 100 per 100,000 of the population in the United States and United Kingdom. MS usually first appears when individuals are in their 30s. Women are affected more frequently than men, by a ratio of almost 3 to 1 (Dobson & Giovannoni, 2019). The cause of MS is unknown. Both genetic and environmental factors seem to influence its occurrence, and some evidence suggests that it might be

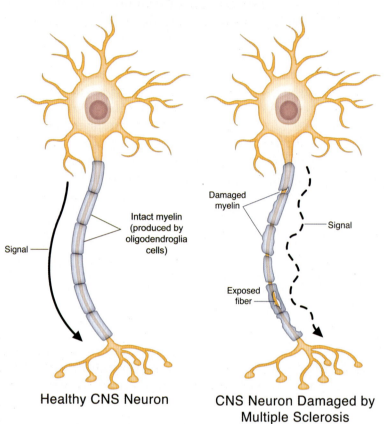

FIGURE 10–1. Multiple sclerosis causes damage to a nerve's myelin sheath in the central nervous system.

an immunologic disorder that is triggered by a virus. Other conditions associated with the disease include obesity and smoking. Reduced exposure to ultraviolet light and low vitamin D also are risk factors, both of which help explain why MS is most prevalent in cold and temperate areas; it is uncommon among individuals living in the tropics.

The myelin degeneration in MS usually appears first as small points of inflammation along axons. Eventually, the inflammation can increase in severity until the myelin and cells that produce it (oligodendrocytes) are destroyed. The amount of affected myelin along the length of an axon can range from only a millimeter to a few centimeters. MS does not directly damage the axon. Instead, the axon remains intact, but the destruction of the protective myelin affects its function by slowing or stopping its ability to conduct neural impulses.

MS can affect myelin almost anywhere in the CNS. Not only can MS affect the myelin-rich white matter areas of the CNS, but it also can attack myelin-covered gray matter in the CNS. Consequently, MS can occur in the brainstem, cerebellum, cerebral hemispheres, and spinal cord. Some patients have symptoms that suggest focal MS lesions in only one area of the brain. For example, a patient's main symptoms might be ataxic in nature, suggesting a focal cerebellar lesion. In contrast, other patients can demonstrate a diffuse collection of symptoms, indicating widespread MS lesions in multiple areas of the CNS.

The symptoms of MS are diverse. Medical textbooks often mention that no two patients with MS have exactly the same symptoms. The general symptoms of MS can be grouped into several broad categories. Visual disturbances are among the most common symptoms of individuals with this disease. These disturbances include double vision (diplopia), impairment of color perception, decreased visual acuity, and impaired central vision (central scotoma). The motor disturbances of MS include chronic feelings of tiredness; weakness in the limbs, particularly in the legs; painful spasticity in the extremities, again particularly in the legs; disturbances of sphincter muscle control; and dysarthria. The sensory disturbances include numbness, burning sensations, itching, and tingling. Depression is another common symptom in MS. A mild dementia might be noted in some advanced cases of the disease. Benedict et al. (2020) reported declines in visual and verbal memory, new learning, and cognitive processing speed, especially in patients over 50 years of age.

The course of MS varies significantly from patient to patient. Wiederholt (2000) described four different ways in which MS progresses:

- About 40% of patients go through relapsing and remitting occurrences of their symptoms during the early stages of the disease. After several years, however, this changes, and the patients begin a slow but steady progression of increasingly more significant symptoms.
- About 20% to 30% of patients maintain a relapsing and remitting course of MS for the duration of their lives. They never experience a steadily progressive increase in symptoms.
- About 10% to 20% of patients have a steady progression of symptoms from the onset of the disease.
- About 20% of patients experience only one or two relapsing and remitting occurrences of symptoms during their lifetimes. They are otherwise unaffected by the disease.

Speech Characteristics of Multiple Sclerosis

Although MS can cause many types of dysarthria, most individuals with this disease do not demonstrate obvious motor speech deficits. In their study of 168 individuals with MS, Darley et al. (1972) found that 59% of their subjects had no evidence of dysarthria, as would be judged by an average listener. Moreover, 28% had an overall deviant speech rating of only "minimal." Taken as a whole, these data indicate that 87% of the subjects with MS had adequate speech or only minor speech deficits. Nonetheless, some of the subjects who were judged to have essentially normal speech still demonstrated a few problems, primarily in controlling the loudness of their voice and in producing a clear phonation. Darley et al. summarized their findings by stating that the most prominent speech errors in individuals with MS are deficits of loudness control, harshness, and impaired articulation. Table 10–1 lists all the speech deficits noted in the study by Darley et al. Piacentini et al. (2014) reported similar results in their qualitative study of 163 patients with MS. Their result showed that 35% of the patients reported having dysarthria, nearly all of them with mild severity. Duffy (2020) suggested that ataxic and spastic dysarthria are the two most common pure dysarthrias found in MS and that ataxic-spastic is the most common mixed dysarthria associated with this

TABLE 10–1 The 10 Most Common Speech Production Errors in Individuals With Multiple Sclerosis

Rank	Speech Production Errors
1	Impaired loudness control
2	Harsh voice quality
3	Imprecise articulation
4	Impaired emphasis (scanning speech)
5	Decreased vital capacity
6	Hypernasality
7	Inappropriate pitch level
8	Breathiness
9	Increased breathing rate
10	Sudden articulatory breakdowns

Source: From "Dysarthria in Multiple Sclerosis," by F. L Darley, J. R. Brown, and N. P. Goldstein, 1972, *Journal of Speech and Hearing Research, 15*, p. 236. Copyright 1972 by American Speech-Language-Hearing Association. Reprinted with permission.

disease. Duffy also mentioned that MS has the potential to cause nearly any type of pure dysarthria and most combinations of mixed dysarthria. Given that MS can affect so many different portions of the nervous system, it should not be surprising that there can be numerous types of dysarthria associated with it.

Multisystems Atrophy

Multisystems atrophy is another progressive condition that can cause mixed dysarthria. It is not a single disorder, however. Multisystems atrophy actually is a group of degenerative disorders, some of which include parkinsonian symptoms. Although there are many disorders classified under the multisystems umbrella, only three are discussed in this textbook—Shy-Drager syndrome, progressive supranuclear palsy, and olivopontocerebellar atrophy.

Shy-Drager Syndrome

Shy-Drager syndrome is a degenerative neurologic disease that primarily affects neurons in the brainstem, basal ganglia, and autonomic nervous system. It usually first appears in middle age and progresses slowly. It is often fatal several years after its onset. Dementia does not develop in patients with Shy-Drager syndrome, and its cause is unknown.

Parkinson-like symptoms are among the many signs of this syndrome. Bradykinesia, akinesia, and rigidity can all be present, but tremor is often absent or could be greatly reduced in intensity as compared with the other forms of parkinsonism. Unfortunately, L-dopa and other antiparkinson drugs are ineffective in treating the parkinsonian symptoms of this disorder. Some of the other symptoms of Shy-Drager syndrome include mild spasticity in the limbs, face, or neck, which is caused by bilateral degeneration of upper motor neurons. Damage to the autonomic nervous system can result in problems in regulating blood pressure, impotence, bowel and bladder dysfunction, and poor pupillary reaction to light. This syndrome also can affect the cerebellum or its control circuits and cause signs of ataxia.

Several combinations of mixed dysarthria have been noted in cases of Shy-Drager syndrome (Linebaugh, 1979). The three most common are spastic-ataxic-hypokinetic, hypokinetic-ataxic, and ataxic-spastic mixed dysarthria. These combinations of dysarthria reflect neurologic degeneration in the basal ganglia, upper motor neurons, and cerebellum.

Progressive Supranuclear Palsy

This rare multisystems degenerative disorder has a prevalence of 6 per 100,000 population (Coughlin & Litvan, 2020). Progressive supranuclear palsy causes the degeneration of neurons in the brainstem, basal ganglia, and cerebellum. It often appears in late middle age and follows a steadily progressive course. The cause of progressive supranuclear palsy is unknown. The median age of onset is 63 years (Gerstenecker et al., 2019), and it is usually fatal after 6 to 7 years. The most characteristic symptom is the gradual restriction of voluntary eye movements, which makes it difficult for these patients to walk down stairs, read, or notice objects in their peripheral vision. Problems with walking and neck rigidity are the most obvious parkinsonian symptoms of this disease, but a generalized rigidity can develop as the disease progresses. Bilateral upper motor neuron involvement can result in mild spasticity of the limbs, face, or neck. Other symptoms of progressive supranuclear palsy include dementia, dysphagia, involuntary closing of the eyelid (blepharospasm), and dysarthria.

Several types of dysarthria are associated with progressive supranuclear palsy. In summarizing the findings of several studies, Duffy (2020) stated that hypokinetic, spastic, and mixed hypokinetic-spastic dysarthria are the most common dysarthrias in this disease. In addition, he reported that ataxic dysarthria also can be present in progressive supranuclear palsy, frequently in conjunction with either hypokinetic or spastic dysarthria.

Olivopontocerebellar Atrophy

This disorder causes the gradual deterioration of neurons in the inferior olivary nucleus, pons, and cerebellum. The inferior olivary nucleus is a collection of neuron-cell bodies in the brainstem near the cerebellar peduncles.

Olivopontocerebellar atrophy is a rare disease, and the cause is unknown. Familial links have been clearly established in some cases. This disorder usually occurs when individuals are in their 30s or 40s. The symptoms include ataxic disturbances of balance, uncoordinated movements of the arms and legs, tremors, numbness in the extremities, muscle spasms, problems with bowel and bladder control, and dysarthria. Involuntary choreic movements and mild dementia have been noted in some individuals. Olivopontocerebellar atrophy has no cure; it progresses quite slowly and leads to death about 15 years after the onset of symptoms in familial cases and after 6 years in sporadic cases.

Because various areas of the brain are affected by this disease, the dysarthria associated with it is most frequently of the mixed type. It could have components of ataxic, spastic, flaccid, or hypokinetic dysarthria (Duffy, 2020), although little research has been conducted into the speech deficits of this disorder.

Amyotrophic Lateral Sclerosis

ALS is a disease that results in the progressive degeneration of motor neurons (Figure 10–2). Its cause is unknown. The prevalence of ALS is between 4.1 and 8.4 per 100,000 population worldwide, but these numbers vary according to geographical location. It can develop in individuals as young as 20 or as old as 90; however, the median age of onset is between 51 and 66 years (Longinetti & Fang, 2019). Men are affected more frequently than women by a ratio of 2 to 1. There are two primary subdivisions of ALS: familial

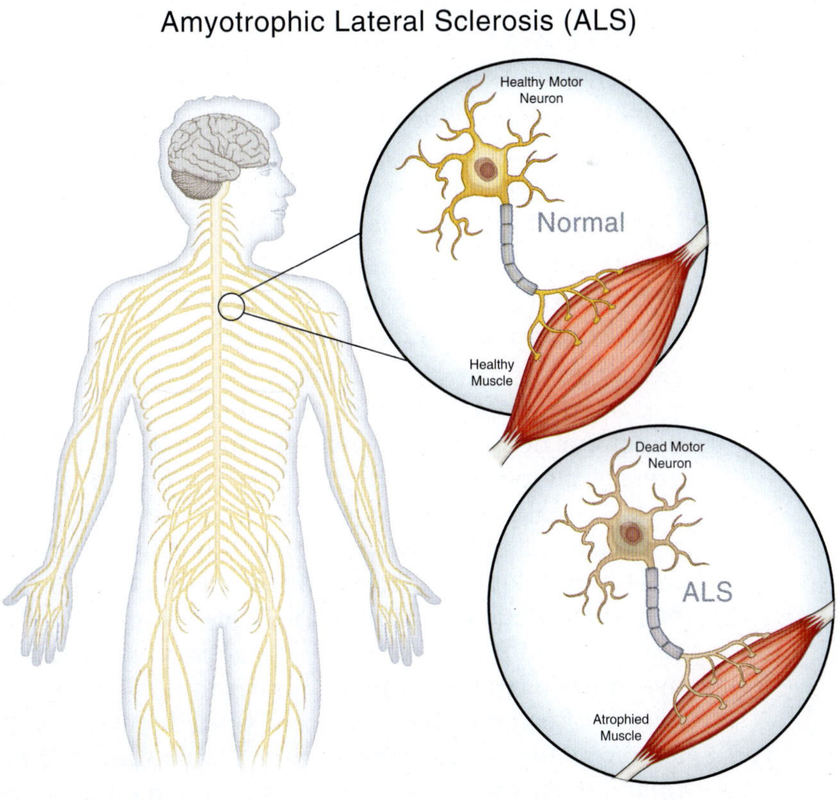

FIGURE 10–2. Amyotrophic lateral sclerosis causes the death of upper and lower motor neurons.

ALS (10% of cases) and sporadic ALS (90%). In nearly all patients, this disease is relentlessly progressive and is fatal within the first few months or years after onset, although 10% survive for about 10 years or longer. Most patients die from complications of pneumonia and respiratory failure.

ALS can affect motor neurons in any of four areas of the motor system—in the spinal nerves at the point where they join the spinal cord (the anterior horn cells of the spinal cord), in the cranial nerves where they join the brainstem (the cranial nerve nuclei), in the upper motor neurons of the corticospinal tracts, and in the upper motor neurons of the corticobulbar tracts. Depending on which motor neurons are affected first, patients with ALS initially might demonstrate one of the four possible clusters of symptoms listed here:

- Patients with spinal nerve involvement will demonstrate weakness in their arms and legs, loss of muscle tone, muscle atrophy, and decreased reflexes.
- Patients with cranial nerve involvement will demonstrate flaccid dysarthria, a reduced gag reflex, tongue atrophy, dysphagia, and facial and oral weakness.
- Patients with involvement of the upper motor neurons of the corticospinal tract will demonstrate weakness and spasticity in the arms and legs, increased reflexes, and painful muscle cramps in the extremities.
- Patients with involvement of the upper motor neurons of the corticobulbar tract will demonstrate spastic dysarthria, hyperactive gag reflexes, facial and oral weakness, and dysphagia.

As mentioned, early in the course of ALS, only one or two of the motor neuron groups will be affected, but as the disease progresses, all four groups are likely to be involved. In the end stages of ALS, weakness and muscle atrophy prevent nearly all attempts at movement. Most patients with ALS maintain their cognitive abilities throughout the course of the disease, although studies indicate that some deficits might be present. For example, Rippon et al. (2006) found that 12 of their 40 patients with ALS showed cognitive impairments on a number of neuropsychologic tests, including deficits of naming, free recall, and word fluency (e.g., "I want you to tell me all the words you can think of that start with the letter 'M'"). In addition, it was once assumed that dementia is not a symptom of this disease, but studies over the past few decades have shown that an associated dementia might co-occur in ALS (Masrori & Van Damme, 2020). Interestingly, bodily sensations, eye movements, and bladder control remain essentially intact in patients with this disease.

Speech Characteristics of Amyotrophic Lateral Sclerosis

The type of dysarthria that appears in individuals with ALS depends on which motor neurons are affected by the disorder. Those with lower motor neuron involvement will demonstrate flaccid dysarthria. Conversely, those with predominantly upper motor neuron involvement will demonstrate spastic dysarthria. When the disease progresses to the point at which both upper and lower motor neurons are affected, patients with ALS will demonstrate flaccid-spastic mixed dysarthria. The pure dysarthrias probably will be present only in the disease's initial, mild stages. The mixed dysarthria condition will predominate throughout most of the disorder.

In their study of 30 subjects with ALS, Darley et al. (1969a, 1969b) found that the subjects' speech errors reflected the combined characteristics of flaccid and spastic dysarthria. The three most prominent errors in their subjects' speech were imprecise consonant production, hypernasality, and harsh vocal quality. The ranking of 10 speech characteristics of their subjects with ALS is presented in Table 10–2.

TABLE 10–2 The 10 Most Common Speech Production Errors in 30 Individuals With Amyotrophic Lateral Sclerosis

Rank	Speech Production Errors
1	Imprecise consonants
2	Hypernasality
3	Harsh voice quality
4	Slow rate
5	Monopitch
6	Short phrases
7	Distorted vowels
8	Low pitch
9	Monoloudness
10	Excess and equal stress

Source: From "Clusters of Diagnostic Patterns of Dysarthria," by F. L. Darley, A. E. Aronson, and J. R. Brown, 1969, *Journal of Speech and Hearing Research, 12*, p. 254. Copyright 1969 by American Speech-Language-Hearing Association. Adapted with permission.

However, a simple ranking of speech errors does not accurately express the devastating effects of ALS on speech production. Perhaps Darley et al. (1975) presented the best description of the speech of an individual with ALS as they concluded their discussion of this disorder:

> The speech gestalt distinctive of ALS, then, consists of grossly defective articulation of both consonants and vowels, often rendering the speech unintelligible; laborious, extremely slow production of words in very short phrases; marked hypernasality coupled with severe harshness and strained-strangled squeezing out of low-pitched tones; and complete disruption of prosody, with monotony suppressing meaningfulness and intervals between words and phrases becoming excessive. (p. 235)

Wilson's Disease

Wilson's disease is another disorder that can cause a mixed dysarthria. It is a very rare hereditary disease that prevents the normal metabolism of dietary copper. Although small amounts of copper are a necessary nutritional mineral, individuals with Wilson's disease cannot metabolize it properly. Instead of being excreted, excessive amounts of copper are deposited in the corneas of the eyes, kidneys, liver, and brain (especially in the basal ganglia). The buildup of copper in these organs produces a unique collection of cognitive, motor, and psychiatric symptoms. The first signs of Wilson's disease usually appear when the affected individuals are in their teens or 20s. The early symptoms include clumsiness, mild decreases in cognitive abilities, and subtle personality changes. The later symptoms include rigidity, bradykinesia, tremor, limb ataxia, dementia, dysphagia, and dysarthria. Dystonic and choreic movements have also been observed in cases of Wilson's disease. The psychiatric symptoms of this disorder—including emotional lability, severe depression, mania, and behaviors having schizophrenic characteristics (Hermann, 2019)—can be significant. Incidentally, the copper deposited in the eye creates a brown-colored ring around the edges of the cornea that can be seen under certain lighting conditions.

Fortunately, effective treatments are available for nearly all individuals with this disease. The most common treatment is oral doses of penicillamine. This drug is able to reduce the copper deposits in the body and often leads to dramatic improvements in all symptoms. However, permanent damage can occur if the treatment is not initiated quickly enough. If left untreated, Wilson's disease can be fatal within 2 or 3 years after the first appearance of symptoms. In untreated cases, death usually occurs from liver failure.

Speech Characteristics of Wilson's Disease

Ever since Wilson's disease was first documented, numerous researchers have commented that dysarthria is a common feature of this disorder (Darley et al., 1975). In fact, dysarthria could be one of the earliest signs of Wilson's disease. Berry, Darley, et al. (1974) conducted the most extensive study of the dysarthria associated with this disease, analyzing the speech of 20 subjects with Wilson's disease. The results showed that reduced stress, monopitch, and monoloudness were the three most prominent speech errors in the subjects. The researchers noted that hypokinetic dysarthria is one of the most noticeable dysarthrias in Wilson's disease. The results also revealed speech errors that were characteristic of ataxic and spastic dysarthria. Overall, the study found that many individuals with Wilson's disease demonstrate an ataxic-spastic-hypokinetic mixed dysarthria, with any one of these three components possibly being more prominent than the others. Furthermore, it was noted that any of these components might appear alone in some individuals with Wilson's disease, reflecting a pure rather than a mixed dysarthria. The ranking of speech errors in this study is presented in Table 10–3.

In an interesting addendum to this study, Berry, Aronson, et al. (1974) followed 10 subjects with Wilson's disease during 3 years of treatment with low-copper diets and penicillamine. The researchers

TABLE 10–3 The 10 Most Common Speech Production Errors in 20 Individuals With Wilson's Disease

Rank	Speech Production Errors
1	Reduced stress
2	Monopitch
3	Monoloudness
4	Imprecise consonants
5	Slow rate
6	Excess and equal stress
7	Low pitch
8	Irregular articulatory breakdowns
9	Hypernasality
10	Inappropriate silences

Source: From "Dysarthria in Wilson's Disease," by W. R. Berry, F. L. Darley, A. E. Aronson, and N. P. Goldstein, 1974, *Journal of Speech and Hearing Research, 17,* p. 175. Copyright 1974 by American Speech-Language-Hearing Association. Reprinted with permission.

obtained pretreatment and posttreatment measures of speech production to measure any changes in the subjects' dysarthria during the treatment period. Although the subjects still had some dysarthric qualities in their speech at the end of the treatment period, significant improvements occurred in nearly all areas of speech production, especially intelligibility. Overall, the improvements were remarkable. Duffy (2020) suggested that changes in speech during the medical treatment of Wilson's disease could serve as an indicator of treatment effectiveness.

Friedreich's Ataxia

Friedreich's ataxia is an inherited, progressive disorder that causes neuron degeneration in the cerebellum, brainstem, and spinal cord (in particular). As mentioned briefly in Chapter 7, this rare disorder first becomes evident when individuals are 10 to 15 years of age (Tai et al., 2018). It is untreatable and usually is fatal within 15 years after the initial appearance of the symptoms. Death is often the result of heart failure or coma. The early symptoms of Friedreich's ataxia are unsteadiness and clumsiness, with ataxia being present in the movements of the arms and legs (Delatycki & Bidichandani, 2019). Mild dysarthria also could be an early symptom. As the disorder progresses, weakness and muscle atrophy become evident in the arms and legs, with most patients eventually losing the ability to walk independently. Visual deficits and sensorineural hearing loss also can occur in the later stages. Dementia develops in some individuals with Friedreich's ataxia.

Although Friedreich's ataxia can cause pure ataxic dysarthria, mixed dysarthria is also common. Joanette and Dudley (1980) found what appeared to be an ataxic-spastic mixed dysarthria in their 22 patients with this disorder. In his discussion of the speech pathology of Friedreich's ataxia, Duffy (2020) suggested that ataxic dysarthria is the most common dysarthria associated with this disease, but other types could be present, especially spastic dysarthria. In addition, he concluded that ataxic-spastic mixed dysarthria is probably the most prevalent of the mixed dysarthrias in this disorder.

Treatment of Mixed Dysarthria

Without doubt, treating mixed dysarthria can be a challenge. There could be so many speech errors that many clinicians are not sure where to start. The general rule in treating mixed dysarthria is to first treat the component that is most severely affecting speech production. As an illustration of this, imagine a patient with flaccid-ataxic mixed dysarthria in which the flaccid characteristics are impairing intelligibility more noticeably than the ataxic characteristics. The first steps of treatment would concentrate on the flaccid elements. Once these had been addressed sufficiently, treatment could then shift to the ataxic characteristics of the dysarthria. However, this is only a general treatment principle, and there will be situations in which it will not be particularly helpful, such as when the various elements of a mixed dysarthria are contributing equally to the patient's speech production difficulties.

When the elements of a mixed dysarthria are affecting speech production equally, Dworkin (1991) suggested that treatment be sequenced according to which of the components of speech production (i.e., respiration, articulation, phonation, resonation, and prosody) are being affected most by the dysarthria. He recommended that errors of respiration be treated first, then resonation, followed by phonation, then articulation, and finally prosody. Thus, if a patient with mixed dysarthria is demonstrating equal measures of monopitch, imprecise consonant production, and hypernasality, the recommended treatment sequence would be resonation first, articulation second, and prosody third.

The reason for completing the treatments in this order is based on how the different components of speech support each other. For example, respiration is addressed first because it is the foundation for all other speech components. Without adequate respiratory support, resonation, phonation, articulation, and prosody are all impaired to one degree or another. For instance, it would be difficult to treat a phonatory problem if a patient's respiration was too weak to create adequate phonation. Likewise, it would impossible to treat many prosodic problems if deficits of resonation, articulation, and so forth had not been addressed beforehand.

In a situation in which there is more than one problem within a single component of speech production, treatment usually should address the most severe problem first. An example of this is a patient who has more than one deficit of prosody, perhaps someone who has very prolonged intervals between syllables and moderately excessive loudness variations. Because both of these are prosodic errors, Dworkin's recommended treatment sequence does not apply. Nevertheless, the most likely treatment choice would be to treat the error that is most affecting the patient's prosody. If the clinician and patient make the judgment that the prolonged syllable interval is the more serious problem, treatment would concentrate on that first. However, this treatment choice assumes that deficits of respiration, resonation, phonation, and articulation have been ruled out as the cause of the prosodic problems.

There will be special exceptions to this rule of treating the most severe error first. For example, a patient might have a strong preference for what needs to be treated initially; perhaps it is something that is personally very annoying or frustrating. Maybe a patient's attention or memory deficit makes working on a particular type of speech production error extremely difficult, but he or she is able to make progress on another type of speech error. In situations such as these, it might be appropriate to choose the less severe speech production deficit for treatment, based on the unique circumstances that might be present.

Augmentative Communication for Patients with ALS

In many of the progressive neurologic disorders discussed in this chapter, the patient will reach the point at which intelligible verbal communication is no longer possible. This will occur for about 75% of individuals with ALS (Saunders et al., 1981) and about 4% of individuals with MS (Beukelman et al., 1985). When verbal speech becomes impossible, the most appropriate option is some type of augmentative communication. Beukelman and Mirenda (2005) described five communicative stages through which a patient with ALS will pass as the disease progresses. For each stage, they discussed the responsibilities of speech-language pathologists working with a person with ALS. Clinicians should remember that there is no typical timetable for when a given patient will move from one stage to another. As mentioned earlier, the full progression of ALS is quite variable, ranging from months to decades. Some patients with ALS will spend weeks or months at one of these stages; others will spend years.

1. No Detectable Speech Disorder. During this first stage, patients and families can be given general facts about the communication deficits associated with ALS. Because of the high likelihood that augmentative communication will be needed eventually, patients should start learning the basics of these systems in this early stage of the disease. For example, patients should learn what communication methods are available and any special features that make them unique. However, Beukelman and Mirenda (2005) cautioned that at this first stage, it might be premature and counterproductive to give too many details about the challenges augmentative communication ultimately will present to a patient with ALS.

2. **Obvious Speech Disorder with Intelligible Speech.** In this second stage, patients begin to demonstrate speech errors that most listeners can easily detect, but their intelligibility remains high. Beukelman and Mirenda (2005) suggested that speech pathologists should become more actively involved in advising a patient and family on how to maximize the intelligibility of the patient's speech. For example, family members should be told about avoiding conversation in noisy settings and how to ensure that listeners understand when a topic of conversation is being changed. It also might be appropriate for a patient to be introduced to voice amplification at this time, if he or she will be speaking in conversational groups. The preliminary steps of assessing and choosing augmentative communication systems should be started at this stage.

3. **Reduction in Speech Intelligibility.** When patients reach this point, their dysarthria is clearly interfering with speech intelligibility. Many of the treatments for flaccid or spastic dysarthria that were presented in Chapters 5 and 6 can help increase or maintain a patient's intelligibility, at least temporarily. For example, speaking with a more open-position mouth, breath group duration, palatal lift, reduced rate of speech, and exaggeration of consonants might be appropriate treatments for a patient's dysarthric deficits. Beukelman and Mirenda (2005) also recommended that augmentative communication systems be in place for patients in this third stage of the disease.

4. **Residual Natural Speech and Augmentative Communication.** In this fourth stage, patients with ALS rely heavily on augmentative communication to supplement their residual intelligible speech. In fact, Beukelman and Mirenda (2005) stated that augmentative communication now becomes the primary method of communication. At this stage, the speech pathologist is involved in assessing the adequacy of the augmentative communication systems, such as determining whether a system is the best match for a patient's remaining motor capabilities or whether the physical position of a system maximizes the patient's ability to use it. Speech pathologists also will be involved in training family members and friends on the best methods of communicating with someone who is using an augmentative communication device.

5. **Loss of Useful Speech.** At this final stage, patients with ALS have lost nearly all of their intelligible speech and depend almost exclusively on augmentative communication systems to make their wants and needs known. In addition to using

sophisticated electronic devices, Beukelman and Mirenda (2005) recommended that a collection of low-tech augmentative procedures also be used to maximize a patient's ability to communicate. These include simple yes–no communication methods, eye-pointing techniques, and eye blinks.

Summary of Mixed Dysarthria

- Mixed dysarthria can occur when damage involves more than one portion of the motor system. For example, when the lower motor neurons and the cerebellum are damaged, the result can be a flaccid-ataxic mixed dysarthria.
- Depending on the extent and location of the neurologic damage, nearly any combination of pure dysarthrias can be the components of a mixed dysarthria.
- Within a mixed dysarthria, it is possible for one of the components to be more noticeable than the other(s).
- There are many conditions that can cause mixed dysarthria, including head injury, stroke, brain tumor, and numerous degenerative or infectious diseases.
- ALS and MS are the two most well-known degenerative disorders that can cause mixed dysarthria.
- The general treatment sequence for mixed dysarthria is to first treat the portion that is contributing most to a patient's speech production deficits.
- If the elements of a mixed dysarthria are contributing equally to the patient's problems, Dworkin (1991) recommended treating the components of speech production in this sequence: respiration, resonation, phonation, articulation, and finally prosody.

Study Questions

1. Define mixed dysarthria in your own words.
2. Describe how multiple strokes could lead to mixed dysarthria.
3. Damage to which anatomical sites would be likely to cause an ataxic-hypokinetic-spastic mixed dysarthria?

4. Why do many clinicians find mixed dysarthria to be a challenge to diagnose?
5. Why can MS result in almost any type of dysarthria?
6. What are the three multisystems atrophy disorders that were discussed in this chapter, and what type of dysarthria can they cause?
7. Describe the four areas of the motor system that can be affected by ALS.
8. What type of mixed dysarthria is most associated with the latter stages of ALS?
9. What is the cause of Wilson's disease?
10. What treatment sequence did Dworkin (1991) recommend when all components of a mixed dysarthria are contributing equally to a patient's speech production errors?

Chapter 11

Apraxia of Speech

Definition of Apraxia of Speech
Overview of the Apraxias
Neurologic Basis of Apraxia of Speech
   The Motor Speech Programmer
Causes of Apraxia of Speech
Speech Characteristics of Apraxia of Speech
   Articulation
   Prosody
   Respiration
   Resonance
   Phonation
Assessment of Apraxia of Speech
Differential Diagnosis of Apraxia of Speech
   Diagnostic Characteristics of Apraxia of Speech
      Primary Clinical Characteristics
      Nondiscriminative Clinical Characteristics
      Clinical Characteristics Usually Found in Other Disorders
      Clinical Characteristics Ruling Out Apraxia of Speech
Additional Diagnostic Considerations
   Differentiating Between Apraxia of Speech and Aphasia
   Differentiating Between Apraxia of Speech and Dysarthria
Treatment of Apraxia of Speech
   General Principles of Treating Apraxia of Speech
   Specific Treatments
      The Eight-Step Continuum Treatment
      Sound Production Treatment
      Darley, Aronson, and Brown's Procedure
      Melodic Intonation Therapy
      PROMPT
Summary of Apraxia of Speech
Study Questions

Definition of Apraxia of Speech

The following definition of apraxia of speech by McNeil et al. (2009) is perhaps the most detailed and complete at the current time. It includes characteristics of this disorder that have been understood for a number of years, as well as a few that are fairly new. The well-known components include traits such as prosodic errors, slow rate of speech, and awkward timing and placement of articulatory movements. It also mentions that listeners might perceive these awkward movements as being phoneme substitutions. In addition, it states that pure apraxia of speech (without a co-occurring aphasia or dysarthria) is rare. Each of these has been a recognized characteristic of apraxia for some time. This definition also contains at least one assertion that could be surprising—that the apraxic speech errors are relatively consistent for both type and location during repeated productions of the same word or phrase.

> Apraxia of Speech is a phonetic-motoric disorder of speech production. It is caused by inefficiencies in the translation of well-formed and filled phonologic frames into previously learned kinematic information used for carrying out intended movements. These inefficiencies result in intra- and interarticulator temporal and spatial segmental and prosodic distortions. It is characterized by distortions of segment and intersegment transitionalization and coarticulation resulting in extended durations of consonants; vowels; and time between sounds, syllables and words. These distortions are often perceived as sound substitutions and as the misassignment of stress and other phrasal and sentence-level prosodic abnormalities. Errors are relatively consistent in location within the utterance and invariable in type. It is not attributable to deficits of muscle tone or reflexes, nor to primary deficits in the processing of sensory (auditory, tactile, kinesthetic, proprioceptive), or language information. In its extremely infrequently occurring isolated form, it is not accompanied by the above listed deficits of basic motor physiology, perception, or language. (McNeil et al., 2009, p. 264)

Because this definition is detailed and complex, it might be helpful to review and paraphrase its key points in a simple list.

1. When our cognitive system selects a word for speech production, the word's phonological representations are combined to form a phonological word "frame." These frames contain the necessary movement patterns needed to

accurately produce the sequence of phonemes in words and sentences.

2. However, these frames need to be transformed into a neural-motor code that can be carried out by the speech musculature. In cases of apraxia of speech, correct phonological frames are poorly transformed into movement patterns for speech.
3. This results in speech that has both timing and movement errors for sounds, syllables, and words.
4. The timing problem causes speech that is slow, with lengthened productions of vowels, consonants, or both.
5. In addition, the timing problem causes pauses between phonemes, syllables, words, and phrases.
6. The movement problem causes distorted productions of vowels and consonants.
7. These distortions can sometimes sound like phoneme substitutions, but they actually are distortions of the correct target sound. (However, real substitutions can occur in apraxia of speech.)
8. These timing and movement problems contribute significantly to prosody errors in connected speech.
9. On repeated utterances, articulation errors in apraxia of speech are generally consistent for type of error (distortion, substitution, omission) and for location.
10. Apraxia of speech errors are not caused by muscle, sensory, or language deficits.

Many earlier definitions of apraxia of speech mentioned that apraxic speech errors are variable from trial to trial. For example, Miller (1986) wrote that, "[Individuals with apraxia of speech] can be said to have difficulty in consistently realizing speech sounds. Sometimes they say a sound or word correctly, and other times they do not" (p. 99). Recent research has suggested that this traditional concept might not be correct. A number of studies have reported that inconsistent articulation errors are more characteristic of patients with phonemic paraphasias than of those with apraxia of speech (McNeil et al., 1995; Shuster & Wambaugh, 2003; Wambaugh et al., 2004). This change to a key traditional characteristic of apraxia of speech has sparked research and discussions (Haley et al., 2018; Haley et al., 2021; Haley et al., 2013; Ziegler et al., 2012). Certainly more studies are needed to examine this and other questions. Until these types of issues are settled, apraxia will remain a rich area of research.

Overview of the Apraxias

Like the dysarthrias, **apraxia** of speech is a neurologic deficit in the production of speech sounds. However, unlike the dysarthrias, the errors in apraxia of speech are not caused by muscle weakness, abnormal muscle tone, reduced range of movement, or decreased muscle steadiness. Rather, the errors in this disorder are caused by a deficit in the ability to accurately sequence the movements needed to produce speech sounds.

As was mentioned in Chapter 1, the term *apraxia* comes from the Greek word *praxis,* which refers to performance of an action. Apraxia literally means without action. In fact, it probably is more accurate to describe this disorder as dyspraxia (which means disordered action) because, strictly speaking, individuals with apraxia of speech are not without movement; they can move their tongue, lips, velum, and other parts of the speech mechanism. Their problem is with the selecting and sequencing of movements needed to produce speech. Because apraxia has become such a common word for describing this disorder, though, it is the one that is used in this chapter.

There are several types of apraxia, of which apraxia of speech is only one subcategory. The two main types of apraxia are ideational apraxia and ideomotor apraxia. **Ideational apraxia** is the inability to make use of an object or gesture because the individual has lost the knowledge (or idea) of the object's or gesture's function. In other words, individuals with ideational apraxia cannot make proper use of an object or gesture because they no longer know its purpose. A patient of Luria's (1972) who had a head injury gave a good example of ideational apraxia when describing an event that occurred in a hospital:

> I was lying in bed and needed a nurse. How was I to get her to come over? All of a sudden I remembered you can beckon to someone and so I tried to beckon to the nurse—that is, move my left hand lightly back and forth. But she walked right on by and paid no attention to my gesturing. I realized then that I'd completely forgotten how to beckon to someone. It appeared I'd even forgotten how to gesture with my hands so that someone could understand what I meant. (p. 45)

Ideational apraxia is an uncommon disorder that can result from damage to the left parietal lobe. It often goes undetected because its symptoms can be masked so easily by an accompanying disorder such as aphasia. It also is difficult to detect because it often resolves quickly when caused by a stroke (Miller, 1986). This disorder has been noted in advanced cases of Alzheimer's disease as well (Cassidy, 2016; Vakkila & Jehkonen, 2023).

The second main type of apraxia is **ideomotor apraxia**. In contrast to ideational apraxia, which is a disturbance in the conception of an object or gesture, ideomotor apraxia is a disturbance in the performance of the movements needed to use an object, make a gesture, or complete a sequence of individual movements; apraxia of speech is one of the ideomotor apraxias. Individuals with ideomotor apraxia have not lost their knowledge of an object's or gesture's function; instead, they have a deficit in the ability to carry out the motor plan needed to use an object or make a gesture. When asked to use a common object such as a toothbrush, an individual with ideomotor apraxia may demonstrate the general pattern of movements required to brush the teeth, indicating that he or she understands the purpose of the toothbrush; for instance, the individual will hold the toothbrush properly and move it toward the mouth. However, the separate movements needed to actually brush the teeth might be out of sequence. Perhaps the up-and-down motion of brushing the front teeth becomes the back-and-forth movement of brushing the molars or vice versa. The individual's attempts to revise and correct these out-of-sequence movements result in tooth brushing that is halting, slow, and awkward.

Ideomotor apraxia has been studied extensively since it was first described in the 1900s, and numerous characteristics of this disorder have been noted. The following is a list of the more well-known symptoms of ideomotor apraxia. It should be noted, however, that these symptoms are likely to be present in cases of pure ideomotor apraxia. When additional motor, language, or cognitive deficits accompany the apraxia, these symptoms might be masked by these other problems and will not necessarily be as evident as these descriptions might suggest.

- Ideomotor apraxia typically affects voluntary movements more often than spontaneous or automatic movements. For example, if asked to wave goodbye on command, an individual with ideomotor apraxia might not be able to successfully sequence the movements needed to accurately complete the action. Even if the action is complete, the overall movements could be effortful and clumsy. However, if the individual were actually leaving a social situation, a goodbye hand wave would be smooth and effortless. Another example of this might involve a movement such as a smile. An individual with ideomotor apraxia might not be able to smile promptly when asked to do so, but a moment later a spontaneous smile might appear without difficulty.

- Movement sequencing is easier when actually manipulating a real object as compared with only pantomiming its use. For example, an individual with ideomotor apraxia will probably be more successful in showing how to drink from a cup when actually given a cup, as compared with only pretending to have one.

- Completing a movement sequence is easier when given a gestural command (imitation), as compared with being given a verbal command. In other words, individuals with ideomotor apraxia might not be able to round their lips when they are asked to do so, but they might be successful when a clinician demonstrates the movement.

- The movement sequencing errors in ideomotor apraxia can sometimes be inconsistent on repeated attempts of the same action. An example of this occurred when one of the author's patients was asked to make the gesture for hitchhiking. Her first attempt resulted in the slow, clumsy formation of a fist. With additional effort, she was slowly able to protrude her thumb to complete the gesture. When asked immediately to do it again, her initial movement was to bring her fingertips together in a pincer-like action, and it again took much effort for her to move her hand into the correct "thumbs up" position.

There are at least three subcategories of ideomotor apraxia. The first is **limb apraxia**. This is the inability to sequence the movements of the arms, legs, hands, or feet during a voluntary action, although the concept behind the action and the general motor plan appears to be accurate. The earlier toothbrush example is an illustration of this type of apraxia. Limb apraxia is most often the result of left hemisphere damage. In a majority of cases, it affects both the right and left limbs, although hemiplegia might hide its effects on one side of the body. This disorder is usually assessed by having the individual pantomime a variety of well-known movements, such as hammering a nail, shaving, putting a key in a lock, and combing hair.

A second subcategory of ideomotor apraxia is **nonverbal oral apraxia**. This type of apraxia is also known as buccofacial apraxia, facial apraxia, orofacial apraxia, or lingual apraxia. As its name implies, nonverbal oral apraxia is a deficit in the ability to sequence nonverbal, voluntary movements of the tongue, lips, jaw, and other associated oral structures. The orofacial movements affected by this disorder might include protruding the tongue, whistling, biting the lower lip, and puffing out the cheeks. When asked to perform tasks such as these, an individual with this type of apraxia might grope for the correct position of the mouth, delay performing the action, only partially complete the movement, or perform the movement slowly and awkwardly. Occasionally, some individuals with nonverbal oral apraxia have trouble performing voluntary movements that are only partially associated with the oral mechanism. For example, they might have trouble taking a deep breath when asked to do so, or they might be unable to swallow on command.

Nonverbal oral apraxia is commonly seen in individuals with left hemisphere damage, and it can often co-occur with aphasia. Although this disorder can be puzzling and even distressing to the patient, it does not affect spontaneous or reflexive orofacial movements, meaning that the individual will still be able swallow while eating, breathe deeply when out of breath, smile at a joke, and make other spontaneous movements of the oral mechanism. Because individuals with this disorder usually are able to perform these important automatic oral movements without difficulty, nonverbal oral apraxia is usually thought to have little clinical significance (Wertz et al., 1991). For the speech-language pathologist, this type of apraxia is of interest primarily because it can co-occur with the third subcategory of ideomotor apraxia, apraxia of speech.

Apraxia of speech is a deficit in the ability to select and time-sequence the motor commands needed to correctly position the articulators during the voluntary production of phonemes. Because most speech is a voluntary motor task, apraxia of speech can have serious effects on a patient's ability to communicate verbally. Apraxia of speech is a disorder specific to the movements needed to produce phonemes, and it can co-occur with limb or nonverbal oral apraxia. The distinction between nonverbal oral apraxia and apraxia of speech is evident in the names of these two disorders. Nonverbal oral apraxia is a disturbance in the sequencing of oral movements that are unrelated to speech production, such as licking the lips, blowing out a match, and moving the tongue from side to side. Apraxia of speech, as already stated, is a timing and movement disturbance in the oral-pharyngeal muscles during speech production. Although it is common for an individual to have a co-occurrence of these two apraxias, both can appear more or less separately. For example, some individuals might have apraxia of speech but not have obvious symptoms of nonverbal oral apraxia, and other individuals could have nonverbal oral apraxia but not obvious symptoms of apraxia of speech.

Apraxia of speech is usually caused by damage to the left frontal lobe, especially when the damage occurs near Broca's area.

Because apraxia of speech is so often associated with damage to the left hemisphere, cases of pure apraxia of speech are actually quite rare. In the majority of cases, apraxia of speech co-occurs with aphasia, usually Broca's aphasia. Ziegler et al. (2022) found that 44% of patients with chronic aphasia also had some degree of apraxia of speech. In addition, it is common for it to co-occur with unilateral upper motor neuron dysarthria (Duffy, 2020). The simultaneous occurrence of these disorders can make it difficult for a beginning clinician to separate the motor speech errors of apraxia from the language and articulation errors of a co-occurring aphasia and dysarthria. The remainder of this chapter is designed to make it easier for the inexperienced clinician to identify the symptoms of apraxia of speech and treat them appropriately.

Neurologic Basis of Apraxia of Speech

As with so many of the functions of the CNS, the method by which motor commands are sequenced for speech is not well understood. This lack of understanding is a reflection of how complex the task of motor speech programming is. For instance, sequencing the motor commands of speech production requires input from many different areas of the brain. The language centers provide the linguistic information that is to be spoken, including the phonemes that need to be sequenced correctly. The basal ganglia, cerebellum, and thalamus provide motor and sensory input about the planned speech movements. The limbic system and right hemisphere provide information about the emotional context of the intended utterance. All of this information needs to be integrated and processed so that an intended message can be transformed into a sequence of neural impulses that will contract the appropriate muscles at the correct times. The enormity of this task was illustrated by Darley et al. (1975), who calculated that for every second a person is talking, a total of 140,000 neuromuscular contractions and relaxations occur in the speech production muscles. The neurologic "mechanism" thought to control this remarkable process is called the motor speech programmer.

The Motor Speech Programmer

The **motor speech programmer** is a neural network in the brain that sequences the motor movements needed to produce speech accurately. It is thought to accomplish this by first analyzing the linguistic, motor, sensory, and emotional information of a planned speech act. It obtains this information through its many neural connections with the cognitive, language, emotional, and motor planning areas of the brain and then sequences that information into a neural code that represents the muscular contractions needed to produce the phonemes, words, and phrases in the intended utterance. If that neural code is sequenced correctly and is received intact at the neuromuscular junction, the muscles will contract in the proper sequence, and the resulting speech will be produced fluently. Included in this neural code are the stress and intonational patterns that are used to convey the communicative intent of the speaker. Through the sensory information received by the motor speech programmer, the code also reflects the immediate circumstances of the oral-motor structures. For example, if the speaker is chewing gum, the neural code must be modified accordingly to ensure clear articulation of the utterance despite the material in the mouth.

Although numerous writers have described the models of the motor speech programmer (Darley et al., 1975; Duffy, 2020; Guenther, 2016; McNeil et al., 2009), it is actually a rather nebulous cerebral structure. Unlike Broca's and Wernicke's areas, the motor speech programmer has not been precisely localized in the brain. Research has indicated that it resides near the **perisylvian area** of the left hemisphere (Figure 11–1), where it has close associations with the language and motor centers of the brain. The motor

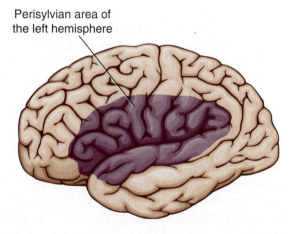

FIGURE 11–1. The perisylvian area of the left hemisphere. Damage to this area (particularly the anterior portion of it) is often associated with apraxia of speech.

speech programmer has especially close ties to the ventral premotor cortex (which includes Broca's area). This area seems to play an important role in transforming the neural code into an accurate representation of the intended utterance. The motor speech programmer is a remarkable entity. It gives humans the ability to rapidly and accurately sequence speech movements, and when it is damaged, apraxia of speech can be the result.

Causes of Apraxia of Speech

Disorders that damage the motor speech programmer have the potential to cause apraxia of speech. In practical terms, this means that apraxia of speech is the result of injury to the perisylvian area of the left hemisphere of the brain. Although the left perisylvian area is the most common site of a lesion in cases of apraxia of speech, it is not the only one. Injuries to the insula and the basal ganglia also have been associated with apraxia of speech. The specific conditions known to cause apraxia of speech include stroke, degenerative disease, trauma, and tumor, with the most frequent cause being stroke. In a retrospective study at the Mayo Clinic of 155 quasi-randomly selected cases, Duffy (2005) reported that strokes caused 49% of the cases of apraxia of speech. Most of these strokes affected the perisylvian area of the left hemisphere, primarily the frontal and parietal lobes. Some cases of apraxia of speech also involved damage to the temporal lobe, but in each of these instances, frontal- or parietal-lobe damage was present as well.

The second most common cause of apraxia of speech in the Mayo study (in 27% of the cases) was degenerative disease, including Alzheimer's disease, primary progressive aphasia, and Creutzfeldt-Jakob disease. Although diseases such as these are usually associated with diffuse brain damage, Duffy (2005) indicated that at least in the early stages, their effects can be focal and result in apraxia of speech or other disorders associated with distinct lesions.

Trauma was the third most frequent cause of this disorder in the Mayo study, resulting in 14% of the cases. Surgical trauma in the left frontal lobe was the most common type of trauma that resulted in apraxia of speech. Aneurysm repair, removal of a tumor, and hemorrhage evacuation were some of the surgical procedures noted in the study. Although a few cases of closed head injury also resulted in apraxia of speech, most were the result of the more focal trauma of surgery. The remaining cases were caused by tumors in the left frontal lobe, seizure disorder, undetermined etiology, or multiple causes, such as a left hemisphere stroke and dementia. Duffy

(2005) cautioned about generalizing the results of this retrospective study to the overall population because it was not a scientific sample of patients.

Speech Characteristics of Apraxia of Speech

Studies of apraxia of speech have revealed many speech production errors that are unique to this disorder. Most researchers agree that apraxia of speech is a disorder primarily of articulation and prosody, although instrument-based studies have revealed problems in other areas of speech production, such as respiration. In general, individuals with this disorder are often described as having speech that is slow, labored, and halting. They could demonstrate instances of articulatory groping, which are trial-and-error attempts at finding the correct articulatory positions for target phonemes. Such groping might be especially noticeable at the beginning of an utterance or word. Traditional definitions of apraxia of speech indicate that these individuals frequently will be inconsistent in their speech errors, perhaps making one error on a first attempt at a word and then making a different error on a second attempt. However, as mentioned at the beginning of this chapter (McNeil et al., 2009), some research suggests that the articulation errors in apraxia of speech are fairly consistent for both location and type on repeated trials. In severe cases of this disorder, affected individuals might be nearly mute because they cannot voluntarily produce any sounds. Others with severe apraxia of speech might be able to produce only a few "stock" (stereotypic) phrases.

The following sections present the specific characteristics of apraxia of speech. Not all of these characteristics will be present in the speech of each individual with this disorder. Several factors influence how many aspects will be present. For example, the severity of the apraxia will influence how many of these characteristics might actually appear in a patient's speech (Miller, 1986). Individuals at the most severe and mild ends of the disorder typically will demonstrate fewer examples of these characteristics than persons in the moderate range of severity. A co-occurring disorder, such as aphasia or dysarthria, also can affect how many of these characteristics will be present because the additional condition could mask the apraxic speech errors. An example of this could be when a patient has severe Broca's aphasia and moderate apraxia of speech. The aphasia will restrict the patient's verbal expression so severely that few, if any, opportunities will arise for a demonstration of the apraxic speech errors. Watch the PluralPlus Apraxia of

Speech Case 1 and 2 videos for examples of patients with moderate and severe cases of this disorder.

Articulation

Articulation errors are the most common problem in apraxia of speech. These errors arise from deficits in the patient's ability to smoothly sequence the oral movements needed to produce fluent speech. The following list of articulation errors is a compilation of those reported by Darley et al. (1975), Duffy (2020), and Wertz et al. (1991) in individuals with apraxia of speech. It is not a complete listing, but it concentrates on the errors most likely to be encountered by the typical clinician.

- Substitutions of one phoneme for another might appear to be more common than distortions, omissions, additions, or repetitions. However, instrumentation or narrow transcription of these substitution errors often reveals that they actually are distortions of the target phoneme.
- Placement errors are the most frequent type of substitution error, followed in order of commonality by manner, voicing, and oronasal errors.
- The substitution of a voiceless phoneme for a voiced phoneme is more common than a substitution of a voiced phoneme for a voiceless.
- Some substitution errors can be perseverative (Viking is pronounced "Viving").
- Fricatives and affricates generally are more often in error than stops, nasals, semivowels, or vowels.
- Consonant clusters are more likely to be in error than single consonants, and single consonants are more often in error than vowels.
- The position of a phoneme within a word does not always determine whether it will be in error. When it does, however, phonemes in the initial position of a word are more likely to be in error than those in the medial or final position.
- Phonemes that appear infrequently in speech are more often in error than frequently appearing phonemes.
- Articulation is more accurate on real words as compared with nonsense words.
- Articulation errors are more common on multisyllabic words than on single-syllable words.

- The farther the distance between the points of articulatory contact, the higher the rate of articulation errors. For example, "puh-tuh-kuh" is typically more difficult than "puh-puh-puh."
- The voluntary production of speech (e.g., describing a picture) is more difficult than automatic speech (e.g., counting 1 to 20) or reactive speech (e.g., swearing), although this might not always be true for individuals with severe apraxia of speech. As mentioned previously, these individuals could have apraxia to such a significant degree that they are nearly mute for all types of speech.
- Sounds produced with the lips or with the tongue on the alveolar ridge are often easier to produce than sounds produced elsewhere.

Prosody

The prosody of individuals with apraxia of speech is frequently abnormal, but it is not exactly clear how apraxia affects prosody. Wertz et al. (1991), Duffy (2020), and others have offered several possibilities for how apraxia and prosody interact. One possibility is that prosody is disrupted by the patients' attempts to compensate for the articulatory errors in their speech. For example, the slow speech rate and equal syllable stress that are noted in apraxia of speech could be the result of patients purposely trying to maintain the best articulation possible while speaking. Another possibility is that the many articulation deficits of this disorder make normal prosody extremely difficult. For instance, a patient who repeatedly stops an utterance, revises the articulation of a target sound, and then restarts the utterance will have great difficulty maintaining normal prosody. A final possibility for the interaction of apraxia and prosody is that prosodic errors are an integral part of apraxia of speech, just as the articulatory errors are. In other words, the prosodic errors in apraxia of speech are the direct result of a patient's motor sequencing deficit and not merely a reaction to it. Duffy (2020) indicated that instrumentation studies have provided some evidence for this third possibility, although the other two might be true as well. Wertz et al. (1991) concluded that, "prosodic disturbances probably reflect the effects of the primary motor deficit as well as the effort to compensate" (p. 69). The following is a list of the more obvious prosodic errors that might be present in patients with apraxia of speech:

- The rate of connected speech is slower than normal.
- Equal stress is often placed on all syllables in an utterance.

- Silent pauses can occur at the initiation of a word, between syllables, or between words. These pauses might be the result of articulatory groping or because the syllables and words are being produced individually, instead of being produced with the normal fluent blending of one syllable into another.
- The normal variations of pitch and loudness in utterances might be reduced.

Respiration

Apraxia has been shown to affect respiration. As mentioned previously, some individuals with apraxia of speech might not be able to take a deep breath on command. When attempting this task, they will demonstrate the same halting, effortful movements seen in their articulation. Instrumentation has revealed more subtle respiration deficits in patients with apraxia. In a study of five subjects with apraxia, Keatley and Pike (1976) found that the amount of abnormal respiratory function was related to the severity of the subjects' apraxia of speech. The most severely affected subject demonstrated abnormal performance on 10 of the 13 measures of respiratory function. It is important to note, however, that these were voluntary respiratory tasks and that reflexive respiration is not affected by apraxia.

Resonance

Hypernasality and hyponasality are seldom significant problems in apraxia of speech. Although little research into the velar movements of individuals with this disorder has been conducted, the few studies that have been completed suggest that disturbed resonance in apraxia of speech seldom reaches the point at which it is perceptible. For example, Itoh et al. (1979) found that although velar movements can be inconsistent on repetitive movements, the general movement pattern of the velum usually remains within normal limits. This might be why Haley et al. (2019) found that "nasal ambiguity" made up only 5% of the distortion errors produced by their patients with both aphasia and apraxia of speech.

Phonation

Individuals with mild or moderate apraxia of speech seldom demonstrate isolated deficits of phonation. When they do have difficulties with phonation, it is usually in conjunction with an articulation problem. For example, there might be a delay in initiating the phonation of the first phoneme in a word, but this delay is part of the individual's groping for the correct articulatory position for that phoneme. In some cases of severe apraxia of speech, however, patients will have significant deficits in their ability to phonate. For instance, they might be unable to complete such a "simple" phonatory task as prolonging a vowel. In these instances, the patients' motor speech sequencing is so disrupted that both voluntary and spontaneous attempts at phonation are unsuccessful. Duffy (2020) reported that such severe phonatory deficits usually occur in the first 1 or 2 weeks after the onset of the apraxia. If they continue beyond this period, such phonatory deficits usually indicate the presence of a co-occurring disorder, such as severe aphasia or akinetic mutism.

It is rare for a patient with apraxia of speech to have phonatory deficits that are more severe than accompanying articulatory problems. Individuals with severe apraxia of speech who cannot prolong a vowel very likely have co-occurring articulatory problems that are just as severe as their phonatory deficits. However, Marshall et al. (1988) described a remarkable patient who was an exception. Their patient had a left hemisphere stroke after the repair of a cerebral aneurysm. The patient's resulting speech and language deficits did not resemble those of Broca's aphasia, dysarthria, or apraxia of speech. Rather, he demonstrated the omission of syllables and words and had numerous stuttering-like dysfluencies. For example, when greeted by someone he had seen only once before, he said, "Face mem [remember], not name mem [remember]." Eventually, it was determined that the patient had a laryngeal apraxia that prevented the normal integration of phonation with the other components of speech production, especially articulation. The accuracy of this diagnosis was confirmed when the patient was taught to use an electrolarynx. With this device providing the voicing for his speech, he communicated normally, using correct articulation, syntax, and grammatical morphemes. Sieron et al. (1995) reported a similar case of laryngeal apraxia in a 51-year-old patient who demonstrated aphonia and disrupted respiration only while speaking. All other respiratory, speech, and language abilities were intact.

Assessment of Apraxia of Speech

Patients in whom apraxia of speech is suspected need to be thoroughly assessed with a motor speech evaluation such as that in Appendix 3–1. All items on the evaluation should be administered, not just those related to apraxia of speech. However, while conducting the motor speech evaluation, clinicians will want to pay particular attention to those tasks that provide especially useful diagnostic information for this disorder, including the following:

- One common assessment procedure for apraxia of speech is the **sequential motion rate (SMR)** task, especially as compared with the patient's performance on the **alternating motion rate (AMR)** task. Many individuals with mild or moderate apraxia of speech can complete the AMR task accurately because it involves only one movement sequence with only one place of articulatory contact. However, they will be unable to complete the SMR task as accurately because it requires the sequencing of multiple articulatory positions in three different locations within the mouth. A difference in their performance on these two tasks might be evident.
- Conversational speech and reading aloud are particularly useful tasks for determining the effects of the apraxia on prosody, as well as for highlighting pauses and prolonged transitions between words and phrases. Note also the intrusion of a schwa during pauses in connected speech.
- Repeating words of increasing length (e.g., fan–fancy–fantastic) can be especially difficult for some patients with apraxia of speech.
- Reading or repeating low-frequency, multisyllabic words in isolation or in sentences also can be difficult for these patients.

Differential Diagnosis of Apraxia of Speech

Once the assessment is completed, the clinician must analyze the results to determine the kinds of errors that are present in the patient's speech. This is perhaps the most important part of diagnosing apraxia of speech. The analysis must be complete and correct because the patient's speech errors need to be compared with the errors that are most closely associated with apraxia. The diagnosis can be made only when it is determined that a significant number of the patient's speech errors match those known to occur in apraxia of speech.

Diagnostic Characteristics of Apraxia of Speech

In their review of apraxia of speech treatment studies, Wambaugh et al. (2006a) developed four categories of behaviors to determine which participants in the studies had been correctly diagnosed. By matching the written descriptions of the studies' participants to the behaviors listed in these categories, Wambaugh and colleagues were able to estimate the accuracy of the diagnoses in the original studies. Clinicians also can use these four categories to assist in the diagnosis of their patients. The first category, primary clinical characteristics, contains those behaviors that (as a whole) are almost exclusively found in individuals with apraxia of speech. The second category, nondiscriminative clinical characteristics, contains those behaviors that often can be observed in apraxia of speech but also are found in other disorders. The third category contains behaviors that usually are found in disorders other than apraxia of speech. The fourth category consists of behaviors that rule out the presence of apraxia of speech.

Primary Clinical Characteristics

The following six behaviors are indicative of apraxia of speech when, as a group, they are present in a patient's speech:

- The patient demonstrates prosody abnormalities.
- The patient has a slow speech rate characterized by lengthened productions of vowels, consonants, or both.
- The patient has a slow speech rate with pauses between phrases, words, syllables, or phonemes. These pauses might often be filled with a schwa.
- The patient produces consonants and vowels that are distorted.
- The patient has phoneme substitutions that are distorted.
- The patient demonstrates articulation errors during repeated utterances that generally are consistent for type of error (omission, distortion, substitution) and for location.

Nondiscriminative Clinical Characteristics

The following behaviors are only suggestive of apraxia of speech when they are found in a patient's speech because they also can be found frequently in other disorders, such as fluent aphasia. By themselves, these behaviors should not be used to make the diagnosis of apraxia of speech.

- The patient has short periods of error-free speech.
- The patient's automatic, overlearned speech (e.g., counting 1 to 10) is produced better than propositional speech (e.g., describing the prior day's activities).

- The patient self-corrects errors and shows other signs of error awareness.
- The patient has difficulty initiating speech.
- The patient's speech errors increase as word length increases.
- The patient has perseverative errors or movements.
- The patient demonstrates articulatory groping, either visually, audibly, or both.

Clinical Characteristics Usually Found in Other Disorders

The following behaviors are more likely to be found in other disorders and therefore should not be used to make the diagnosis of apraxia of speech.

- The patient demonstrates a difference between expressive and receptive speech and language abilities.
- The patient has transposition errors on phonemes or syllables.
- The patient has anticipatory articulation errors.
- The presence of limb apraxia or nonverbal oral apraxia does not necessarily indicate a diagnosis of apraxia of speech.

Clinical Characteristics Ruling Out Apraxia of Speech

These three behaviors are exclusionary characteristics; they do not occur in the speech of patients with apraxia of speech. Their presence in a patient's utterances indicates that apraxia of speech would not be the correct diagnosis.

- The patient demonstrates a fast rate of speech.
- The patient has a normal rate of speech.
- The patient demonstrates normal prosody.

Clinicians can use these four categories of behavioral characteristics to assist in the diagnosis of apraxia of speech. After carefully analyzing the patient's speech characteristics through a motor speech evaluation and comparing them with the items in these four diagnostic categories, the following guidelines can be used to determine whether apraxia of speech is the likely diagnosis.

- A patient demonstrating all six of the primary characteristics has a high probability of having apraxia of speech.

- A patient primarily demonstrating the nondiscriminative characteristics and most of the primary characteristics has a moderate probability of having apraxia of speech.
- A patient primarily demonstrating the four characteristics associated with other disorders has a low probability of having apraxia of speech.
- A patient demonstrating any of the "ruling out" characteristics does not have apraxia of speech.

Additional Diagnostic Considerations

Before making the final diagnosis of apraxia of speech, it is important to rule out other conditions that can cause movement difficulties similar to those seen in apraxia. Brookshire (2015) discussed four such conditions. The first is muscle weakness, which can produce slow, labored movements in affected body parts. Such effortful movements could sometimes resemble the movements of apraxia. The first step in making the differential diagnosis between weakness and apraxia is determining which movements are affected. When muscle weakness is the cause of the movement difficulty, all movements of the affected body part will reflect the weakness. However, in cases of apraxia, the problem exists only with the voluntary movements of the affected body part; automatic and spontaneous movements usually will be performed normally. In a case of true apraxia of speech, for example, the patient might be able to spontaneously produce a very clear "hello" when greeting a clinician at the beginning of a treatment session. But later, in the middle of the treatment session, the patient's voluntary attempts to say "hello" might be filled with distorted or substituted phonemes, revisions, or other apraxic errors. If the patient's articulation errors were the result of weakness, all attempts at saying hello would show evidence of the imprecise articulation.

Sensory loss is the second condition that needs be examined carefully before confirming a diagnosis of apraxia. Brookshire (2015) noted that sensory loss does not necessarily cause a movement disorder, but it can contribute to slowed or clumsy movement of an affected body part. For example, sensory loss in oral structures can contribute to imprecise articulation of speech sounds, as anyone who has had local numbing for dental treatment can attest. When there is sensory loss in suspected cases of apraxia, it is important for the clinician to determine whether the movement difficulties are caused by the sensory loss or the apraxia. As in cases of muscle weakness, Brookshire indicated that when sensory loss is contributing to a movement deficit, the problem will be present in both volitional and automatic actions. When caused by apraxia, it will, for the most part, be present only in volitional actions.

A comprehension deficit is the third factor that must be ruled out in suspected cases of apraxia. The clinician needs to be sure that what appears to be an apraxic error is not actually the patient's inability to understand the instructions for the task. To determine whether the inability to complete the task is due to apraxia or poor comprehension, Brookshire (2015) suggested that the clinician demonstrate the target movement for the patient and ask questions about the movement, such as, "Am I drinking from a glass?" or "Am I rounding my lips?" If the answers to the questions are correct, the clinician can assume that the patient understands the task and has knowledge of what is represented by the movements. Any movement difficulties noted during the patient's subsequent attempts at the task can be presumed to be unrelated to a comprehension deficit.

Incoordination is the fourth condition that can sometimes be confused with the movement difficulties of apraxia. When individuals show signs of incoordination, such as in cases of cerebellar ataxia, they have movements that are slow and awkward. Although they usually do not have problems sequencing the individual steps of a movement, their clumsy movements sometimes mimic the halting, effortful movements seen in apraxia. To rule out incoordination in suspected cases of apraxia, Brookshire (2015) once again suggested that clinicians determine whether the movement difficulty is present only in voluntary movements or whether it is seen in all movements, both voluntary and automatic.

Differentiating Between Apraxia of Speech and Aphasia

In addition to distinguishing the errors of apraxia of speech from those of such conditions as muscle weakness and sensory loss, clinicians often need to distinguish between apraxia of speech and aphasia. At least three situations present difficulties for clinicians making a differential diagnosis between these two disorders. The first is making a diagnosis between a patient with pure apraxia of speech and a patient either with aphasia alone or with aphasia and apraxia of speech. As mentioned at the beginning of this chapter, apraxia of speech can appear without any co-occurring aphasia. When it is present without aphasia, it is said to be pure apraxia of speech. Although pure apraxia of speech is very rare, clinicians might encounter it occasionally. To determine whether a patient has pure apraxia of speech or aphasia (either with or without an accompanying apraxia), it is important to remember that in pure apraxia of speech, the patient's auditory comprehension, reading, and writing will be largely unaffected by whatever caused the apraxia. This means that these three language modalities will be far more functional than the patient's verbal expression ability, which will demonstrate the articulation and prosody deficits of apraxia of speech. In contrast, aphasia will affect all four language modalities to one degree or another. The candidates for a diagnosis of pure apraxia of speech are patients who demonstrate the motor sequencing errors of apraxia of speech and have unaffected auditory comprehension, reading, and writing abilities. Only careful diagnostic testing of speech and language abilities will identify patients with pure apraxia of speech.

The second situation that clinicians might find especially challenging is distinguishing between the errors of apraxia of speech and the literal paraphasic errors of aphasia. Literal paraphasic errors are the incorrect placement of one phoneme or more into a word. These errors most often are heard in individuals with fluent aphasia and, accordingly, are thought to be caused primarily by damage to Wernicke's area. In most instances, literal paraphasic errors consist of the transposition of phonemes or syllables in a word, the addition of extra phonemes to a syllable, or the substitutions of phonemes or syllables (Brookshire, 2015). At first glance, apraxia of speech and literal paraphasias can appear to be nearly identical because they both seem to involve a few of the same phoneme-based errors. A closer examination, however, can reveal definite distinctions. Kent (1976) described a number of differences between apraxic errors and literal paraphasias:

- Patients with apraxia of speech often have anterior brain damage and right hemiparesis. Patients with aphasia who produce literal paraphasias often have posterior brain damage and do not have hemiparesis.
- Patients with apraxia of speech usually have a co-occurring Broca's aphasia. Patients who produce literal paraphasias usually have Wernicke's or conduction aphasia.
- Patients with apraxia of speech usually have disturbed prosody, often because they are frequently stopping or slowing their speech as they search for correct articulatory positions. Patients with aphasia usually produce their literal paraphasic errors in a flow of speech that has normal prosody.
- Patients with apraxia of speech might have difficulty initiating speech because they are searching for the correct articulatory

position of the first word in an utterance. Patients with aphasia who produce literal paraphasias typically do not have as much trouble initiating an utterance.

- The phoneme and syllable substitutions in apraxia of speech are usually close to the intended sounds. For example, a /b/ might be substituted for a /d/. The substitutions in literal paraphasias can be far off target from the intended sounds, such as a nasal consonant being used in place of a stop consonant, or perhaps even a vowel being substituted for a consonant.

The following are several additional factors to consider when attempting to distinguish apraxia of speech from literal paraphasias (McNeil et al., 2009).

- Phoneme distortions often are present in cases of apraxia of speech; they are rare in the speech of patients with literal paraphasias.
- Self-initiated efforts at fixing articulation errors usually do not result in improvements in apraxia of speech. In cases of literal paraphasia, these self-repair efforts often can result in improved articulation.
- In apraxia of speech, patients often have prolonged transitions when moving from phoneme to phoneme and from word to word (even when the words are articulated correctly); they also often prolong vowels in multisyllabic words and sentences. Patients with literal paraphasias demonstrate much more normal movement transition times in their speech.
- An overall slow speech rate for phrases and sentences is found in cases of apraxia of speech, even when the words are produced correctly. In cases of literal paraphasias, the speech rate is within normal limits during error-free utterances.
- When patients with apraxia of speech attempt to increase their speech rate, phoneme production errors also increase, often quite noticeably. Patients with literal paraphasias usually can increase their speech rate and maintain accurate phoneme production.

Keeping these distinctions in mind, a thorough analysis of a patient's errors should reveal those that are apraxic and those that are literal paraphasias, at least in a majority of instances. But even the most knowledgeable clinician will not be able to identify every error correctly. It might be best to look primarily for a strong trend one way or the other when trying to determine whether a patient's phoneme-based errors are caused by apraxia or fluent aphasia.

The third challenging diagnostic situation is distinguishing apraxic speech errors from the nonfluent language errors of Broca's aphasia. This can be an especially difficult task for several reasons. One is that there is little anatomical difference between sites of lesion for apraxia of speech and Broca's aphasia. Although Broca's area is not the exclusive site of lesion for either disorder, lower frontal lobe damage is frequently associated with both conditions. As a result, information on the site of lesion is usually not helpful in determining whether a patient's errors are primarily caused by apraxia or Broca's aphasia. Another reason it is difficult to tell these two disorders apart is that they co-occur so frequently. Most individuals with apraxia of speech also have Broca's aphasia. This results in the general descriptions of both disorders often being similar. Words such as *nonfluent, effortful, halting,* and *disturbed prosody* have been used to describe the speech of individuals with either disorder. Ultimately, it can be difficult in many cases to tell precisely how many of a patient's errors are the result of apraxia or of Broca's aphasia. Sometimes, the best a clinician can do is assess a patient's speech and language abilities as completely as possible and then make an estimate as to the severity of the apraxia in comparison to the Broca's aphasia. If one condition is so severe as to mask the other, the clinician might want to take Rosenbek's (1978) advice that, "diagnosis of some patients with severe apraxia [and aphasia] may have to wait until the outcome of therapy is determined" (p. 193). In other words, it might be necessary to wait until treatment of the more obvious disorder reveals the hidden disorder.

Differentiating Between Apraxia of Speech and Dysarthria

Beginning clinicians also might find it difficult to separate the errors of apraxia of speech from those of dysarthria. A key to successfully accomplishing this task is a careful examination of the patient's speech and comparison of those results with the characteristics of both disorders. With a little experience, accurately distinguishing the errors of these two disorders is not as challenging as it might seem, as shown by the following.

- The speech errors in apraxia tend to increase as word length and complexity increase. The speech errors in dysarthria usually are fairly constant irrespective of word length and complexity.
- In apraxia of speech, muscle range of motion, tone, coordination, and strength are within normal limits. At least one

of these muscle qualities is impaired in nearly all cases of dysarthria.
- Apraxia of speech primarily affects articulation and prosody. Dysarthria can affect respiration, phonation, and resonance, in addition to articulation and prosody.
- Apraxia of speech can result in articulatory groping, usually on the first phoneme of a word. Effortful searching for articulatory positions is unusual in dysarthria.
- Apraxia of speech usually occurs after damage to the perisylvian area of the language-dominant hemisphere. Dysarthria, in contrast, can be the result of damage to such diverse parts of the nervous system as upper and lower motor neurons, the cerebellum, and the basal ganglia.
- Apraxia of speech co-occurs much more frequently with aphasia than dysarthria does.
- Patients with apraxia of speech often produce automatic speech and emotional speech with few errors. Patients with dysarthria typically demonstrate the same speech errors regardless of whether an utterance is overlearned or emotional in nature.

Treatment of Apraxia of Speech

Nearly all treatments for apraxia of speech are behaviorally based procedures that help affected individuals improve their ability to select and sequence speech sounds correctly. Unlike some of the treatments for dysarthria, prosthetic and medical interventions for apraxia of speech are rare. Most well-known treatments use intensive one-on-one sessions in which the clinician and patient work on a sequence of tasks that progress from simple to complex verbal productions of target words and phrases. The treatment sessions for apraxia of speech tend to be time-intensive, repetitive, and highly structured. Because of this, a patient's first impression of these treatments can be negative. However, there is a significant amount of evidence indicating that treatment for apraxia of speech can be effective, particularly if an accompanying aphasia is not too severe (Ballard et al., 2015; Munasinghe et al., 2023; Wambaugh, 2021; Wambaugh et al., 2006a, 2006b). This section of the chapter examines the general concepts underlying apraxia treatment. It also presents the individual steps of several treatment programs.

These steps are presented primarily to provide an idea of how the treatment sessions within a given program might be conducted. If you are preparing to treat individuals with apraxia of speech, you are encouraged to seek out the original sources.

General Principles of Treating Apraxia of Speech

Darley et al. (1975) stated that the goal of treating apraxia of speech is to help the patient relearn the motor sequences needed to produce phonemes accurately. Most researchers who have studied apraxia treatment have described the general principles that are important in helping their subjects relearn speech movements (Darley et al., 1975; Duffy, 2020; McNeil et al., 2017; Rosenbek et al., 1973; Wambaugh et al., 2006a, 2006b; Wertz et al., 1991). The similarity of these principles from writer to writer is striking. Their overall agreement suggests that a core set of factors actually can facilitate the relearning of speech movements. The following list is a collection of six such principles that seem to be essential to managing apraxia of speech.

- Not all individuals with apraxia of speech are appropriate candidates for treatment. Duffy (2020) indicated that some patients with severe aphasia and apraxia of speech might be too aphasic to benefit from apraxia treatment. If a patient's language impairments are so severe that functional speech production is impossible, what will be the benefit of treating the apraxia? In this situation, it might be best to postpone the apraxia treatment until the patient's language abilities improve sufficiently to allow for better speech production. If the language abilities do not improve to this degree, apraxia treatment would not be appropriate. Perhaps the therapy time would be better spent on continued language treatment or enhancing nonverbal communication skills through the use of gestures and augmentative communication procedures.
- Patients and families need to understand the characteristics of apraxia and the rationale for the treatment tasks. Wertz et al. (1991) stressed the importance of counseling patients and families about the nature of this disorder and the treatment process. They reported that it can be especially important to help patients and families understand the reasons behind the treatment tasks clinicians ask the patients to complete. For example, patients and families need to know why treatment

usually begins with syllables or short words, why there is so much repetition, and why progress could be slow.

- Repetitive and intensive drill work is an essential part of most treatment programs. To relearn the motor sequences of intelligible speech, patients with apraxia of speech need to practice and rehearse the movements of speech production over and over again. The repetitive nature of this treatment is largely a consequence of the brain injury—individuals with such an injury typically need to work harder and longer than those without a brain injury to relearn a task (Rosenbek et al., 1973).

- The treatment should be sequenced carefully so that the patient is able to maintain a high success rate. This means that patients begin with easy activities and progress to more difficult ones only when they are able to continually be accurate on the tasks. Wertz et al. (1991) said that the success rate in treatment could vary. For example, a typical patient will make many more errors in the very beginning of a treatment program than later, when they are more familiar with a task. In this situation, what constitutes an adequate success rate for the beginning of treatment will differ from what will be acceptable later in treatment.

- Patients should learn to monitor their own speech. The importance of this is stressed by numerous writers (Duffy, 2020; Rosenbek et al., 1973; Wertz et al., 1991). It is a great asset for individuals with apraxia of speech to be able to listen for their own errors and self-correct them. Feedback from the clinician can facilitate this ability in many patients. When the clinician gives information on what is an acceptable production of a target syllable, word, or phrase, patients are better able to judge what is correct or incorrect. It is not unusual, however, to find many patients who can make accurate judgments about their verbal productions without help from the clinician.

- Treatment should concentrate on functional and useful words as soon as possible. Rosenbek et al. (1973) noted that because patients with apraxia of speech have lived most of their lives using verbal communication normally, it is important that they begin speaking meaningful words as early in a treatment sequence as possible. Although recognizing that some treatment needs to begin at the single-phoneme level, Wertz et al. (1991) stated that meaningful stimuli are more reinforcing than nonsense words and that it is easier for patients to judge the accuracy of their productions when real words are being spoken.

Finally, a few words need to be said about principles of motor learning and apraxia of speech treatment. These principles have been well understood for some time, having been applied to athletics, occupational tasks, and other settings for decades. They have been shown to facilitate (a) the acquisition of new movements, and (b) the adaption of previously mastered movements to new but related actions. Two examples of motor learning principles are massed practice (many repetitions of a desired movement within a single session) and distributed practice (fewer repetitions per session, but many sessions over time). Research has shown that massed practice (also known as blocked practice) is the quickest way to gain a new skill. However, distributed practice is better at ensuring that the skill is maintained over time. Motor learning principles also have shown that the long-term result is even better when distributed practice is combined with task variability, such as adding real-world tasks or settings each time the new movement is practiced.

Principles of motor learning have been incorporated into apraxia of speech treatments since the 1970s. McNeil et al. (2017) noted, for example, that early apraxia of speech studies regularly recommended intensive and repetitive work over numerous sessions. Motor learning principles are still being incorporated into treatment studies today. In their review of apraxia of speech treatments since 2012, Munasinghe et al. (2023) found 19 studies that incorporated some aspect of motor learning into treatments or analyses of the results.

Specific Treatments

A number of specific treatments for apraxia of speech have been developed over the past few years. In their review of apraxia treatment research, Wambaugh et al. (2006a, 2006b) divided these procedures into five categories, based on a treatment's theoretical rationale and the types of therapy activities used in the procedure.

- Articulatory kinematic treatments concentrate on improving the timing and placement of articulatory movements through modeling, positioning of articulators, and repetition. Examples of articulatory kinematic procedures include the Eight-Step Continuum (Rosenbek et al., 1973) and the Sound Production Treatment (Wambaugh & Nessler, 2004), both of which are discussed later in this chapter.
- Rate and rhythm procedures assume that apraxia of speech is primarily the result of articulatory timing errors. By controlling the rate and rhythm of a patient's speech, these treatments

attempt to restore the natural patterns of articulatory movements (Aichert et al., 2021; Jungblut et al., 2014). Rate and rhythm treatments include using a metronome to set the pace of verbal production (Dworkin et al., 1988) and using computers to present stimuli at desired rates (Southwood, 1987).

- Alternative and augmentative communication procedures are usually recommended when the patient's apraxia of speech is so severe that it prevents useful verbal communication. When speech production is this impaired, the clinician works with the patient to create a collection of procedures that meet the individual's day-to-day needs. For instance, drawing, pantomime, and writing might all be combined into a comprehensive communication system for a specific patient (Fawcus & Fawcus, 1990; Yorkston & Waugh, 1989).

- In intersystemic facilitation and reorganization treatment, a patient's stronger methods of communicating are used to assist the production of verbal speech. Raymer and Thompson (1991) combined the verbal production of a word with gestural equivalent, and Skelly et al. (1974) combined speech with Amer-Ind gestures.

- Other types of apraxia treatment do not easily fit into any of the prior four categories. For instance, McNeil et al. (1976) looked at the effects of relaxation; Florance et al. (1980) examined conversational skills.

In reviewing these procedures, Wambaugh et al. (2006a, 2006b) found that there were 30 published studies of articulatory kinematic treatments, 7 of rate and rhythm treatments, 8 of alternative and augmentative communication, 8 of intersystemic reorganization treatments, and 5 studies in the "other" category. Although their analysis indicated that the overall quality of the studies was weak (e.g., few replications, limited internal controls, overreliance on expert opinion), a significant majority of the participants showed measurable improvements in their speech production. The authors concluded that, "Taken as a whole, the AOS [apraxia of speech] treatment literature indicates that individuals with AOS may be expected to make improvements in speech production as a result of treatment, even when AOS is chronic." They also stated that, "The strongest evidence for this conclusion exists for treatments designed to improve articulatory kinematic aspects of speech production" (Wambaugh et al., 2006b, p. lxiii). Follow-up reviews of apraxia of speech research also found that the articulatory kinematic approaches continue to have the best outcomes (Ballard et al., 2015; Munasinghe et al., 2023; Wambaugh, 2021).

This is not to say that the other procedures were ineffective, just that their reviews of the literature found more consistent positive effects when articulatory kinematic treatment activities were used.

The following sections describe a number of these apraxia of speech treatments in more detail. To one degree or another, each of them incorporates the general principles of apraxia treatment mentioned previously. The choice of which procedure to use with a given patient depends on several factors. One is the patient's preference. If a patient is not comfortable with the procedures in a treatment program or has doubts about a program's effectiveness, progress will probably be less than optimal. For example, some patients will enjoy the melody-based drills in melodic intonation therapy (MIT); others will not. Some patients will permit the clinician to perform the "hands-on" manipulations of their oral structures as part of the PROMPT program; others will not. Determining a patient's preference is sometimes a trial-and-error process, and clinicians need to be willing to modify or drop a treatment procedure that is not working with a particular patient.

Another factor in choosing one of these techniques is the severity of the apraxia. Some programs seem to concentrate on the more severely involved patients (e.g., PROMPT, MIT); others might be appropriate for patients with milder concerns because of the ease with which certain steps can be skipped or modified (e.g., Sound Production Treatment, Eight-Step Continuum). Familiarity with numerous treatment programs and procedures will facilitate the clinician's choice of which treatment to use with different severity levels.

Finally, the clinician's preference can be a factor in determining which program will be used. All clinicians develop a predilection for certain treatment techniques. Sometimes this preference is based on what best suits an individual's clinical style; sometimes it is just the result of learning which is the more effective treatment procedure. Clinicians need to be convinced of a particular treatment's effectiveness, just as patients do. This knowledge of what works best is acquired partly by reading about the programs and partly by gaining practical experience with them.

The Eight-Step Continuum Treatment

This articulatory kinematic procedure was developed by Rosenbek et al. (1973). It is an eight-step sequence of structured activities that moves the patient from repeating target phonemes with the clinician to independent productions of utterances in role-playing situations. One key element of this treatment is integral stimulation—a procedure developed in the 1950s as an articulation treatment for children. It requires the patient to carefully watch the clinician's face while listening to him or her verbally produce a target word. The combined presentation of a verbal and visual model can significantly enhance an apraxic patient's own attempts at a verbal production. In the Eight-Step Continuum Treatment, often the clinician directly cues the patient to "Watch me and listen to me" before presenting the stimulus.

Another key element of the Eight-Step Continuum Treatment is careful selection of target sounds and words. The authors listed five principles that will facilitate the patient's progression through the treatment steps.

1. Begin with the easiest speech sounds and then move to the more difficult ones. Vowels, nasals, and stops are the easier sounds; fricatives, affricates, and consonant clusters are more difficult.
2. As the patient begins to sequence sounds together, gradually increase the distance between points of articulatory contact in the target words. For example, the first target words or syllables might only contain bilabial consonants; the next might have both bilabials and lingua-alveolar sounds; the next could have bilabial and velar sounds.
3. Choose the initial phonemes of target words carefully. Words that begin with vowels, nasals, or stops are more likely to be produced correctly than words beginning with fricatives, affricates, or consonant clusters.
4. Gradually increase the length of the target words. It is best to start with short words that have repeating syllables, such as B-B, so-so, and ta-ta. Once these are mastered, systematically begin using longer words that have more complex syllable structure.
5. When choosing real words for treatment, start with words that appear more often in day-to-day speech (i.e., high-frequency words).

Once these principles are incorporated into the selection of initial target syllables or words, the treatment sequence is ready to begin. While guiding the patient through the eight treatment steps, the clinician should keep in mind several general rules:

- Move through the steps at a pace that keeps the patient successful.
- Repetitive drill will be necessary to help the patient relearn the motor sequences needed to produce volitional speech.

- Use functional, useful words in treatment as soon as possible.
- Encourage the patient to self-correct errors.
- Teach compensatory strategies to facilitate speech, such as prolonging vowels, slowing rate, and pausing when needed.

The actual treatment steps in this program follow a logical sequence that moves from maximal to minimal cueing by the clinician. The following list is a summary of what the clinician and patient do in each of the eight steps. Not all patients need to start on Step 1 or move through every step. Some will be able to skip steps, depending on the severity of their deficits.

1. The clinician tells the patient to "Watch me" and "Listen to me" and says the target word. They then say the target word in unison.
2. The clinician tells the patient to "Watch me" and "Listen to me" and says the target word. Then, while the clinician silently mouths the word, the patient says the word aloud.
3. The clinician tells the patient to "Watch me" and "Listen to me" and says the target word. The patient then repeats the word independently.
4. The clinician tells the patient to "Watch me" and "Listen to me" and says the target word. The patient then repeats the word several times independently.
5. The clinician presents the target word written on paper, and the patient says the word while looking at it.
6. The clinician presents the target word written on paper, removes it, and then the patient says the word.
7. The patient says the word in response to a question from the clinician. For example, if the target word were the patient's name, the clinician would ask, "What is your name?" The patient would then say his or her name.
8. Role playing with the clinician, family, or friends is used to evoke the target word in an appropriate conversational context.

Sound Production Treatment

Wambaugh and colleagues developed an apraxia treatment that combined components of the Eight Step Continuum technique with articulatory placement cueing, phonetic tasks, and extensive modeling (Wambaugh et al., 1998). Like the Eight Step Continuum,

Sound Production Treatment (SPT) is an articulatory kinematic procedure. It contains a four-step treatment hierarchy and is unique in several ways. First of all, skipping steps in the treatment hierarchy is actually built into the treatment procedure. The clinician can omit steps in the treatment sequence depending on how well the patient produces the target sounds. For example, if the patient produces a target word correctly in the first step, that trial is complete, and the patient can move on to the next word. The benefit of this is that it allows the treatment to progress at a faster pace than it would otherwise. A second unique feature of SPT is that it combines phonetic treatment tasks with traditional motor sequencing activities. The phonetic tasks are included because some studies have suggested that apraxia of speech is a phonetic-level disorder, as well as a motor sequencing disorder. Because it incorporates motor and phonetic tasks in the treatment hierarchy, SPT could enhance a patient's productions of target phonemes. The third unique aspect is the amount of research that has been conducted on this procedure: STP is the most well-researched treatment for apraxia of speech (Wambaugh et al., 2006a, 2006b).

The SPT hierarchy presented here is Wambaugh and Nessler's (2004) modification of the original procedure. In contrast to the original procedure, this version begins working immediately on target sounds, and it requires the patient to repeat the target words more frequently. In the following description of the SPT treatment sequence, it is assumed that the patient is working on the phoneme /m/ and that the clinician has prepared a list of five target words containing that target sound (*mutt, me, mum, mow,* and *man*).

Step 1 (Saying the Word)—The clinician says the first word (*mutt*) and asks the patient to repeat it. If *mutt* is repeated correctly, the patient is asked to repeat the word five more times independently. Once the five repetitions are completed successfully, the next word containing /m/ (*me*) is presented, and Step 1 is started again.

If *mutt* is not repeated correctly, the clinician explains what was wrong and says, "Let's try a different word." The clinician now presents a word that is a minimal pair for *mutt* (e.g., *but*) and asks the patient to repeat it. If the patient repeats *but* correctly, the clinician says, "Good, let's go back to the other word" and moves to Step 2 using *mutt*.

If the minimal pair word (*but*) is not repeated correctly, the clinician says, "Watch me and listen to me and say the word with me." The clinician then says, *but* three times, while the patient attempts to repeat the word in unison. Regardless of whether these productions of *but* are correct or incorrect, the clinician moves on to Step 2 with the original word (*mutt*).

Step 2 (Show the Letter)—The clinician presents a card with a large M (the target sound) written on it. The clinician then asks the patient to repeat the word *mutt*. If the patient's production is correct, the clinician asks for five independent repetitions of *mutt* and then goes to Step 1 with next word on the list (*me*). If incorrect, the clinician moves to Step 3.

Step 3 (Watch Me and Listen to Me)—The clinician says, "Watch me and listen to me and say the word with me," and then says *mutt* three times. The patient attempts to say the word in unison with the clinician. If correct, the clinician asks the patient to repeat the word five times independently and then goes to Step 1 with the next word on the list. If the patient cannot correctly produce *mutt* by looking and listening, the clinician moves to Step 4.

Step 4 (Articulatory Placement Cueing)—When the patient cannot say the target word by looking and listening, the clinician provides a combination of verbal, visual, or tactile cues on how to produce the target sound. In the current example, the cues would show or describe how the lips need to be together to produce /m/ and how the sound needs to travel through the nose, rather than through the mouth. After giving the cue(s), the patient is asked again to look and listen to the clinician and say the word (*mutt*) three times in unison. If the productions in unison are correct, the patient is asked to repeat the word five times independently. If the productions in unison are incorrect, the clinician and patient stop working on *mutt* for the time being and go to Step 1 using the next word on the list (*me*).

This written description of SPT might make the process seem more complicated than it actually is. Beginning clinicians are encouraged to thoroughly rehearse its treatment steps with a friend or colleague before attempting it with a patient. With practice, SPT sessions can progress at a comfortable pace, and the individual steps have a logical hierarchy of cueing. Incidentally, when the patient is independently repeating a stimulus word five times during one of the SPT steps, Wambaugh recommended giving feedback on only about 60% of the patient's attempts. The primary reason for this is that too much feedback can interrupt the patient's concentration and inadvertently impose a delay between the separate attempts at saying the word, something that can make the task more difficult for the patient. Furthermore, Wambaugh et al. (2017) found that random presentation of stimulus words in SPT is moderately more effective than block presentation. For example, if a patient were working on the phonemes /v/, /m/, and /t/, each with 10 target words as stimuli, block presentation would be working on all the /v/ words first, then all the /m/ words, and finally all the /t/ words. Random presentation would be working on all 30 target words in random order. The study's results showed that although both methods increased speech accuracy for targeted phonemes, there was a 12% greater improvement for random practice 2 weeks after treatment and 8% at 10 weeks.

Darley, Aronson, and Brown's Procedure

Darley et al. (1975) described another articulatory kinematic approach to helping individuals with apraxia of speech relearn the motor sequences for speech production. No controlled studies show this technique's effectiveness, but anecdotal clinical reports indicate that it could be useful for patients with severe apraxia. For instance, its first steps are designed for a patient who is having difficulty with voluntary phonations, tongue protrusions, and other simple oral movements. Darley et al. called these beginning procedures "initiating speech activities."

1. Encourage the patient to prolong an "ah." If this is not possible, see whether the patient can cough voluntarily. If so, then try to shape the cough into a prolonged exhalation or sigh. If these are not successful, see whether the patient can hum a familiar song or complete an automatic, open-ended phrase, such as "The sky is _____," or "Open the _____."
2. When a phonation is produced, the patient is asked to say that sound repeatedly, using different durations and levels of loudness. Then the patient should be encouraged to try shaping the phonation into several vowel sounds, such as "ee," "oh," "oo," and so forth.
3. Once vowels are being produced, the patient is asked to imitate the clinician's model of /m/. Darley et al. (1975) recommended using a mirror to facilitate the volitional closing of mouth for the /m/. When this consonant is produced, the patient is asked to begin forming syllables with /m/ in the initial position, such as *me*, *moe*, and *moo*.
4. Slightly more complicated production of consonant–vowel (CV) syllables can be encouraged by having the patient alternate between syllables with open and closed vowels, such as *moe-me, moe-me, moe-me*. This also can be accomplished by using syllables that have /w/ in the initial position.

Once these tasks are accomplished, the patient should be ready for the next portion of this treatment program, which is called "Using Automatic Responses." For these tasks, it is assumed that the patient is able to produce some automatic phrases, such as counting or other overlearned word sequences. Darley et al. (1975) recommended that patients attempt to recite automatic responses so that they can regain the experience of producing speech easily. A list of recommended automatic responses is:

- Counting from 1 to 10.
- Reciting the days of the week or months of the year.
- Common expressions such as "hello," "how are you?" "fine," "very well," "thank you," "I don't know," and so forth.
- Well-known materials including nursery rhymes, phrases from television commercials, and opening lines from famous poems.
- Singing well-known songs.

The next step, called "Phonemic Drill," is a return to working on volitional speech production. It is hoped that by this stage the patient is beginning to attempt some utterances spontaneously, although they might be filled with apraxic errors. Darley et al. (1975) recommended using the integral stimulation "watch and listen" method of presenting these phonemic drill tasks to the patient.

1. The first step is to choose an easy phoneme such as /m/. The patient is asked to hum the /m/ after the clinician demonstrates what to do.
2. Then the patient adds a series of vowels to the /m/, such as *my, moe, maw, moo, may,* and *me*. These words are practiced 10 to 20 times each.
3. These CV words are then doubled, so that *me* becomes *me-me* and *may* becomes *may-may*. The patient again practices saying these words 10 to 20 times each.
4. The next step is to add /m/ to the end of the CV words. For example, *mom, moom,* and *meem* would be some of the words created for this step.
5. The patient next begins saying actual words. Choose words that begin with /m/ and have other easy phonemes in them. Darley et al. (1975) suggested words such as *more, man, mine, moon, mare, mat, map,* and *mum*. As with all of these steps, the words are practiced at least 10 to 20 times each.
6. Producing two-word phrases is the next step. Both words in the phrases should begin with /m/. Examples of words for this step include *my mom, my mail, miss me, much more,* and *make me*.

7. Now the patient produces two-word phrases that end with /m/, such as *come home, name him, lame lamb, dumb bum,* and so forth.

8. This step has the patient say two-word phrases in which /m/ is in the initial position of the first word and in the final position of the second. Examples would include *make him, my home, must name, my name, meet them,* and *Mary's room.*

9. The final step is having the patient produce longer phrases that include multisyllabic words, such as *moment by moment, my morning meeting, made much money, Monday morning,* and *among my memories.*

From here, the patient moves to productions of other consonants in words, using the same sequence as with the /m/. Eventually, the patient will be asked to use the consonants he or she has mastered in words that contain the same vowel, such as *me, she, we, tea, bee, fee,* and *key.* Ultimately, the goal is to incorporate these words into phrases and then into sentences.

Melodic Intonation Therapy

MIT (Helm-Estabrooks et al., 1989) would be classified as a rate-and-rhythm type of apraxia treatment. It is based on the observation that many individuals with aphasia or apraxia of speech can sing the words of a song much better than they can say the same words in conversation. Many clinicians have worked with patients who could sing the words of a well-known song intelligibly, but when asked to say the words, they could not. One theory for this phenomenon is that singing is accessed through the undamaged right hemisphere. It is thought that singing the words of a song somehow allows the right hemisphere to facilitate the function of the damaged left hemisphere, resulting in better verbalizations in song than in conversation. MIT was designed to capitalize on this by blending rhythm and melody into the volitional speech of individuals with aphasia or apraxia of speech. In the MIT program, the rhythm and melody aspects of the program are emphasized primarily in the beginning steps of the program. The patient's intonation is then modified into a more natural prosody in the final steps.

The authors identified the most successful treatment candidates for this program—those who (a) experienced a stroke, (b) have nonfluent aphasia or otherwise restricted verbal output, (c) have good auditory comprehension, (d) demonstrate poor articulation and repetition abilities, and (e) are motivated and have an adequate attention span. Patients with large lesions in Wernicke's area or co-occurring right hemisphere damage are unlikely to benefit from the MIT program.

The MIT program is divided into three levels, with each level containing several individual steps. In the first two levels, the patient works on producing short, high-frequency words and phrases. The third level concentrates on longer, more complex utterances. The overall sequence of treatment is to first incorporate melodic intonation into the target utterances, then gradually shift to saying the words with exaggerated prosody, and finally saying the words with normal prosody. The following is a summary of the MIT treatment sequence.

Elementary Level

1. First the clinician demonstrates the melody by humming and singing the target word. The clinician taps the patient's hand on each syllable of the word or phrase. The patient does not respond, but only listens carefully.
2. The clinician and patient sing the target word and tap out the syllables together.
3. The clinician and patient begin by singing and tapping the word together, but the clinician stops about halfway through. The patient is required to complete the word alone.
4. The clinician sings and taps the target first; the patient then repeats it immediately.
5. When the patient repeats the word from Step 4, the clinician immediately asks a question such as, "What did you say?" The patient attempts to say the target word in response to this question.

Intermediate Level. The four steps of this level follow the general sequence found in the elementary level, except that delays of several seconds are inserted between the clinician's presentation of the target word and the patient's response. The length and complexity of the target words and phrases in this level are approximately the same as in the elementary level.

Advanced Level. The five steps in this portion of the program also concentrate on the delayed repetition of target phrases, as was done in the intermediate level. However, the melody used in the patient's utterances in the prior levels is now modified to match more closely normal speech intonation through a procedure called speech-song. The authors described speech-song as being similar to choral reading, in that the rhythm and stress of the target phrase are exaggerated. The words are not actually sung in a melody. In the final step, the clinician asks a question, the patient waits about 6 s, and then answers with the correct target phrase using normal intonation.

PROMPT

PROMPT, an acronym for Prompts for Restructuring Oral Muscular Targets, is an articulatory kinematic treatment approach. It was developed originally as a treatment for childhood apraxia of speech. The PROMPT program uses a combination of proprioceptive, pressure, and kinesthetic cues that show patients how to sequence their oral movements for speech (Square-Storer & Hayden, 1989). The clinician provides these cues by touching the patient's face and manually guiding the articulators to the appropriate positions needed to produce the target sounds. These "hands-on" cues are designed to provide the patients with sensory information regarding place of articulatory contact, extent of jaw opening, voicing, relative timing of syllables, manner of articulation, and coarticulation. The basic premise of PROMPT is that clinicians are acting as external motor speech programmers when they guide a patient's articulators through the correct motor sequence to produce a target sound. PROMPT identifies numerous contact points around the mouth, under the chin, and on the neck, where clinicians place their fingers and hands to guide the articulators into the proper positions for speech production. The overall sequence of a PROMPT treatment is to first have the clinician say the target syllable, word, or phrase. The patient then attempts to say the word. If correct, the next word is presented. If incorrect, the clinician finds the correct contact points for the phonemes of the word and moves the patient's articulators passively. The patient is then asked to try saying the word again with the clinician simultaneously moving the articulators into the correct positions for the word's phonemes. Some of the cues are simple and can be understood by any clinician, such as those for bilabial sounds, voicing, and jaw opening. Many, however, are complex and require special instructions learned from a PROMPT workshop to understand fully. For example, the more dynamic cues, such as those for coarticulation or phrases, can be quite intricate. Nevertheless, PROMPT has been effective in helping some patients with co-occurring severe Broca's aphasia and apraxia of speech use a core vocabulary of a few words and phrases (Bose et al., 2001; Freed et al., 1997; Square et al., 1985; Square et al., 1986).

Summary of Apraxia of Speech

- Apraxia of speech is a disorder of motor sequencing for speech production, wherein the timing and accuracy of movements is disturbed. It is not caused by muscle weakness, abnormal muscle tone, reduced range of movement, or decreased muscle steadiness.
- Apraxia of speech is a subcategory of ideomotor apraxia, which is defined as a disturbance in the performance needed to complete an action. This contrasts with ideational apraxia, which is a disturbance in the idea or purpose of a movement.
- The neural network thought to control the sequencing of speech movements is called the motor speech programmer. It is an indistinct cerebral structure that seems to be located primarily in the perisylvian area of the brain.
- Apraxia of speech has numerous potential causes, including stroke, degenerative diseases, trauma, and tumor.
- Apraxia of speech is primarily a disorder of articulation and prosody.
- When diagnosing apraxia of speech, it is important to eliminate conditions that can cause speech errors similar to those in apraxia of speech. Brookshire (2015) listed four such conditions: muscle weakness, sensory loss, comprehension deficit, and incoordination.
- Many treatments for apraxia of speech have been developed. The choice of which is best can depend on the severity of the apraxia and the patient's and clinician's personal preferences.

Study Questions

1. Define apraxia of speech in your own words.
2. Describe how apraxia of speech is both similar to and different from dysarthria.
3. How are ideational apraxia and ideomotor apraxia different?
4. Limb apraxia, nonverbal oral apraxia, and apraxia of speech are subcategories of which type of apraxia?
5. What is the difference between nonverbal oral apraxia and apraxia of speech?
6. What is the motor speech programmer?

7. The motor speech programmer receives input from what other parts of the brain?
8. What is the most common cause of apraxia of speech?
9. Why do patients with mild or severe apraxia of speech typically demonstrate fewer apraxic speech errors than patients with moderate apraxia of speech?
10. Apraxia of speech is primarily a disorder of which two components of speech production?
11. What are two of the possible ways in which apraxia of speech affects prosody?
12. When making the diagnosis of apraxia of speech, why must such conditions as weakness and reduced range of movement be eliminated as possible causes of a speech disorder?
13. Why can it be especially difficult to distinguish apraxia of speech from Broca's aphasia?
14. What is one of the most sensitive evaluation tasks for identifying apraxia of speech?
15. What is integral stimulation? Which apraxia treatments have incorporated it into their treatment procedure?

References

Ackermann, H., & Ziegler, W. (1991). Cerebellar voice tremor: An acoustic analysis. *Journal of Neurology, Neurosurgery, and Psychiatry, 54,* 74–76.

Aichert, I., Lehner, K., Falk, S., Späth, M., Franke, M., & Ziegler, W. (2021). In time with the beat: Entrainment in patients with phonological impairment, apraxia of speech, and Parkinson's disease. *Brain Sciences, 11*(11), 1524.

Alfwaress, F. S., Bibars, A. R., Hamasha, A., & Al Maaitah, E. (2017). Outcomes of palatal lift prosthesis on dysarthric speech. *Journal of Craniofacial Surgery, 28*(1), 30–35.

American Psychiatric Association. (2013). *Diagnostic and statistical manual of mental disorders* (5th ed.). https://doi.org/10.1176/appi.books.9780890425596

Andreatta, R. D. (2023). *Neuroscience fundamentals for communication sciences and disorders* (2nd ed.). Plural Publishing.

Andrén, P., Holmsved, M., Ringberg, H., Wachtmeister, V., Isomura, K., Aspvall, K., . . . Mataix-Cols, D. (2022). Therapist-supported internet-delivered exposure and response prevention for children and adolescents with Tourette syndrome: A randomized clinical trial. *JAMA Network Open, 5*(8), e2225614.

Aphorisms of Hippocratic Corpus. (1995). *World's greatest classic books* [CD]. Corel. (Original work published 400 BC)

Bachoud-Lévi, A. C., Ferreira, J., Massart, R., Youssov, K., Rosser, A., Busse, M., . . . Burgunder, J. M. (2019). International guidelines for the treatment of Huntington's disease. *Frontiers in Neurology, 10,* 710.

Ballard, K. J., Wambaugh, J. L., Duffy, J. R., Layfield, C., Maas, E., Mauszycki, S., & McNeil, M. R. (2015). Treatment for acquired apraxia of speech: A systematic review of intervention research between 2004 and 2012. *American Journal of Speech-Language Pathology, 24*(2), 316–337.

Behrman, A., Cody, J., Elandary, S., Flom, P., & Chitnis, S. (2020). The effect of SPEAK OUT! and The LOUD crowd on dysarthria due to

Parkinson's disease. *American Journal of Speech-Language Pathology, 29*(3), 1448–1465.

Benedict, R. H., Amato, M. P., DeLuca, J., & Geurts, J. J. (2020). Cognitive impairment in multiple sclerosis: Clinical management, MRI, and therapeutic avenues. *The Lancet Neurology, 19*(10), 860–871.

Bergin, A., Waranch, H. R., Brown, J., Carson, K., & Singer, H. S. (1998). Relaxation therapy in Tourette syndrome: A pilot study. *Pediatric Neurology, 18,* 136–142.

Berry, W. R., Aronson, A. E., Darley, R. L., & Goldstein, N. P. (1974). Effects of penicillamine therapy and low-copper diet on dysarthria in Wilson's disease (hepatolenticular degeneration). *Mayo Clinic Proceedings, 49,* 405–408.

Berry, W. R., Darley, F. L., Aronson, A. E., & Goldstein, N. P. (1974). Dysarthria in Wilson's disease. *Journal of Speech and Hearing Research, 17,* 169–183.

Berry, W. R., & Sanders, S. B. (1983). Environmental education: The universal management approach for adults with dysarthria. In W. R. Berry (Ed.), *Clinical dysarthria* (pp. 203–216). College-Hill Press.

Beukelman, D. R., Kraft, G., & Freal, J. (1985). Expressive communication disorders in persons with multiple sclerosis: A survey. *Archives of Physical Medicine and Rehabilitation, 66,* 675–677.

Beukelman, D. R., & Mirenda, P. (2005). *Augmentative and alternative communication: Supporting children and adults with complex communication needs* (3rd ed.). Paul H. Brookes.

Beukelman, P. C., Yorkston, K., Hakel, M., & Dorsey, M. (2007). *Speech intelligibility test for Windows.* Institute for Rehabilitation Science and Engineering at Madonna Rehabilitation Hospital.

Bloem, B. R., Okun, M. S., & Klein, C. (2021). Parkinson's disease. *The Lancet, 397*(10291), 2284–2303.

Bose, A., Square, P. A., Schlosser, R., & van Lieshout, P. (2001). Effects of PROMPT therapy on speech motor function in a person with aphasia. *Aphasiology, 15*(8), 767–785.

Boutsen, F., Park, E., Dvorak, J., & Cid, C. (2018). Prosodic improvement in persons with Parkinson disease receiving SPEAKOUT!® voice therapy. *Folia Phoniatrica et Logopaedica, 70*(2), 51–58. https://doi.org/10.1159/000488875

Britton, D., Hoit, J. D., & Benditt, J. O. (2017). Dysarthria of spinal cord injury and its management. *Seminars in Speech and Language, 38*(3), 161–172.

Brodal, P. (2010). *The central nervous system* (4th ed.). Oxford University Press.

Brookshire, R. H. (2015). *Introduction to neurogenic communication disorders* (8th ed.). Mosby.

Bryans, L. A., Palmer, A. D., Anderson, S., Schindler, J., & Graville, D. J. (2021). The impact of Lee Silverman Voice Treatment (LSVT LOUD®)

on voice, communication, and participation: Findings from a prospective, longitudinal study. *Journal of Communication Disorders*, *89*, 106031.

Cannito, M. P., & Marquardt, T. P. (1997). Ataxic dysarthria. In M. R. McNeil (Ed.), *Clinical management of sensorimotor speech disorders* (pp. 217–248). Thieme.

Canter, G. J. (1963). Speech characteristics of patients with Parkinson's disease: I. Intensity, pitch, and duration. *Journal of Speech and Hearing Disorders*, *28*, 221–229.

Carbayo, Á., Sarto, J., Santana, D., Compta, Y., & Urra, X. (2020). Hemichorea as presentation of acute cortical ischemic stroke. Case series and review of the literature. *Journal of Stroke and Cerebrovascular Diseases*, *29*(10), 105150.

Cassidy, A. (2016). The clinical assessment of apraxia. *Practical Neurology*, *16*, 317–322.

Chen, Y., Zhu, G., Liu, D., Liu, Y., Yuan, T., Zhang, X., . . . Zhang, J. (2020). Brain morphological changes in hypokinetic dysarthria of Parkinson's disease and use of machine learning to predict severity. *CNS Neuroscience & Therapeutics*, *26*(7), 711–719.

Chiaramonte, R., Pavone, P., & Vecchio, M. (2020). Speech rehabilitation in dysarthria after stroke: A systematic review of the studies. *European Journal of Physical and Rehabilitation Medicine*, *56*(5), 547–562.

Cole, M. R., & Cole, M. (1971). *Pierre Marie's papers on speech disorders*. Hafner.

Coughlin, D. G., & Litvan, I. (2020). Progressive supranuclear palsy: Advances in diagnosis and management. *Parkinsonism & Related Disorders*, *73*, 105–116.

Dabul, B. (2000). *Apraxia battery for adults* (2nd ed.). Pro-Ed.

Dagenais, P. A., Southwood, M. H., & Lee, T. L. (1998). Rate reduction methods for improving speech intelligibility of dysarthric speakers with Parkinson's disease. *Journal of Medical Speech Language Pathology*, *3*, 143–157.

Darley, F. L. (1983). Foreword. In W. R. Berry (Ed.), *Clinical dysarthria* (pp. xiii–xv). College-Hill Press.

Darley, F. L., Aronson, A. E., & Brown, J. R. (1969a). Clusters of deviant speech dimensions in the dysarthrias. *Journal of Speech and Hearing Research*, *12*, 462–496.

Darley, F. L., Aronson, A. E., & Brown, J. R. (1969b). Differential diagnostic patterns of dysarthria. *Journal of Speech and Hearing Research*, *12*, 246–269.

Darley, F. L., Aronson, A. E., & Brown, J. R. (1975). *Motor speech disorders*. W. B. Saunders.

Darley, F. L., Brown, J. R., & Goldstein, N. P. (1972). Dysarthria in multiple sclerosis. *Journal of Speech and Hearing Research*, *15*, 229–245.

Debrey, S. M., & Goldsmith, D. R. (2021). Tardive dyskinesia: Spotlight on current approaches to treatment. *Focus, 19*(1), 14–23.

Delatycki, M. B., & Bidichandani, S. I. (2019). Friedreich ataxia-pathogenesis and implications for therapies. *Neurobiology of Disease, 132*, 104606.

di Biase, L., Di Santo, A., Caminiti, M. L., Pecoraro, P. M., & Di Lazzaro, V. (2022). Classification of dystonia. *Life, 12*(2), 206.

Dobson, R., & Giovannoni, G. (2019). Multiple sclerosis—A review. *European Journal of Neurology, 26*(1), 27–40.

Downie, A. W., Low, J. M., & Lindsay, D. D. (1981). Speech disorders in parkinsonism: Usefulness of delayed auditory feedback in selected cases. *British Journal of Disorders of Communication, 16*, 135–139.

Dresser, L., Wlodarski, R., Rezania, K., & Soliven, B. (2021). Myasthenia gravis: Epidemiology, pathophysiology and clinical manifestations. *Journal of Clinical Medicine, 10*(11), 2235.

Duffy, J. R. (2005). *Motor speech disorders: Substrates, differential diagnosis, and management* (2nd ed.). Elsevier Mosby.

Duffy, J. R. (2013). *Motor speech disorders: Substrates, differential diagnosis, and management* (3rd ed.). Elsevier Mosby.

Duffy, J. R. (2020). *Motor speech disorders: Substrates, differential diagnosis, and management* (4th ed.). Elsevier Mosby.

Duffy, J. R., & Folger, N. W. (1986, November). *Dysarthria in unilateral central nervous system lesions* [Paper presentation]. American Speech-Language-Hearing Association Annual Meeting, Detroit, MI.

Duffy, J. R., Martin, P. R., Clark, H. M., Utianski, R. L., Strand, E. A., Whitwell, J. L., & Josephs, K. A. (2023). The apraxia of speech rating scale: Reliability, validity, and utility. *American Journal of Speech-Language Pathology, 32*(2), 469–491.

Dworkin, J. P. (1991). *Motor speech disorders: A treatment guide*. Mosby.

Dworkin, J. P., Abkarian, G. G., & Johns, D. F. (1988). Apraxia of speech: The effectiveness of a treatment regimen. *Journal of Speech and Hearing Disorders, 53*(3), 280–294.

Dworkin, J. P., & Johns, D. F. (1980). Management of velopharyngeal incompetence in dysarthria: A historical review. *Clinical Otolaryngology, 5*, 61–74.

Dworkin, J. P., & Meleca, R. (1997). *Vocal pathologies: Diagnosis, treatment, and case studies*. Singular Publishing.

Eggert, G. H. (1977). *Wernicke's works on aphasia: A sourcebook and review*. Mouton.

Enderby, P. M., & Palmer, R. (2008). *FDA-2: Frenchay Dysarthria Assessment: Examiner's manual*. Pro-Ed.

Espil, F. M., Woods, D. W., Specht, M. W., Bennett, S. M., Walkup, J. T., Ricketts, E. J., . . . Piacentini, J. C. (2022). Long-term outcomes of behavior therapy for youth with Tourette disorder. *Journal of the American Academy of Child & Adolescent Psychiatry, 61*(6), 764–771.

Fabbrini, A., & Guerra, A. (2021). Pathophysiological mechanisms and experimental pharmacotherapy for L-dopa-induced dyskinesia. *Journal of Experimental Pharmacology, 13*, 469–485.

Fawcus, M., & Fawcus, R. (1990). Information transfer in four cases of severe articulatory dyspraxia. *Aphasiology, 4*(2), 207–212.

Feinstein, E., & Walker, R. (2020). Treatment of secondary chorea: A review of the current literature. *Tremor and Other Hyperkinetic Movements, 10*(1), 1–14. https://doi.org/10.5334/tohm.351

Finch, E., Rumbach, A. F., & Park, S. (2020). Speech pathology management of non-progressive dysarthria: A systematic review of the literature. *Disability and Rehabilitation, 42*(3), 296–306.

Fleet, J. L., Calver, R., Perera, G. C., & Deng, Z. (2020). Palato-pharyngo-laryngeal myoclonus with recurrent retrograde feeding tube migration after cerebellar hemorrhagic stroke: A case report and review of hypertrophic olivary degeneration. *BMC Neurology, 20*, 1–5.

Florance, C. L., Rabidoux, P. L., & McCauslin, L. S. (1980). An environmental manipulation approach to treating apraxia of speech. In R. H. Brookshire (Ed.), *Clinical aphasiology conference proceedings* (pp. 285–293). BRK.

Frank, M., & Cavanna, A. E. (2013). Behavioural treatments for Tourette syndrome: An evidence-based review. *Behavioural Neurology, 27*(1), 105–117.

Freed, D. B., Marshall, R. C., & Frazier, K. E. (1997). Long-term effectiveness of PROMPT treatment in a severely apractic-aphasic speaker. *Aphasiology, 11*(4/5), 365–372.

Gandhi, P., Tobin, S., Vongphakdi, M., Copley, A., & Watter, K. (2020). A scoping review of interventions for adults with dysarthria following traumatic brain injury. *Brain Injury, 34*(4), 466–479.

Garhnayak, M., Garhnayak, L., & Sahoo, K. K. (2020). Palatal lift prosthesis for velopharyngeal incompetence: A case report. *Indian Journal of Forensic Medicine & Toxicology, 14*(4), 8338–8342.

Garratt, B. R., Hanson, D. G., & Berke, G. S. (1987). Glottographic measures of laryngeal function in individuals with abnormal motor control. In T. Baer, C. Sasaki, & K. Harris (Eds.), *Laryngeal function in phonation and respiration* (pp. 521–532). College-Hill Press.

Garrison, F. H. (1969). *History of neurology* (L. C. McHenry, Jr., Rev.). Charles C. Thomas. (Original work published 1925)

Gerstenecker, A., Grimsley, L., Otruba, B., Cowden, L., Marson, D. C., Gerstenecker, K. T., . . . Roberson, E. D. (2019). Medical decision-making in progressive supranuclear palsy: A comparison to other neurodegenerative disorders. *Parkinsonism & Related Disorders, 61*, 77–81.

Guenther, F. H. (2016). *Neural control of speech*. MIT Press.

Haley, K. L., Cunningham, K. T., Eaton, C. T., & Jacks, A. (2018). Error consistency in acquired apraxia of speech with aphasia: Effects of the analysis unit. *Journal of Speech, Language, and Hearing Research*, *61*(2), 210–226.

Haley, K. L., Cunningham, K. T., Jacks, A., Richardson, J. D., Harmon, T., & Turkeltaub, P. E. (2021). Repeated word production is inconsistent in both aphasia and apraxia of speech. *Aphasiology*, *35*(4), 518–538.

Haley, K. L., Jacks, A., & Cunningham, K. T. (2013). Error variability and the differentiation between apraxia of speech and aphasia with phonemic paraphasia. *Journal of Speech, Language, and Hearing Research*, *56*(3), 891–905.

Haley, K. L., Smith, M., & Wambaugh, J. L. (2019). Sound distortion errors in aphasia with apraxia of speech. *American Journal of Speech-Language Pathology*, *28*(1), 121–135.

Hardcastle, W. J., Barry, R. A., & Clark, C. J. (1985). Articulatory and voicing characteristics of adult dysarthric and verbal dyspraxic speakers: An instrumental study. *British Journal of Communication Disorders*, *20*, 249–270.

Hartman, D. E., & Abbs, J. H. (1992). Dysarthria associated with focal unilateral upper motor neuron lesion. *European Journal of Disorders of Communication*, *27*, 187–196.

Haynes, W. O., & Pindzola, R. H. (2011). *Diagnosis and evaluation in speech pathology* (5th ed.). Allyn & Bacon.

Hegde, M. N., & Freed, D. (2022). *Assessment of communication disorders in adults: Resources and protocols* (3rd ed.). Plural Publishing.

Heilman, K. M., Watson, R. T., & Greer, M. (1977). *Handbook for differential diagnosis of neurologic signs and symptoms*. Appleton-Century-Crofts.

Helm-Estabrooks, N., Nicholas, M., & Morgan, A. R. (1989). *Melodic intonation therapy* [Manual]. Special Press.

Hermann, W. (2019). Classification and differential diagnosis of Wilson's disease. *Annals of Translational Medicine*, *7*(Suppl. 2), S63. https://doi.org/10.21037/atm.2019.02.07

Hirasaki, M., Takagi, D., Umeda, Y., Moriwaki, M., Katagiri, N., Nomoto, A., . . . Fujishima, I. (2023). A case of dysphagia and dysarthria improved by flexible-palatal lift/augmentation combination prosthesis. *Progress in Rehabilitation Medicine*, *8*, 20230006.

Hirose, H. (1986). Pathophysiology of motor speech disorders (dysarthria). *Folia Phoniatria*, *38*, 61–88.

Hollis, C., Pennant, M., Cuenca, J., Glazebrook, C., Kendall, T., Whittington, C., . . . Stern, J. (2016). Clinical effectiveness and patient perspectives of different treatment strategies for tics in children and adolescents with Tourette syndrome: A systematic review and qualitative analysis. *Health Technology Assessment*, *20*(4),1–450, vii–viii. DOI: 10.3310/hta 20040. PMID: 26786936.

Horton, S. K., Murdoch, B. E., Theodoros, D. G., & Thompson, E. C. (1997). Motor speech impairment in a case of childhood basilar artery stroke: Treatment directions derived from physiological and perceptual assessment. *Pediatric Rehabilitation, 1*(3), 163–177.

Hybbinette, H., Östberg, P., & Schalling, E. (2021). Intra-and interjudge reliability of the Apraxia of Speech Rating Scale in early stroke patients. *Journal of Communication Disorders, 89*, 106076.

Hyodo, M., Asano, K., Nagao, A., Hirose, K., Nakahira, M., Yanagida, S., & Nishizawa, N. (2021). Botulinum toxin therapy: A series of clinical studies on patients with spasmodic dysphonia in Japan. *Toxins, 13*(12), 840.

Itoh, M., Sasanuma, S., & Ushijima, T. (1979). Velar movements during speech in a patient with apraxia of speech. *Brain and Language, 7*, 227–239.

Jahanshahi, M. (2000). Factors that ameliorate or aggravate spasmodic-torticollis. *Journal of Neurology, Neurosurgery, and Psychiatry, 68*, 227–229.

Joanette, Y., & Dudley, J. G. (1980). Dysarthric symptomatology of Friedreich's ataxia. *Brain and Language, 10*, 39–50.

Johnson, J. A., & Pring, T. R. (1990). Speech therapy and Parkinson's disease: A review and further data. *British Journal of Disorders of Communication, 25*, 187–192.

Jungblut, M., Huber, W., Mais, C., & Schnitker, R. (2014). Paving the way for speech: Voice-training-induced plasticity in chronic aphasia and apraxia of speech—Three single cases. *Neural Plasticity, 2014*, Article ID 841982, 14 pp. https://doi.org/10.1155/2014/841982

Keatley, M. A., & Pike, P. (1976). An automated pulmonary function laboratory: Clinical use in determining respiratory variations in apraxia. In R. H. Brookshire (Ed.), *Clinical aphasiology conference proceedings* (pp. 98–109). BRK.

Kent, R. (1976). *Study of vocal tract characteristics in the dysarthrias* [Paper presentation]. Veterans Administration Workshop on Motor Speech Disorders, Madison, WI.

Kent, R. D. (2015). Nonspeech oral movements and oral motor disorders: A narrative review. *American Journal of Speech-Language Pathology, 24*(4), 763–789.

Kim, J. Y., Nam, Y., Rim, Y. A., & Ju, J. H. (2022). Review of the current trends in clinical trials involving induced pluripotent stem cells. *Stem Cell Reviews and Reports, 18*(1), 142–154.

Kuehn, D. P. (1997). The development of a new technique for treatment of hypernasality: CPAP. *American Journal of Speech-Language Pathology, 6*(4), 5–8.

Kumar, A., Kumar, V., Singh, K., Kumar, S., Kim, Y. S., Lee, Y. M., & Kim, J. J. (2020). Therapeutic advances for Huntington's disease. *Brain Sciences, 10*(1), 43.

Lazaridis, K., & Tzartos, S. J. (2020). Autoantibody specificities in myasthenia gravis; implications for improved diagnostics and therapeutics. *Frontiers in Immunology, 11,* 212.

Leonhard, S. E., Mandarakas, M. R., Gondim, F. A., Bateman, K., Ferreira, M. L., Cornblath, D. R., . . . Jacobs, B. C. (2019). Diagnosis and management of Guillain–Barré syndrome in ten steps. *Nature Reviews Neurology, 15*(11), 671–683.

Lester-Smith, R. A., Miller, C. H., & Cherney, L. R. (2021). Behavioral therapy for tremor or dystonia affecting voice in speakers with hyperkinetic dysarthria: A systematic review. *Journal of Voice: Official Journal of the Voice Foundation,* S0892-1997. https://doi.org/10.1016/j.jvoice.2021.03.026

Levitt, J. S., Chitnis, S., & Walker-Batson, D. (2015). The effects of the "SPEAK OUT!®" and "LOUD crowd®" voice programs for Parkinson. *International Journal of Health Sciences, 3*(2), 13–19.

Lieto, M., Roca, A., Santorelli, F. M., Fico, T., De Michele, G., Bellofatto, M., . . . Filla, A. (2019). Degenerative and acquired sporadic adult onset ataxia. *Neurological Sciences, 40,* 1335–1342.

Light, J., Edelman, S. B., & Alba, A. (2001). The dental prosthesis used for intraoral muscle therapy in the rehabilitation of the stroke patient: A preliminary research study. *The New York State Dental Journal, 67*(5), 22–27.

Limousin, P., & Foltynie, T. (2019). Long-term outcomes of deep brain stimulation in Parkinson disease. *Nature Reviews Neurology, 15*(4), 234–242.

Linebaugh, C. W. (1979). The dysarthrias of Shy-Drager syndrome. *Journal of Speech and Hearing Disorders, 44,* 55–60.

Linebaugh, C. W. (1983). Treatment of flaccid dysarthria. In W. H. Perkins (Ed.), *Current therapy in communication disorders: Dysarthria and apraxia* (pp. 59–68). Thieme.

Liotti, M., Vogel, D., Ramig, L., New, P., Cook, C., Ingham, R. J., . . . Fox, P. (2003). Hypophonia in Parkinson's disease: Neural correlates of voice treatment revealed by PET. *Neurology, 60,* 432–440.

Liss, J. M., Kuehn, D. P., & Hinkle, K. P. (1994). Direct training of velopharyngeal musculature. *Journal of Medical Speech-Language Pathology, 2*(3), 243–251.

Logemann, J. A., Fisher, H. B., Boshes, B., & Blonsky, E. R. (1978). Frequency and cooccurrence of vocal tract dysfunctions in the speech of a large sample of Parkinson patients. *Journal of Speech and Hearing Disorders, 43,* 47–57.

Longinetti, E., & Fang, F. (2019). Epidemiology of amyotrophic lateral sclerosis: An update of recent literature. *Current Opinion in Neurology, 32*(5), 771.

Louis, E. D., & McCreary, M. (2021). How common is essential tremor? Update on the worldwide prevalence of essential tremor. *Tremor and*

Other Hyperkinetic Movements, 11(1): 28, pp. 1–14. doi: https://doi.org/10.5334/tohm.632

Lowell, S. Y., Kelley, R. T., Dischinat, N., Monahan, M., Hosbach-Cannon, C. J., Colton, R. H., & Mihaila, D. (2021). Clinical features of essential voice tremor and associations with tremor severity and response to octanoic acid treatment. *The Laryngoscope, 131*(11), E2792–E2801.

Lowell, S. Y., Kelley, R. T., Monahan, M., Hosbach-Cannon, C. J., Colton, R. H., & Mihaila, D. (2019). The effect of octanoic acid on essential voice tremor: A double-blind, placebo-controlled study. *The Laryngoscope, 129*(8), 1882–1890.

Luchsinger, R., & Arnold, G. E. (1965). *Voice-speech-language* (G. E. Arnold & E. R. Finkbeiner, Trans.). Wadsworth.

Ludlow, C. L., & Bassich, C. J. (1984). Relationships between perceptual ratings and acoustic measures of hypokinetic speech. In M. R. McNeil, J. C. Rosenbek, & A. E. Aronson (Eds.), *The dysarthrias: Physiology, acoustics, perceptions, management* (pp. 163–196). College-Hill Press.

Ludlow, C. L., Connor, N. P., & Bassich, C. J. (1987). Speech timing in Parkinson's and Huntington's disease. *Brain and Language, 32*, 195–214.

Luria, A. (1972). *The man with a shattered world*. Penguin.

Maas, E. (2017). Speech and nonspeech: What are we talking about? *International Journal of Speech-Language Pathology, 19*(4), 345–359.

Marshall, R. C., Gandour, J., & Windsor, J. (1988). Selective impairment of phonation: A case study. *Brain and Language, 35*, 313–339.

Martino, D., & Hedderly, T. (2019). Tics and stereotypies: A comparative clinical review. *Parkinsonism & Related Disorders, 59*, 117–124.

Marzouqah, R., Huynh, A., Chen, J. L., Boulos, M. I., & Yunusova, Y. (2023). The role of oral and pharyngeal motor exercises in post-stroke recovery: A scoping review. *Clinical Rehabilitation, 37*(5), 620–635.

Masrori, P., & Van Damme, P. (2020). Amyotrophic lateral sclerosis: A clinical review. *European Journal of Neurology, 27*(10), 1918–1929.

McAuliffe, M. J., Fletcher, A. R., Kerr, S. E., O'Beirne, G. A., & Anderson, T. (2017). Effect of dysarthria type, speaking condition, and listener age on speech intelligibility. *American Journal of Speech-Language Pathology, 26*(1), 113–123.

McHenry, M. A. (1998). The ability to effect intended stress following traumatic brain injury. *Brain Injury, 12*(6), 495–503.

McNeil, M. R. (2009). *Clinical management of sensorimotor speech disorders* (2nd ed.). Thieme.

McNeil, M. R., Ballard, K. J., Duffy, J. R., Wambaugh, J. L. van Lieshout, P., Maassen, B., & Terband, H. (2017). Apraxia of speech theory, assessment, differential diagnosis, and treatment: Past, present, and future. In P. van Lieshout, B. Maassen, & H. Terband (Eds.), *Speech motor control in normal and disordered speech: Future developments in theory and methodology* (pp. 195–221). ASHA Press.

McNeil, M. R., Odell, K. H., Miller, S. B., & Hunter, L. (1995). Consistency, variability, and target approximation for successive speech repetitions among apraxic, conduction aphasic, and ataxic dysarthric speakers. *Clinical Aphasiology, 23*, 39–55.

McNeil, M. R., Prescott, T. E., & Lemme, M. L. (1976). An application of electromyographic biofeedback to aphasia/apraxia treatment. In R. H. Brookshire (Ed.), *Clinical aphasiology conference proceedings* (pp. 151–171). BRK.

McNeil, M. R., Robin, D. A., & Schmidt, R. A. (2009). Apraxia of speech: Definition, differentiation, and treatment. In M. R. McNeil (Ed.), *Clinical management of sensorimotor speech disorders* (pp. 249–268). Thieme.

Meidinger, A. L., Miltenberger, R. G., Himle, M., Omvig, M., Trainor, C., & Crosby, R. (2005). An investigation of tic suppression and the rebound effect in Tourette's disorder. *Behavior Modification, 29*(5), 716–745.

Miller, N. (1986). *Dyspraxia and its management.* Aspen.

Mitchell, C., Bowen, A., Tyson, S., Butterfint, Z., & Conroy, P. (2017). Interventions for dysarthria due to stroke and other adult-acquired, nonprogressive brain injury. *Cochrane Database of Systematic Reviews,* 1(1), CD002088. https://doi.org/10.1002/14651858.CD002088.pub3

Moya-Galé, G., & Levy, E. S. (2019). Parkinson's disease-associated dysarthria: Prevalence, impact and management strategies. *Research and Reviews in Parkinsonism, 2019*(9), 9–16.

Munasinghe, T. U., Ariyasena, A. D. K., & Siriwardhana, D. D. (2023). Speech therapy interventions for acquired apraxia of speech: An updated systematic review. *American Journal of Speech-Language Pathology, 32*(3), 1336–1359. https://doi.org/10.1044/2022_AJSLP-21-00236

Muñoz-Vigueras, N., Prados-Román, E., Valenza, M. C., Granados-Santiago, M., Cabrera-Martos, I., Rodríguez-Torres, J., & Torres-Sánchez, I. (2021). Speech and language therapy treatment on hypokinetic dysarthria in Parkinson disease: Systematic review and meta-analysis. *Clinical Rehabilitation, 35*(5), 639–655.

Murdoch, B. E., Chenery, H., Stokes, P., & Hardcastle, W. (1991). Respiratory kinematics in speakers with cerebellar disease. *Journal of Speech and Hearing Research, 34*, 768–780.

Murdoch, B. E., Thompson, E. C., & Theodoros, D. G. (1997). Spastic dysarthria. In M. R. McNeil (Ed.), *Clinical management of sensorimotor speech disorders* (pp. 287–310). Thieme.

Nagao, K., Fujimoto, K., Suito, H., Goto, T., Ishida, Y., Watanabe, M., & Ichikawa, T. (2023). Effect of palatal augmentation prosthesis on speech and swallowing in tongue dysfunction: A literature review. *Journal of Oral Health and Biosciences, 35*(2), 39–46.

Nathan, C. L., Quigley, S., & Spindler, M. (2022). Palato-pharyngo-laryngeal myoclonus with facial involvement after an ischemic stroke. *Movement Disorders Clinical Practice*, *9*(1), 104.

Netsell, R., & Kent, R. (1976). Paroxymal ataxic dysarthria. *Journal of Speech and Hearing Disorders*, *41*, 93–109.

Newland, D. P., Novakovic, D., & Richards, A. L. (2022). Voice tremor and botulinum neurotoxin therapy: A contemporary review. *Toxins*, *14*(11), 773.

Nicolosi, L., Harryman, E., & Kresheck, J. (1983). *Terminology of communication disorders: Speech-language-hearing* (2nd ed.). Williams and Wilkins.

Of the epidemics of Hippocratic Corpus. (1995). *World's greatest classic books* [CD]. Corel. (Original work published 400 BC)

O'Neill, Y. V. (1980). *Speech and speech disorders in Western thought before 1600*. Greenwood Press.

Ono, T., Hamamura, M., Honda, K., & Nokubi, T. (2005). Collaboration of a dentist and speech-language pathologist in the rehabilitation of a stroke patient with dysarthria: A case study. *Gerodontology*, *22*(2), 116–119.

Page, A. D., & Siegel, L. (2017). Perspectives on the psychosocial management of oromandibular dystonia. *Seminars in Speech and Language*, *38*(3), 173–183.

Paja, M. S., & Falk, T. H. (2012, September 9–13). *Automated dysarthria severity classification for improved objective intelligibility assessment of spastic dysarthric speech* [Paper presentation]. International Speech Communication Association Thirteenth Annual Conference, Portland, OR.

Palmer, R., & Enderby, P. (2007). Methods of speech therapy treatment for stable dysarthria: A review. *Advances in Speech Language Pathology*, *9*(2), 140–153.

Park, S., Theodoros, D., Finch, E., & Cardell, E. (2016). Be clear: A new intensive speech treatment for adults with nonprogressive dysarthria. *American Journal of Speech-Language Pathology*, *25*(1), 97–110.

Parkinson, J. (1817). *An essay on the shaking palsy*. Whittingham & Rowland.

Peterson, A. L., Blount, T. H., Villarreal, R., Raj, J. J., & McGuire, J. F. (2022). Relaxation training with and without comprehensive behavioral intervention for tics for Tourette's disorder: A multiple baseline across participants consecutive case series. *Journal of Behavior Therapy and Experimental Psychiatry*, *74*, 101692.

Peterson, A. L., McGuire, J. F., Wilhelm, S., Piacentini, J., Woods, D. W., Walkup, J. T., . . . Scahill, L. (2016). An empirical examination of symptom substitution associated with behavior therapy for Tourette's disorder. *Behavior Therapy*, *47*(1), 29–41.

Peterson, B. S., & Cohen, D. J. (1998). The treatment of Tourette's syndrome: Multimodal, developmental intervention. *Journal of Clinical Psychiatry*, *59*(Suppl. 1), 62–72.

Piacentini, J., Woods, D. W., Scahill, L., Wilhelm, S., Peterson, A. L., Chang, S., . . . Walkup, J. T. (2010). Behavior therapy for children with Tourette disorder: A randomized controlled trial. *JAMA, 303*(19), 1929–1937.

Piacentini, V., Mauri, I., Cattaneo, D., Gilardone, M., Montesano, A., & Schindler, A. (2014). Relationship between quality of life and dysarthria in patients with multiple sclerosis. *Archives of Physical Medicine and Rehabilitation, 95*(11), 2047–2054.

Picheny, M., Durlach, N., & Braida, L. (1985). Speaking clearly for the hard of hearing I: Intelligibility differences between clear and conversational speech. *Journal of Speech & Hearing Research, 28*(1), 96–103.

Pierce, R. S. (1991). Apraxia of speech versus phonemic paraphasia: Theoretical, diagnostic, and treatment considerations. In D. Vogel & M. P. Cannito (Eds.), *Treating disorders speech motor control: For clinicians by clinicians* (pp. 185–216). Pro-Ed.

Przedborski, S., Brunko, E., Hubert, M., Mavroudakis, N., & de Beyl, D. Z. (1988). The effect of acute hemiplegia on intercostal muscle activity. *Neurology, 38*, 1882–1884.

Ramig, L. O. (1995). Voice therapy for neurologic disease. *Otolaryngology and Head and Neck Surgery, 3*, 174–182.

Ramig, L. O., Countryman, S., Thompson, L. L., & Horii, Y. (1995). A comparison of two forms of intensive speech treatment in Parkinson disease. *Journal of Speech and Hearing Research, 38*, 1232–1251.

Rampello, L., Rampello, L., Patti, F., & Zappia, M. (2016). When the word doesn't come out: A synthetic overview of dysarthria. *Journal of the Neurological Sciences, 369*, 354–360.

Raymer, A. M., & Thompson, C. K. (1991). Effects of verbal plus gestural treatment in a patient with aphasia and severe apraxia of speech. In T. E. Prescott (Ed.), *Clinical aphasiology* (Vol. 20, pp. 285–298). Pro-Ed.

Rippon, G. A., Scarmeas, N., Gordon, P. H., Murphy, P. L., Albert, S. M., Mitsumoto, H., . . . Stern, Y. (2006). An observational study of cognitive impairment in amyotrophic lateral sclerosis. *Archives of Neurology, 63*(3), 345–352.

Ropper, A. H. (1987). Severe dysarthria with right hemisphere stroke. *Neurology, 37*, 1061–1063.

Rosenbek, J. C. (1978). Treating apraxia of speech. In D. E. Johns (Ed.), *Clinical management of neurogenic communicative disorders* (pp. 191–242). Little, Brown.

Rosenbek, J. C. (2017). Mind over motor: Motor speech disorder treatment works best when clinicians emphasize the cognitive along with the physical. *The ASHA Leader, 22*(3), 44–49.

Rosenbek, J. C., & LaPointe, L. L. (1985). The dysarthrias: Description, diagnosis, and treatment. In D. F. Johns (Ed.), *Clinical management of neurogenic communication disorders* (pp. 251–310). Little, Brown.

Rosenbek, J. C., LaPointe, L. L., & Wertz, R. T. (1989). *Aphasia: A clinical approach*. College-Hill Press.

Rosenbek, J. C., Lemme, M. L., Ahern, M. B., Harris, E. H., & Wertz, R. T. (1973). A treatment for apraxia of speech. *Journal of Speech and Hearing Disorders, 38*, 462–472.

Rubow, R., & Swift, E. (1985). A microcomputer-based wearable biofeedback device to improve transfer of treatment in parkinsonian dysarthria. *Journal of Speech and Hearing Disorders, 50*, 178–185.

Ruckart, K. W., Moya-Mendez, M. E., Nagatsuka, M., Barry, J. L., Siddiqui, M. S., & Madden, L. L. (2022). Comprehensive evaluation of voice-specific outcomes in patients with essential tremor before and after deep brain stimulation. *Journal of Voice, 36*(6), 838–846.

Sanuki, T. (2023). Spasmodic dysphonia: An overview of clinical features and treatment options. *Auris Nasus Larynx, 50*(1), 17–22. https://doi.org/10.1016/j.anl.2022.05.012

Sapir, S., Spielman, J., Ramig, L. O., Hinds, S. L., Countryman, S., Fox, C., & Story, B. (2003). Effects of intensive voice treatment (the Lee Silverman Voice Treatment [LSVT]) on ataxic dysarthria: A case study. *American Journal of Speech-Language Pathology, 12*(4), 387–399.

Sapir, S., Spielman, J., Ramig, L., Story, B. & Fox, C. (2007). Effects of intensive voice treatment on vowel articulation in dysarthric individuals with idiopathic Parkinson's disease: Acoustic and perceptual findings. *Journal of Speech, Language, and Hearing Research, 50*, 899–912.

Saunders, C., Walsh, T., & Smith, M. (1981). Hospice care in the motor neuron diseases. In C. Saunders & J. Teller (Eds.), *Hospice: The living idea* (pp. 126-147). Edward Arnold.

Scott, S., & Caird, F. I. (1983). Speech therapy for Parkinson's disease. *Journal of Neurology, Neurosurgery, and Psychiatry, 46*, 140–144.

Seideman, M. F., & Seideman, T. A. (2020). A review of the current treatment of Tourette syndrome. *The Journal of Pediatric Pharmacology and Therapeutics, 25*(5), 401–412.

Seikel, J. A., Konstantopoulos, K., & Drumright, D. G. (2020). *Neuroanatomy and neurophysiology for speech and hearing sciences*. Plural Publishing.

Shahrizaila, N., Lehmann, H. C., & Kuwabara, S. (2021). Guillain-Barré syndrome. *The Lancet, 397*(10280), 1214–1228.

Shanker, V. (2019). Essential tremor: diagnosis and management. *BMJ, 366*. http://dx.doi.org/10.1136/bmj.l4485

Shuster, L., & Wambaugh, J. L. (2003, May). *Consistency of speech sound errors in apraxia of speech accompanied by aphasia* [Poster presentation]. Clinical Aphasiology Conference, Orca's Island, WA.

Sieron, J., Westphal, K. P., & Johannsen, H. S. (1995). Apraxia of the Aarynx. *Folia Phoniatrica et Logopaedica: Official Organ of the International Association of Logopedics and Phoniatrics (IALP), 47*(1), 33–38.

Singh, S., & Kent, R. D. (2000). *Singular's illustrated dictionary of speech-language pathology*. Singular Publishing.

Skelly, M., Schinsky, L., Smith, R. W., & Fust, R. S. (1974). American Indian Sign (AMERIND) as a facilitator of verbalization for the oral verbal apraxic. *Journal of Speech and Hearing Disorders, 39*, 445–456.

Smith, W. D. (1994). *Hippocrates: Volume VII*. Cambridge, MA: Harvard University Press.

Solomon, N. P., Makashay, M. J., Helou, L. B., & Clark, H. M. (2017). Neurogenic orofacial weakness and speech in adults with dysarthria. *American Journal of Speech-Language Pathology, 26*(3), 951–960.

Southwood, H. (1987). The use of prolonged speech in the treatment of apraxia of speech. In R. H. Brookshire (Ed.), *Clinical aphasiology conference proceedings* (pp. 277–287). BRK.

Spencer, K., Yorkston, K., & Duffy, J. (2003). Behavioral management of respiratory/phonatory dysfunction from dysarthria: A flowchart for guidance in clinical decision making. *Journal of Medical Speech Language Pathology, 11*(2), xxxix–lxi.

Square, P., Chumpelik, D., & Adams, S. (1985). Efficacy of the PROMPT system of therapy for the treatment of acquired apraxia of speech. In R. Brookshire (Ed.), *Clinical aphasiology conference proceedings* (pp. 319–320). BRK.

Square, P., Chumpelik, D., Morningstar, D., & Adams, S. (1986). Efficacy of the PROMPT system of therapy for the treatment of acquired apraxia of speech: A follow-up investigation. In R. Brookshire (Ed.), *Clinical aphasiology conference proceedings* (pp. 221–226). BRK.

Square-Storer, P., & Hayden, D. (1989). PROMPT treatment. In P. Square-Storer (Ed.), *Acquired apraxia of speech in aphasic adults* (pp. 165–189). Taylor & Francis.

Stoddard-Bennett, T., & Reijo Pera, R. (2019). Treatment of Parkinson's disease through personalized medicine and induced pluripotent stem cells. *Cells, 8*(1), 26.

Strand, E. A., Duffy, J. R., Clark, H. M., & Josephs, K. (2014). The apraxia of speech rating scale: A tool for diagnosis and description of apraxia of speech. *Journal of Communication Disorders, 51*, 43–50.

Strand, E., & Sullivan, M. (2001). Evidence-based practice guidelines for dysarthria: Management of velopharyngeal function. *Journal of Medical Speech-Language Pathology, 9*, 257–274.

Sulica, L. (2010). Clinical characteristics of essential voice tremor: A study of 34 cases. *Laryngoscope, 120*(3), 516–528.

Swigert, N. B. (2010). *The source for dysarthria* (2nd. ed.). LinguiSystems.

Tai, G., Corben, L. A., Yiu, E. M., Milne, S. C., & Delatycki, M. B. (2018). Progress in the treatment of Friedreich ataxia. *Neurologia i neurochirurgia polska, 52*(2), 129–139.

Uziel, A., Bohe, M., Cadilhac, J., & Passouant, P. (1975). Voice and speech disorders in the Parkinsonian syndrome. *Folia phoniatrica*, *27*(3), 166–176.

Vakkila, E., & Jehkonen, M. (2023). Apraxia and dementia severity in Alzheimer's disease: A systematic review. *Journal of Clinical and Experimental Neuropsychology*, *45*(1), 84–103.

Viefhaus, P., Feldhausen, M., Görtz-Dorten, A., Volk, H., Döpfner, M., & Woitecki, K. (2020). Efficacy of habit reversal training in children with chronic tic disorders: A within-subject analysis. *Behavior Modification*, *44*(1), 114–136.

Walshe, M., Peach, R. K., & Miller, N. (2009). Dysarthria impact profile: Development of a scale to measure psychosocial effects. *International Journal of Language & Communication Disorders*, *44*(5), 693–715.

Wambaugh, J. (2021). An expanding apraxia of speech (AOS) treatment evidence base: An update of recent developments, *Aphasiology*, 35(4), 442–461, DOI:10.1080/02687038.2020.1732289

Wambaugh, J., Duffy, J., McNeil, M., Robin, D., & Rogers, M. (2006a). Treatment guidelines for acquired apraxia of speech: A synthesis and evaluation of the evidence. *Journal of Medical Speech-Language Pathology*, *14*(2), xv–xxxiii.

Wambaugh, J., Duffy, J., McNeil, M., Robin, D., & Rogers, M. (2006b). Treatment guidelines for acquired apraxia of speech: Treatment descriptions and recommendations. *Journal of Medical Speech-Language Pathology*, *14*(2), xxxv–lxvii.

Wambaugh, J. L., Kalinyak-Fliszar, M. M., West, J. E., & Doyle, P. J. (1998). Effects of treatment for sound errors in apraxia of speech. *Journal of Speech, Language, and Hearing Research*, *41*, 725–743.

Wambaugh, J. L., & Nessler, C. (2004). Modification of Sound Production Treatment for aphasia: Generalization effects. *Aphasiology*, *18*(5/6/7), 407–427.

Wambaugh, J. L., Nessler, C., Bennett, J., & Mauszycki, S. C. (2004). Variability in apraxia of speech: A perceptual and VOT analysis of stop consonants. *Journal of Medical Speech-Language Pathology*, *12*(4), 221–228.

Wambaugh, J. L., Nessler, C., Cameron, R., & Mauszycki, S. C. (2013). Treatment for acquired apraxia of speech: Examination of treatment intensity and practice schedule. *American Journal of Speech-Language Pathology*, *22*(1), 84–102.

Wambaugh, J. L., Nessler, C., Wright, S., Mauszycki, S. C., DeLong, C., Berggren, K., & Bailey, D. J. (2017). Effects of blocked and random practice schedule on outcomes of sound production treatment for acquired apraxia of speech: Results of a group investigation. *Journal of Speech, Language, and Hearing Research*, *60*(6S), 1739–1751.

Warlow, C. (1991). *Handbook of neurology*. Blackwell.

Watson, P. J., & Hixon, T. J. (2001). Effects of abdominal trussing on breathing and speech in men with cervical spinal cord injury. *Journal of Speech, Language, and Hearing Research, 44*(4), 751–762.

Weismer, G. (2007). Neural perspectives on motor speech disorders: Current understanding. In G. Weismer (Ed.), *Motor speech disorders: Essays for Ray Kent* (pp. 57–92). Plural Publishing.

Wenke, R. J., Cornwell, P., & Theodoros, D. G. (2010). Changes to articulation following LSVT[R] and traditional dysarthria therapy in nonprogressive dysarthria. *International Journal of Speech Language Pathology, 12*(3), 203–220.

Wenke, R. J., Theodoros, D., & Cornwell, P. (2008). The short and long-term effectiveness of the LSVT for dysarthria following TBI and stroke. *Brain Injury, 22*(4), 339–352.

Wenke, R. J., Theodoros, D., & Cornwall, P. (2011). A comparison of the effects of Lee Silverman Voice Treatment and traditional therapy on intelligibility, perceptual speech features, and everyday communication in nonprogressive dysarthria. *Journal of Medical Speech-Language Pathology, 19*, 1–25.

Wertz, R. T., LaPointe, L. L., & Rosenbek, J. C. (1991). *Apraxia of speech in adults: The disorder and its management*. Singular Publishing.

Whelan, B. M., Theodoros, D., Cahill, L., Vaezipour, A., Vogel, A. P., Finch, E., . . . Cardell, E. (2022). Feasibility of a telerehabilitation adaptation of the Be Clear speech treatment program for non-progressive dysarthria. *Brain Sciences, 12*(2), 197.

Wiederholt, W. C. (2000). *Neurology for non-neurologists* (4th ed.). W. B. Saunders.

Woo, A. S. (2012). Velopharyngeal dysfunction. *Seminars in Plastic Surgery, 26*(4), 170–177.

Yokoyama, T., Mukai, T., Kodama, N., Takao, K., Hiraoka, T., Arai, N., . . . Minagi, S. (2022). Protocol: Efficacy of soft palatal augmentation prosthesis for oral functional rehabilitation in patients with dysarthria and dysphagia: A protocol for a randomised controlled trial. *BMJ Open, 12*:e060040. https://doi.org.doi/10.1136/bmjopen-2021-060040

Yorkston, K. M., & Beukelman, D. R. (1981). *Assessment of intelligibility of dysarthric speech*. Pro-Ed.

Yorkston, K. M., Beukelman, D. R., & Bell, K. (1988). *Clinical management of dysarthric speakers*. College-Hill Press.

Yorkston, K., Beukelman, D., Hakel, M., & Dorsey, M. (2007). *Speech Intelligibility Test for Windows*. Institute for Rehabilitation Science and Engineering at Madonna Rehabilitation Hospital.

Yorkston, K. M., Beukelman, D. R., Strand, E. A., & Hakel, M. (2010). *Management of motor speech disorders in children and adults*. Pro-Ed.

Yorkston, K. M., Beukelman, D. R., & Traynor, C. (1984). *Computerized Assessment of Intelligibility of Dysarthric Speech: A computerized assessment tool*. Pro-Ed

Yorkston, K. M., Hakel, M., Beukelman, D. R., & Fager, S. (2007). Evidence for effectiveness of treatment of loudness, rate or prosody in dysarthria: A systematic review. *Journal of Medical Speech-Language Pathology, 15*(2), xi–xxxvi.

Yorkston, K. M., Miller, R. M., Strand, E. A, & Britton, D. (2012). *Management of speech and swallowing in degenerative diseases* (3rd ed.). Pro-Ed.

Yorkston, K. M., Spencer, K. A., Duffy, J. R., Beukelman, D. R., Golper, L. A., Miller, R. M., . . . Sullivan, M. (2001). Evidence-based practice guidelines for dysarthria: Management of velopharyngeal function. *Journal of Medical Speech-Language Pathology, 9*(4), 257–273.

Yorkston, K. M., & Waugh, P. F. (1989). Use of augmentative communication devices with apractic individuals. In P. Square-Storer (Ed.), *Acquired apraxia of speech aphasic adults* (pp. 267–283). Erlbaum.

Yoshida, K. (2022). Botulinum toxin therapy for oromandibular dystonia and other movement disorders in the stomatognathic system. *Toxins, 14*(4), 282.

Young, A., & Spinner, A. (2022). *Velopharyngeal insufficiency*. StatPearls Publishing.

Youssef, G. Y. S., Anter, A., & Hassen, H. E. (2015). The effects of the Lee Silverman Voice Treatment program and traditional dysarthria therapy in flaccid dysarthria. *Advanced Arab Academy of Audio-Vestibulogy Journal, 2*(1), 5.

Yu, L., Li, Y., Zhang, J., Yan, C., Wen, F., Yan, J., . . . Cui, Y. (2020). The therapeutic effect of habit reversal training for Tourette syndrome: A meta-analysis of randomized control trials. *Expert Review of Neurotherapeutics, 20*(11), 1189–1196.

Yuan, F., Guo, X., Wei, X., Xie, F., Zheng, J., Huang, Y., . . . Wang, Q. (2020). Lee Silverman Voice Treatment for dysarthria in patients with Parkinson's disease: A systematic review and meta-analysis. *European Journal of Neurology, 27*(10), 1957–1970.

Ziegler, W., Aichert, I., & Staiger, A. (2012). Apraxia of speech: Concepts and controversies. *Journal of Speech, Language, and Hearing Research, 55*(5), S1485–S1501.

Ziegler, W., Aichert, I., Staiger, A., Willmes, K., Baumgaertner, A., Grewe, T., . . . Breitenstein, C. (2022). The prevalence of apraxia of speech in chronic aphasia after stroke: A Bayesian hierarchical analysis. *Cortex, 151*, 15–29.

Zraick, R. I., & LaPointe, L. L. (1997). Hyperkinetic dysarthria. In M. R. McNeil (Ed.), *Clinical management of sensorimotor speech disorders* (pp. 249–260). Thieme.

Glossary

abduction Moving away from the midline, such as in abduction of the vocal folds.

ablative procedures Surgical techniques that remove, eradicate, or separate tissue.

acetylcholine Neurotransmitter at several sites in the nervous system, including at the neuromuscular junction and in the basal ganglia.

action tremor Tremor that is present only when an affected body part is being moved actively, such as when an arm and hand are outstretched. When the body part is at rest, the tremor is absent or greatly reduced in intensity.

adduction Moving toward the midline, such as in the adduction of the vocal folds.

afferent neurons Neurons that convey neural impulses from the periphery to the central nervous system.

akinesia Delay in the initiation of movements; one of the most common characteristics of parkinsonism.

alternating motion rate (AMR) Rapid repetition of a single movement; usually obtained by timing patients as they repeat a syllable, such as "puh, puh, puh," as quickly, evenly, and clearly as possible.

amyotrophic lateral sclerosis (ALS) Degenerative neurologic disease that ultimately affects upper and lower motor neurons; cognition remains intact as the disease progresses.

anatomy Study of the parts of the body and how the parts are related in structure.

aneurysm "Ballooning" of a blood vessel at a point of weakness; aneurysms are subject to rupture.

anoxia A lack of oxygen to tissue.

anterior In the front or forward part.

aphasia Acquired language deficit that affects verbal production, auditory comprehension, reading, and writing.

aphonia Loss or absence of voice.

apraxia Deficit in the ability to sequence the correct movements needed to carry out a familiar action.

apraxia, ideational Inability to use an object or gesture because the individual has lost the knowledge of the object's or gesture's function.

apraxia, ideomotor Disturbance in the ability to sequence the movements needed to use an object or perform a gesture; in contrast to ideational apraxia, the individual retains knowledge of the object's or gesture's function.

apraxia, limb Deficit in the ability to sequence familiar movement of the limbs; a subcategory of ideomotor apraxia.

apraxia, nonverbal oral Deficit in the ability to sequence oral movements that are not related to speech production.

apraxia of speech Deficit in the ability to sequence the movements of the articulators, resulting mainly in problems of articulation and prosody.

articulation Movement of the speech mechanism for the production of phonemes, syllables, and words.

articulators Components of the speech mechanism, usually said to be the lips, tongue, jaw, and velum; however, the vocal folds also can be considered to be one of the articulators in that they are used to produce /h/, which is often described as a glottal fricative phoneme.

association cortex Portions of the cerebral cortex that interpret and integrate sensory information from the primary cortex.

astrocytes Cells with fibrous processes that make up the connective tissue in the central nervous system.

ataxia Deficits in the timing, force, range, and direction of voluntary movement; ataxia is caused by damage to the cerebellum or its control circuits.

ataxic dysarthria A dysarthria caused by damage to the cerebellum or to the neural tracts that connect the cerebellum to the central nervous system.

autosomal dominant cerebellar ataxia of late onset A degenerative disease that can lead to ataxic dysarthria and other motor deficits.

axon Single long extension of a neuron that conducts neural impulses away from the cell body.

basal ganglia Collection of subcortical gray matter structures that play an important role in the refinement of movements.

bilateral Pertaining to both sides of an anatomical structure.

bradykinesia Neurologic deficit that results in movements that are slow and have reduced range of motion; often seen in parkinsonism.

brainstem Portion of the brain that connects the cerebral hemispheres with the spinal cord. It consists of the midbrain, pons, and medulla.

breathy voice quality A disorder of phonation caused by incomplete adduction of the vocal folds, often associated with vocal fold paralysis or paresis.

bulbar Pertaining to the brainstem, in particular to the medulla.

caudate nucleus A part of the basal ganglia; it is important in refining planned movements.

cell body The part of a cell that contains the nucleus; it is responsible for regulating a cell's metabolic processes.

central nervous system (CNS) Brain and spinal cord.

central sulcus The sulcus that separates the frontal lobe and parietal lobe.

cerebellar ataxia A movement disorder caused by damage to the cerebellum; it is characterized by incoordination and irregular muscle contraction.

cerebellar control circuits The neural tracts that send information to and from the cerebellum; see *cerebellar peduncles*.

cerebellar peduncles Three bundles of neural tracts that connect the cerebellum with the rest of the central nervous system.

cerebellum The part of the brain that is attached to the back of the brainstem and is responsible for coordinating movements.

cerebral anoxia The loss of oxygen to brain tissue, often caused by reduced blood flow through the capillaries in the brain.

cerebral cortex Outermost layer of the cerebrum.

cerebrovascular accident (CVA) Interruption of blood flow to the brain; also known as a stroke.

cerebrum The primary part of the brain; it is the largest portion of the central nervous system.

chorea Hyperkinetic movement disorder that results in involuntary movements that often are "dance-like" in appearance and usually affects many parts of the body, including the head, limbs, and torso.

chronic drug-induced dystonia A hyperkinetic movement disorder caused by long-term use of antipsychotic drugs.

collateral Small branch from an axon that enables a neuron to transmit its impulses to neurons not normally reached directly by the axon.

contralateral Pertaining to the opposite side.

coronal section Dividing a body part into front and back halves.

cortex External layer, usually used to describe the surface of the cerebrum.

corticobulbar tract Tract of upper motor neurons that course from the cortex to the brainstem; one of the tracts in the pyramidal system; it carries primarily motor impulses for skilled, voluntary movements.

corticospinal tract Tract of upper motor neurons that course from the cortex to the spinal cord; one of the tracts in the pyramidal system; it carries primarily motor impulses for skilled, voluntary movements.

cranial nerve nuclei Sites in the brainstem where the cell bodies of lower motor neurons in the cranial nerves are located.

cranial nerves Twelve pairs of nerves that branch from the brain; mostly from the brainstem.

decomposition of movement A characteristic of ataxia where movements are performed in a series of jerky actions, with each motion seeming to be a separate component.

decussation of the pyramids Place in the medulla where most axons in the corticospinal tract cross to the contralateral side of the body.

deep brain stimulation A surgical treatment for severe idiopathic Parkinson's disease in which the basal ganglia is electrically stimulated, thereby reducing many of the motor deficits found in that disorder.

delayed auditory feedback (DAF) Electronic biofeedback effect, in which a device delays individuals' perception of their speech; sometimes used to slow the rate of speech in individuals with parkinsonism.

dendrites Short extensions from the neuron cell body that receive impulses from other neurons.

diplophonia Simultaneous phonation of two sounds, usually the result of hyperadducted vocal folds that cause vibrations in the false and true vocal folds.

direct activation system Another name for the pyramidal system.

dopamine Important neurotransmitter in the central nervous system, with considerable localization in the basal ganglia.

dorsal Pertaining to the back.

dysarthria Impaired production of speech because of disturbances in the neuromuscular control of the speech mechanism.

dystonia A hyperkinetic movement disorder that causes sustained involuntary contractions of muscle groups, body parts, or large areas of the body.

efferent neurons Neurons that convey neural impulses from the central nervous system to the periphery.

equal and excess stress Equalization of stress that typically is variable in normal speech and placement of excessive stress on words or syllables that are typically unstressed.

essential tremor A benign hyperkinetic movement disorder that causes action tremors in affected body parts. It is a relatively common condition that can be found in about 4% of the population and usually appears later in life. When this condition affects the larynx, it is called essential voice tremor.

extrapyramidal system Complex collection of upper motor neuron tracts that are "extra" to the pyramidal system; these tracts are responsible for controlling posture, reflexes, and muscle tone.

fasciculations Small spontaneous contractions of muscle tissue, often seen after lower motor neuron damage.

final common pathway Another name for lower motor neurons; so named because there is no further pyramidal or extrapyramidal influence on a motor impulse once it has started traveling along a lower motor neuron.

flaccid Weak or soft.

flaccid dysarthria A dysarthria caused by damage to lower motor neurons.

Friedreich's ataxia A rare degenerative condition that affects the cerebellum, brainstem, and spinal cord; it can cause mixed dysarthria.

frontal Pertaining to the forehead; also, located in the front.

frontal association area A part of the association cortex; it is important in the planning and initiation of movement.

frontal lobe The most anterior part of the cerebrum, ranging from the frontal pole to the central sulcus.

ganglion Collection of neuron cell bodies in the peripheral nervous system; also small cystic tumors.

Gilles de la Tourette's syndrome A hyperkinetic movement disorder characterized by motor and vocal tics.

glial cells The cells that provide the supporting structure of the nervous system.

globus pallidus A part of the basal ganglia, important in refining planned movements.

glottal stop Stop sound that is produced by the rapid release of subglottic air pressure at the vocal folds.

glottis Space between the true vocal folds.

gray matter Neural tissue that is rich with neuron cell bodies, which are gray in color.

Guillain-Barré syndrome Peripheral neuropathy that causes the acute inflammation of the myelin sheath around axons; also known as acute idiopathic polyneuritis.

gyrus Convoluted ridge on the surface of the brain; in contrast to a "groove" on the surface of the brain (sulcus).

harsh vocal quality A disorder of phonation caused by abnormally tight adduction of the vocal folds.

hemangioblastomas Brain tumors composed of proliferated blood vessels.

hemiballism Violent motor movements of one side of the body; caused by damage to the subthalamic nucleus.

hemifacial spasm A hyperkinetic movement disorder that causes involuntary movements on one side of the face.

Hippocrates Greek physician; called historic father of modern medicine.

Hippocratic Corpus Collection of Greek medical texts probably written in the fourth and fifth centuries BC.

hyper- Prefix: excessive; above; more than normal.

hyperkinetic disorders Movement disorders characterized by involuntary movements that interfere with voluntary movements.

hyperkinetic dysarthria A dysarthria caused by involuntary movements that interfere with speech.

hypernasality Excessive amounts of nasal resonance on nonnasal phonemes.

hypo- Prefix: too little; below; less than normal.

hypokinetic Class of movement disorders characterized by reduced and restricted movements; seen commonly in parkinsonism.

hypokinetic dysarthria A dysarthria caused by dysfunction in the basal ganglia, usually associated with idiopathic Parkinson's disease.

hyponasal Speech with too little nasal resonance on nasal phonemes.

idiopathic Spontaneous occurrence of a pathologic condition with an unknown or obscure cause.

idiopathic sporadic late-onset cerebellar ataxia A degenerative disease that affects the cerebellum; it can cause ataxic dysarthria.

indirect activation system Another name for the extrapyramidal system.

inferior peduncle A large neural tract that transmits body sensations to the cerebellum.

inhalatory stridor Phonation on inhalation caused by the incomplete abduction of one or both vocal folds.

innervation Supply of nerve fibers functionally linked with a body part.

innervation ratio Relative number of muscle fibers innervated by one axon; a low innervation ratio (e.g., 25 fibers innervated by 1 axon) is seen in body parts that perform fine, skilled movements.

instrumental analysis Use of electronic or computerized instruments in the analysis of disorders, including motor speech disorders.

intention tremor Tremor that becomes more evident as the affected body part approaches a target, such as in reaching for an object.

internal capsule Subcortical site in the cerebrum where descending upper motor neurons are squeezed together as they pass between the thalamus and the basal ganglia.

interneurons Neurons that are between two other neurons; they often play a role in mediating communication between the two other neurons.

intonation Changes in pitch and stress that have communicative intent, such as the rising intonation of a question or the drop in intonation at the end of a statement.

ipsilateral Pertaining to the same side.

irregular articulatory breakdowns An articulation disorder where the speaker will unexpectedly misarticulate syllables within a word, usually associated with ataxic dysarthria.

lateral sulcus A prominent sulcus in the cerebrum that separates the frontal and parietal lobes from the temporal lobe.

L-dopa A chemical precursor of dopamine; used to treat the effects of parkinsonism.

Lee Silverman Voice Treatment an intensive treatment program in which patients with parkinsonism are guided through a daily schedule of maximum effort in their phonations.

limbic system Collection of interconnected structures in the brain that helps control emotions.

lobe Well-defined area of an organ.

low-grade astrocytoma Tumors consisting of neuroglial cells; these types of tumors are graded according to increasing amounts of malignancy.

lower motor neurons Neurons in the cranial and spinal nerves that transmit motor impulses to muscles, organs, or glands; also known as the final common pathway.

mandible Jaw.

medial Pertaining to the midline or middle.

medulla A part of the brainstem.

meninges Three membranes that cover the brain and spinal cord, namely the dura mater, arachnoid, and pia mater.

metastatic tumors Tumors that have been transferred to a secondary location via the circulation of pathogenic cells.

microglia Glial cells that are migratory and remove waste products from nerve tissue.

midbrain A part of the brainstem.

middle peduncle A large neural tract that sends information from the association cortex to the cerebellum.

monoloudness Reduced vocal loudness variation during speech.

monopitch Reduced vocal pitch variation during speech.

motor neurons Neurons that transmit motor impulses.

motor speech programmer Neural "mechanism" in the language-dominant hemisphere of the brain that creates the motor code needed to smoothly sequence and perform the complex movements of speech production; the motor speech programmer is an as-yet ill-defined neurologic structure.

motor strip Another name for the primary motor cortex or the precentral gyrus.

motor system Portion of the nervous system responsible for voluntary and involuntary body movements.

multisystems atrophy A collection of degenerative diseases that often have parkinsonism as one of the symptoms. Because they usually affect more than one area of the motor system, they often cause a mixed dysarthria.

muscular dystrophy A progressive disease that causes the degeneration of muscle tissue.

myasthenia gravis Disease that causes the destruction of acetylcholine receptors in muscle tissue, resulting in the rapid fatigue of muscle contractions.

myelin White, fatty covering around axons; myelin acts as insulation.

myo- Prefix: pertaining to muscle tissue.

nasal emission Audible or measurable escape of air through the nasal cavity during the production of nonnasal phonemes, usually most evident on voiceless stop and fricative consonants.

nerves Bundles of neurons in the peripheral nervous system; nerves carry impulses between the central nervous system and some other part of the body.

neural tract Bundle of neurons in the central nervous system; neurons in a neural tract convey similar types of impulses; this contrasts with nerves, which often carry both sensory and motor impulses.

neuroleptic Pertaining to the effects of antipsychotic drugs on cognition and behavior.

neurology Study of the nervous system and the disorders associated with the nervous system.

neuromuscular junction The point where the ends of lower

motor neuron axons (terminal boutons) make synaptic contact with muscle tissue.

neurons Nervous system cells that can conduct and transmit electrochemical impulses.

neurotransmitter Chemical released by the terminal boutons of an axon that either excite or inhibit the firing of an adjoining neuron.

occipital lobe The most posterior lobe of the cerebrum; important in the processing of visual sensations.

oligodendroglia Glial cells that provide the myelin sheath around axons in the central nervous system.

olivopontocerebellar degeneration A progressive, degenerative disease that affects neurons in the brainstem and cerebellum.

optic nerve A cranial nerve (II) that originates in the retina; it sends visual sensations to the occipital lobe.

overarticulation Purposeful, exaggerated articulation of consonant phonemes; can often improve the intelligibility in speakers with dysarthria.

pacing board Device that has numerous finger-width grooves along its length; sometimes can be used to slow the rate of speech of individuals with hypokinetic dysarthria.

palatal lift Intraoral prosthetic device that is attached to a dental retainer to facilitate the elevation of the velum during speech; used to treat incomplete velopharyngeal closure.

palatopharyngolaryngeal myoclonus A myoclonic movement disorder that causes rhythmic, involuntary contractions of palatal, pharyngeal, and laryngeal muscles.

palilalia The compulsive repetition of an individual's own speech.

palsy Paralysis; also unchecked tremor.

parietal association area A part of the association cortex.

parietal lobe The upper central lobe of the cerebrum, extending from the central sulcus to the occipital lobe; important for the integration of sensations from the body.

parkinsonism Collection of neurologic disorders with symptoms of tremor, bradykinesia, akinesia, muscular rigidity, and disturbed postural reflexes.

perceptual analysis Use of a clinician's perceptions to analyze and evaluate motor speech disorders.

peri- Prefix: around; near.

peripheral nervous system (PNS) Cranial and spinal nerves.

perisylvian area Area around the Sylvian fissure of the brain.

pharyngeal flap procedure Surgical attachment of a flap of tissue from the pharynx to the velum; used to treat incomplete velopharyngeal closure.

phonation Production of acoustic energy by the vibration of the vocal folds.

phonatory incompetence The inability to fully adduct the vocal folds, usually associated with vocal fold paralysis or paresis.

physiology Study of the function of the parts of a living organism.

polio Acute viral infection that attacks the cell bodies of lower motor neurons.

pons A part of the brainstem.

postcentral gyrus Another name for the primary sensory cortex.

posterior pharyngeal wall augmentation Injection of Teflon paste or hyaluronic acid into the posterior pharyngeal wall to create a small bulge, which lessens the distance the velum must travel before velopharyngeal closure is made.

postural reflexes Reflexive movements that allow for the normal execution of such movements as walking, rising from a chair, or reaching for an object; the swinging of the arms while walking is an example of a postural reflex.

precentral gyrus Another name for the primary motor cortex.

premotor area Area of the frontal lobe that plays a role in the refinement of movements; the premotor area is especially important in controlling visually guided movements.

primary auditory cortex The area of the cortex that first receives auditory sensation from the inner ear.

primary cortex Areas of the cerebral cortex that first receive sensory impulses from the body; however, the primary motor cortex is an exception; the primary motor cortex receives planned movements from cortical and subcortical areas of the brain.

primary dystonia A dystonia that is not a secondary symptom of another disorder.

primary motor cortex The area of the cortex that transmits refined, skilled voluntary movements to muscles; also known as the precentral gyrus and the motor strip.

primary sensory cortex The area of the cortex that first receives sensory impulses from the body; also known as the postcentral gyrus and the sensory strip.

primary visual cortex The area of the cortex that first receives visual sensations from the optic tract.

progressive bulbar palsy A progressive, degenerative disease that can affect lower and upper motor neurons; sometimes considered a subtype of amyotrophic lateral sclerosis.

prosody Melody of speech, which conveys meaning within an utterance through the use of intonation and stress.

pseudobulbar Condition whose symptoms mimic those seen after damage to the brainstem but is actually caused by another factor.

pseudobulbar affect Uncontrolled laughing or crying that occurs independently of the emotions actually felt by an individual; among motor speech disorders, it is most common in spastic dysarthria.

punch drunk encephalopathy Brain damage associated with repeated blows to the head, characterized by slowed cognitive function, dysarthria, and uncoordinated movement.

putamen A part of the basal ganglia; it is important in the refining of planned movements.

pyramidal system Upper motor neuron pathways that convey motor impulses for skilled, voluntary movements; the pyramidal system is divided into the corticobulbar and corticospinal tracts.

range of movement Distance that a body part can move when its muscles are contracted.

reflex Rapid, involuntary action in response to a stimulus.

resonance Placement of oral or nasal tonality onto phonemes during speech.

respiration "Power supply" of speech production; respiration provides the subglottic air pressure that is turned into acoustic energy by the speech production mechanism.

resting tremor Tremor that occurs when the affected body part is still; the tremor will typically disappear when the body part is actively being moved; resting tremor is common in parkinsonism.

reticular formation Specialized, complex collection of neurons in the brainstem that regulates arousal, respiration, and blood pressure; through its connections with the extrapyramidal system, the reticular formation plays an important role in postural reflexes.

reticulospinal tract An extrapyramidal tract; it transmits neural impulses that influence reflexes, muscle tone, and posture.

rigidity Abnormal increase in muscle tone. Rigidity differs from spasticity in that the increased muscle tone is constant. In spasticity, there are increasing and decreasing amounts of muscle tone as the affected body part is moved passively.

rubrospinal tract An extrapyramidal tract; it transmits neural impulses that influence reflexes, muscle tone, and posture.

scanning speech Term often used by medical doctors to describe the slow and deliberate production of syllables and words in cases of ataxic dysarthria.

Schwann cells Glial cells that produce the myelin sheath around axons in the peripheral nervous system.

sensory neurons Neurons that transmit sensory impulses through the nervous system.

sensory strip Another name for the primary sensory cortex or the postcentral gyrus.

sensory tricks Idiosyncratic actions that individuals with dystonia use to temporarily inhibit the involuntary muscular contractions of the disorder; examples include touching the chin to stop a focal mandibular dystonia or holding a piece of candy in the mouth to suppress a focal tongue dystonia.

sequential motion rate (SMR) Rapid repetition of a sequence of movements; usually obtained by timing patients as they repeat syllables, such as "puh, tuh, kuh," as quickly, evenly, and clearly as possible.

spasmodic dysphonia A hyperkinetic movement disorder that causes involuntary contractions of the laryngeal muscles. There are three subcategories of this disorder: adductor spasmodic dysphonia, abductor spasmodic dysphonia, and mixed spasmodic dysphonia.

spasmodic torticollis A hyperkinetic movement disorder that causes an involuntary turning of the head. In some cases, it can affect articulation and prosody.

spastic dysarthria A dysarthria associated with bilateral upper motor neuron damage to the pyramidal and extrapyramidal tracts.

spasticity Abnormal increase in muscle tone. Spasticity differs from rigidity, in that the increased muscle tone is inconsistent as an affected body is moved passively. Initially, there will be an increase in muscle tone during a passive movement, but it can then disappear completely as the movement continues. In rigidity, the increased muscle tone is constant throughout all movements.

spinal nerves Thirty-one pairs of nerves that branch from the spinal cord. Spinal nerves innervate most of the body's muscles.

strained-strangled vocal quality A disorder of phonation caused by abnormally tight adduction of the vocal folds, considered to be more severe than harsh vocal quality.

stress Changes in the pitch, loudness, and duration of syllables that give a word added importance or to clarify meaning.

striatum A part of the basal ganglia, composed of the putamen and the caudate nucleus.

substantia nigra Subcortical gray matter structure whose neurons provide the neurotransmitter dopamine to the striatum; the degeneration of these neurons causes the symptoms of idiopathic Parkinson's disease.

sulcus Groove in the surface of the brain.

superior peduncle A large tract of axons that transmit information from the cerebellum to the central nervous system.

supplementary motor area Area of the brain's frontal lobe that is important in the refining of motor movements, especially in movements that require complex actions of both hands.

synaptic cleft Microscopic gap between the terminal boutons of an axon and the dendrites of an adjoining neuron.

tardive dyskinesia Delayed appearance of choreic movements after prolonged ingestion of certain neuroleptic (antipsychotic) drugs.

tardive dystonia Delayed appearance of dystonic movements after long-term use of certain antipsychotic drugs.

temporal association area Part of the association cortex; important for the processing of sound and the formation of memories.

temporal lobe The lower lobe of the cerebrum, separated from the frontal lobe by the lateral sulcus.

terminal boutons Small projections at the end of an axon that make synaptic connections with muscles, organs, glands, or other neurons.

terminal ramifications Same as terminal boutons.

thalamus Subcortical gray matter structure through which all sensory information passes as it travels to the cortex and other areas of the brain; the thalamus plays a poorly understood role in the refinement of planned movements.

tic Involuntary, compulsive movement that is properly coordinated, such as eye blinks and shoulder shrugs. Unlike other hyperkinetic movement disorders, tics are unique in that they can be suppressed voluntarily for a time.

tracts Bundles of axons in the central nervous system that have the same origin, transmit the same information, and terminate in the same general location.

tremor Involuntary, repetitive quivering of a body part.

tumor Uncontrolled and progressive growth of tissue as a result of cell multiplication.

unilateral Pertaining to one side.

unilateral upper motor neuron dysarthria A dysarthria caused by unilateral damage to upper motor neurons; it is primarily a disorder of articulation.

upper motor neurons Neurons in the central nervous system that ultimately make synaptic connections with the lower motor neurons of the cranial and spinal nerves. The neurons that make up the pyramidal and extrapyramidal systems are upper motor neurons.

velopharyngeal incompetence Incomplete closure of the velopharyngeal port, usually resulting in hypernasal resonance.

ventral Pertaining to the front.

vermis The deep sulcus that separates the two hemispheres of the cerebellum.

visual association area Part of the association cortex; important in the planning of visually guided movements.

vital capacity Total air that can be exhaled from the lungs after a full inhalation.

voice stoppage The stopping of phonation during connected speech due to tight adduction of the vocal folds.

voice tremor Involuntary, rhythmic contractions of laryngeal muscles, producing an audible distortion of phonation.

weak pressure consonants Stop, fricative, and afficate phonemes that are distorted because of the inability to properly impound air in the oral cavity, usually due to weakness in the lips, tongue, or velum.

white matter Myelin-covered axons that course through the central nervous system; so named because myelin is white in color.

Wilson's disease Condition marked by the inability to metabolize dietary copper, which is deposited in the cornea of the eye, the brain, and other organs; Wilson's disease most often results in a mixed dysarthria.

Index

Note: Page numbers in **bold** indicate non-text material.

A

ABA-2 (Apraxia Battery for Adults-Second Edition), 65–67
Abdominal binder (girdle), 141
Abducens nerve (cranial nerve VI), **21**
Abduction, 122, 353
Ablative procedures, 223, 225, 353
Abscess, bacterial, 196
Accessory nerve (cranial nerve XI), **21**, 101, 111, **112**
Acetylcholine, 25, 213, 353
Acoustic motor speech examination, **91–93**
Action tremors, 256–257, 353
Adduction, 61, 353
Affect, pseudobulbar, 156–157, 361
Afferent neurons, 24, 353
Affricate consonants, 221, 306
Akinesia, 212–213, 219, 353
Alphabet boards, 228, **229**
ALS. *See* Amyotrophic lateral sclerosis
Alternating motion rate (AMR), 69, 81, 353
  in apraxia of speech, 67, 82, 310
  in ataxic dysarthria, 200
  examination form, **92–93**
  in hyperkinetic dysarthria, 264
  in hypokinetic dysarthria, 223
  in spastic dysarthria, 159
  standardized tests, 67–68
  in unilateral upper motor neuron dysarthria, 178, 181
Alternative and augmentative communication procedures, 322
Alzheimer's disease, 216, 254
AMR. *See* Alternating motion rate
Amyotrophic lateral sclerosis (ALS), 11, **283**, 283–286
  augmentative communication for patients with, 290–292
  definition, 353
  familial, 283–284
  mixed dysarthria in, 276
  spastic dysarthria in, 151
  speech characteristics, **285**, 285–286
  sporadic, 284
  symptoms of, 284
Anatomy, 3, 353
Ancient Greece, 3–6
Aneurysms, 353
Anoxia
  cerebral, 152, 218, 355
  definition, 353
Anticholinergic drugs, 224–225

Aphasia
　Broca's, 305–306, 317
　case reports from ancient
　　Greece, 4–5
　case reports from the Middle
　　Ages and Renaissance, 7
　definition, 353
　differential diagnosis, 314–317
Aphonia, 222, 353
Apraxia(s)
　overview, 298–302
　definition, 2, 298, 353
　ideational, 298–299, 333, 353–354
　ideomotor, 299–300, 333, 354
　laryngeal, 309
　limb, 300
　nonverbal oral, 12–13, 82–83,
　　94, 300–301, 354
　standardized tests for, 65–68
Apraxia Battery for Adults-Second
　Edition (ABA-2), 65–67
Apraxia of speech, 13, 59, 295–334
　assessment of, 309–310
　case reports from the Middle
　　Ages and Renaissance, 7
　causes, 304–305, 333
　clinical characteristics, 311–312
　definition, 2, 296–297, 354
　diagnostic characteristics,
　　310–313
　diagnostic considerations,
　　313–318
　diagnostic guidelines, 312–313
　differential diagnosis, 310–318,
　　333
　neurologic basis, 302–304, **303**,
　　333
　overview, 301–302
　pure, 296
　speech characteristics, 305–309
　testing for, 83–84, **95–96**
　treatment of, 318–333
Apraxia of Speech Rating Scale
　(ASRS), 67–68
Arteriosclerotic parkinsonism, 218
Articulation, 62
　in apraxia of speech, 306–307
　in ataxic dysarthria, 197–198

in chorea, 251–252
definition, 354, 360
in dystonia, 262–263
evaluation of, 81–82
examination form, **92–93**
in flaccid dysarthria, 121
in hypokinetic dysarthria,
　220–221, 223
irregular breakdowns, 197–198,
　262–263, 358
overarticulation, 139–140, 163,
　206–207, 231–232
in spastic dysarthria, 153–154, 159
undershoot, 221
in unilateral upper motor
　neuron dysarthria, 170,
　177–179, 183–184
Articulation treatments, 161–164,
　205–207
　behavioral, 227–232
　traditional, 138–140, 162–164,
　　231–232
Articulators, 62, 354
Articulatory kinematic procedures
　for apraxia of speech, 321–322
　Darley, Aronson, and Brown's
　　procedure, 328–330
　Eight-Step Continuum, 321,
　　323–325
　PROMPT program, 323, 332
　Sound Production Treatment
　　(SPT), 321, 323, 325–328
ASRS (Apraxia of Speech Rating
　Scale), 67–68
Assessment of Intelligibility of
　Dysarthric Speech, 64
Association cortex, 28–32, 354
　four areas of, 30, **30**
Astrocytes, 24, 354
Astrocytoma, low-grade, 195–196,
　358
Ataxia, 37, 186, 354
　cerebellar. *See* Cerebellar ataxia
　Friedreich's. *See* Friedreich's
　　ataxia
Ataxic dysarthria, 11, 185–208
　causes, **60**, 192–196, 207
　definition, 186, 354

key evaluation tasks for, 200–201
neurologic basis, 186–191
speech characteristics, **60**, 196–200, **197**, 207
treatment of, 201–207
Ataxic speech, 13
Atrophy
multisystems, 281–283, 359
muscle, 124
Auditory-perceptual evaluations, 78–85
Augmentative communication
for apraxia of speech, 322
for patients with ALS, 290–292
Automatic responses, 328–329
Automatic speech, 307
Autosomal dominant cerebellar ataxia of late onset, 193, 354
Axon(s), 22, **23**, 24–25, 354

B

Bacterial abscess, 196
Basal ganglia, 32–35, **33, 34**, 354
control circuit, 213–215, **214**, 243, **244**
in hyperkinetic dysarthria, 246
in parkinsonism, 213–215, **214**
Behavioral treatments
for dystonia, 267–268
for Huntington's disease, 266–267
for hypernasality, 133–134, 166–167
for parkinsonism, 223, 226–239
for tic disorders, 268–270
Bernard of Gordon, 7
Bilateral damage, 149
Biofeedback, instrumental, 233–234
Bite blocks, 268
Blood–brain barrier, 224
Botulinum toxin (Botox), 257, 265–266
Bradykinesia, 211–212, 219, 354
Brain, **17**, 17–18, **18**, 27
landmarks of the cerebrum, **33**
landmarks on the lateral surface, **19**, 19–20

Brain tumors, 175–177
Brainstem, 18, **18**, 20–22, **21, 189**, 354
Brainstem stroke, 115–116
Breath holding, 135
Breathy voice quality, 354
in flaccid dysarthria, 122, 124
in hypokinetic dysarthria, 222
Broca's aphasia, 305–306, 317
Broca's area, **19**, 301, 303
Buccofacial apraxia, 300–301
Bulbar palsy, 13, 157
progressive, 119, 361

C

Case reports
from ancient Greece, 3–6
from the Middle Ages and Renaissance, 6–7
Caudate nucleus, 32, **33**, 213, 243, **244**, 354
CBIT (Comprehensive Behavioral Intervention for Tics), 270
Cell body, 22, **23**, 354
Central nervous system (CNS), 16–17, **17**, 27, 355
Central sulcus, **19**, 19–20, 355
Cerebellar ataxia, 192
autosomal dominant, of late onset, 193, 354
definition, 355
idiopathic sporadic late-onset, 193, 357
Cerebellar control circuits, 191, 355
Cerebellar dysarthria. *See* Ataxic dysarthria
Cerebellar peduncles, 187–189, **188, 189**, 355
Cerebellar speech, 13
Cerebellum, 18, **18**, 22, 32, 35–37, **36**, 187, **188**
definition, 355
neural pathways to/from, 187–191, **190**
and speech, 191–192
Cerebral anoxia, 152, 218

Cerebral cortex, 20, 355
Cerebral ventricles, 8, **9, 188**
Cerebrovascular accident (CVA), 115, 355
Cerebrum, **18**, 18–20, 27
   definition, 355
   landmarks of, **33**
Charcot, Jean-Martin, 11, **11**
Chorea
   causes of, 250
   characteristics of, 264
   definition, 355
   hemichorea, 249
   hyperkinetic dysarthria of, 247–254, **252**, 264, 270
   speech errors in, 250–254, **252**
   Sydenham's, 247
Chronic drug-induced dystonia, 355
Chunking utterances into syntactic units, 137, 165, 205, 239
Clonazepam, 265
CNS (central nervous system), 16–17, **17**, 27, 355
Cognitive-linguistic load, 127
Cogwheel resistance, 212
Collaterals, 22
Communication, augmentative
   for apraxia of speech, 322
   for patients with ALS, 290–292
Comprehensive Behavioral Intervention for Tics (CBIT), 270
Computerized Assessment of Intelligibility of Dysarthric Speech, 64
Confusion, language of, 7
Connected speech
   analysis of, 84–85
   examination form for, **96–97**
Consonant clusters, 306
Consonants
   affricate, 221, 306
   exaggerating, 139–140, 163, 182–183, 206–207, 231–232
   fricative, 220–221
   imprecise, 121, 159, 223, 251–252, 262–263
   stop, 220
   weak pressure, 120, 364
Continuous positive airway pressure (CPAP) activity, 132
Contrastive stress drills, 137, 165, 204, 238–239
Conversational speech, 69
   in apraxia of speech, 67, 310
   in ataxic dysarthria, 200–201
   average loudness, 234
   in flaccid dysarthria, 124
   in hyperkinetic dysarthria, 264
   in hypokinetic dysarthria, 223
   in spastic dysarthria, 159
   in unilateral upper motor neuron dysarthria, 181
Coronal section, 355
Cortex
   bilateral areas of, 28
   definition, 355
Corticobulbar tract, 41, **43**, 48, 355
Corticospinal tract, 25, 41, **42**, 48, 355
Cranial nerve II (optic nerve), **21**, 25, 360
Cranial nerve III (oculomotor nerve), **21**
Cranial nerve IV (trochlear nerve), **21**
Cranial nerve V. *See* Trigeminal nerve
Cranial nerve VI (abducens nerve), **21**
Cranial nerve VII. *See* Facial nerve
Cranial nerve VIII (vestibulocochlear nerve), **21**
Cranial nerve IX (glossopharyngeal nerve), **21**, 77, 101, 107, **108**
Cranial nerve X. *See* Vagus nerve
Cranial nerve XI (accessory nerve), **21**, 101, 111, **112**
Cranial nerve XII. *See* Hypoglossal nerve
Cranial nerves, 17, **17**, 47–48, **49**
   definition, 355
   nuclei, **21**, 22, 48, 355

of speech production, 101–113, 142
Creutzfeldt-Jakob's disease, 254
Cued reading material, 203–204
Cueing, 203–204
   articulatory placement, 327, 332
   for complete inhalation, 141–142, 237
CVA (cerebrovascular accident), 115, 355

D

Da Vigo, Giovanni, 8–9
Da Vinci, Leonardo, 8, **9**
DAF (delayed auditory feedback), 228–229
Darley, Aronson, and Brown's procedure, 328–330
Decomposition of movement, 197, 355
Decussation of the pyramids, 41, 355–356
Deep brain stimulation, 223, 225–226, 257, 266, 356
Degenerative diseases, 193–194, 304
Delayed auditory feedback (DAF), 228–229, 356
Dementia, 216, 218
Dendrites, 22, **23**, 356
Depression, 216
Descending motor tracts, 40–47
Differences, recognizing, 125
Diplophonia, 79–80, 124, 356
Diplopia (double vision), 279
Direct activation system, 41, 356
Dopamine, 25
   definition, 356
   reduction of, 33–34, 213–215, **214**, 217, 239, 245
Double vision (diplopia), 279
Drooling, 157
Drug-induced dystonia, 260
   chronic, 355
Dysarthria, 13
   case reports from ancient Greece, 5–6
   causes and characteristics, 59, **60**
   cerebellar. *See* Ataxic dysarthria
   definition, 2, 356
   differentiation from apraxia of speech, 317–318
   hyperkinetic. *See* Hyperkinetic dysarthria
   hypokinetic. *See* Hypokinetic dysarthria
   mixed. *See* Mixed dysarthria
   neuromuscular. *See* Flaccid dysarthria
   spastic. *See* Spastic dysarthria
   standardized tests for, 63–65
   unilateral upper motor neuron. *See* Unilateral upper motor neuron dysarthria
Dysarthria Impact Profile, 64–65
Dyskinesia, L-dopa-induced, 245–246
Dysphonia, spasmodic, 260–261, 265–266, 362–363
Dystonia
   behavioral treatment for, 267–268
   causes of, 259–261
   characteristics of, 265
   chronic drug-induced, 355
   definition, 356
   drug-induced, 260, 355
   focal, 258
   generalized, 258
   hemidystonia, 258
   hyperkinetic dysarthria of, 257–264, **262**, 265, 270
   multifocal, 258
   oromandibular, 259, 268
   primary, 259, 361
   segmental, 258
   speech errors in, 261–264, **262**
   tardive, 260, 363

E

Easy-onset phonation, 160, 268
Efferent neurons, 24, 356
Effortful closing techniques, 233

Eight-Step Continuum Treatment, 321, 323–325
  general rules for, 324–325
  principles that facilitate progression, 324
  summary steps, 325
Encephalitis, 217
Encephalopathy, punch drunk, 218, 361
Equal and excess stress, 198, 356
Essential (or organic) tremor, 256–257, 265–266, 356
Evaluation, 55–97
  auditory-perceptual, 78–85
  examination form, **87–97**
  key tasks for ataxic dysarthria, 200–201
  key tasks for flaccid dysarthria, 123–124
  key tasks for hyperkinetic dysarthria, 264–265
  key tasks for hypokinetic dysarthria, 223
  key tasks for spastic dysarthria, 158–159
  key tasks for unilateral upper motor neuron dysarthria, 181
  learning to evaluate, 127
  standardized tests for apraxia, 65–68
  standardized tests for dysarthria, 63–65
  stress testing, 69, 82, **93**
  testing for apraxia of speech, 83–84, **95–96**
  testing for nonverbal oral apraxia, 82–83, **94**
Exercise(s)
  for ataxic dysarthria, 204–206
  contrastive stress drills, 137, 165, 204, 238–239
  for flaccid dysarthria, 138–140
  for hypokinetic dysarthria, 230–232, 238
  intelligibility drills, 138–139, 162, 182, 205–206, 231
  jaw-stretching tasks, 230–231
  lip-stretching tasks, 162, 230
  minimal contrast drills, 140, 163–164, 183, 207, 232
  nonspeech, 132
  optimal breath group, 238
  for phonation deficits, 160
  phonemic drills, 329–330
  pitch range, 136–137, 164, 204–205
  for spastic dysarthria, 162–164
  stress and intonation, 204–205
  stretching tasks, 230–231
  tongue-stretching tasks, 161–162, 230
  for unilateral upper motor neuron dysarthria, 182–183
  velar strengthening, 132
  yawn-sigh, 160
Exhalation
  slow and controlled, 201, 237
  speaking immediately on, 141, 201–202, 237
Expiratory board, 141
Exposure response prevention, 270
Extrapyramidal system, 40–41, 44–47, **45, 46**
  definition, 356
  in spastic dysarthria, 148

F

Facial apraxia, 300–301
Facial muscle evaluation, 72–74, **88**
Facial nerve (cranial neve VII), 101, 103–107
  assessment of, 72–73
  branches, 103–105, **105**
  root, **21**
  treatment for damage to, 138–142
  upper motor neuron innervation of, 105–107, **106**
Familial amyotrophic lateral sclerosis, 283–284
Familial tremor, 256
Fasciculations, 75, 356

Fat injection, 130
Feedback
  instrumental biofeedback, 233–234
  visual, 166
Final common pathway, 101, 356
Finger or hand tapping, 203, 228
Flaccid dysarthria, 48, 99–143
  causes, **60**, 114–119, 142
  definition, 100–101, 356
  differential diagnosis, 157–158
  key evaluation tasks, 123–124
  neurologic basis, 101–114
  recommended textbooks, 128
  respiratory weakness in, 140–142
  vs spastic dysarthria, 157–158
  speech characteristics, **60**, 119–123, **120**, 124, 142
  treatment of, 128–142
Frenchay Dysarthria Assessment-2, 63
Fricative consonants, 220–221, 306
Friedreich's ataxia, 193–194, 288, 356
Frontal association area, 30, **30**, 31, 357
Frontal lobe, 18, **19**, 357

G

Gag reflex, 77, 124
Galen, 8
Ganglion, 48, 357
Geste antagoniste, 258–259
Gilles de la Tourette's syndrome, 255–256, 266, 269–270, 357
Glial cells, 24, 357
Globus pallidus, 32, **33**, 213, **244**, 357
Glossopharyngeal nerve (cranial nerve IX), **21**, 77, 101, 107, **108**
Glottal stop, 78, 357
Glottis, 357
Goal setting, 126
Gray matter, 20, **33**, 357

Guillain-Barré syndrome, 117–118, **118**, 276, 357
Gyrus, 18, 357

H

Habit reversal training, 269
Haloperidol, 265
Hand or finger tapping, 203, 228
Hard glottal attack, 135, 233
Harsh vocal quality, 357
  in ataxic dysarthria, 199–200
  in hypokinetic dysarthria, 222
  in spastic dysarthria, 154
  in unilateral upper motor neuron dysarthria, 179–181
Head and neck relaxation, 160
Head injury, traumatic
  in ataxic dysarthria, 195
  in hypokinetic dysarthria, 217–218
  in spastic dysarthria, 151
  traumatic brain injury (TBI), 134, 177
  in unilateral upper motor neuron dysarthria, 177
Head turning, 135–136
Hemangioblastomas, 196, 357
Hemiballism, 249, 357
Hemichorea, 249
Hemidystonia, 258
Hemifacial spasm, 254, 357
Hippocrates, 4, **4**, 357
Hippocratic Corpus, 3–6, 357
Historical review, 1–13
Holding breath, 135
Huntington's chorea, 34–35
Huntington's disease, 33–35, 248–249
  behavioral treatment for, 266–267
  mixed dysarthria in, 276
Hyaluronic acid, 130, 166
Hyperkinetic disorders, 34–35, 357
Hyperkinetic dysarthria, 35, 241–271
  causes, **60**, 246–264, 270
  of chorea, 247–254, **252**, 264, 270

Hyperkinetic dysarthria *(continued)*
  definition, 242–243, 357
  of dystonia, 257–264, **262**, 265, 270
  key evaluation tasks for, 264–265
  of myoclonus, 254–255, 264
  neurologic basis, 243–246
  speech characteristics, **60**, 250–254, **252**, 261–264, **262**, 270
  treatment of, 265–271
Hyperkinetic movements, 245–246
Hypernasality
  in apraxia of speech, 308
  in ataxic dysarthria, 199
  in chorea, 253
  definition, 357
  in dystonia, 263–264
  in flaccid dysarthria, 120
  in hypokinetic dysarthria, 222–223
  mild, 133–134, 166–167
  in spastic dysarthria, 155, 159, 165
  treatment of, 130–134, 165–167
Hyperreflexes, 124
Hypoglossal nerve (cranial nerve XII), 101–102, 111–113, **113**
  assessment, 74–75
  root, **21**
  treatment of damage to, 138–142
Hypokinetic dysarthria, 34, 209–240
  causes, **60**, 215–218, 239
  definition, 210, 357
  key evaluation tasks for, 223
  neurologic basis, 210–215
  speech characteristics, **60**, 218–223, **219**, 239
  treatment of, 223–240
Hyponasality, 253, 308
Hypothyroidism, 195
Hypotonia, 199

I

Ideational apraxia, 298–299, 333, 353–354
Ideomotor apraxia, 299–300, 333, 354
Idiopathic Parkinson's disease, 215–216, 239
Idiopathic sporadic late-onset cerebellar ataxia, 193, 357
Indirect activation system, 44, 357
Infections, 196
Inferior peduncle, 187–189, **188, 189, 190,** 357
Inhalation, cueing for, 141–142, 237
Inhalatory stridor, 78, 124, 357
Initiating speech activities, 328
Innervation, 41–42, 357
Innervation ratio, 53, 357
Instrumental analysis, 56–57, 357
Instrumental biofeedback, 233–234
Intelligibility drills
  for ataxic dysarthria, 205–206
  for flaccid dysarthria, 138–139
  for hypokinetic dysarthria, 231
  for spastic dysarthria, 162
  for unilateral upper motor neuron dysarthria, 182
Intelligible speech, 291
Intention tremors, 37, 357
Internal capsule, 41, **176**, 358
Interneurons, 24, 358
Intersystemic facilitation and reorganization treatment, 322
Intonation, 62, 358
Intonation exercises, 204–205
Intonation profiles, 137, 164–165, 205, 238
Irregular articulatory breakdowns, 197–198, 262–263, 358

J

Jaw muscles, 72–74
Jaw-stretching tasks, 230–231

L

L-dopa, 216, 223, 224, 358
L-dopa-induced dyskinesia, 245–246

Lanfranc, 7
Language of confusion, 7
Laryngeal apraxia, 309
Laryngeal function, 77–78, **90**
Larynx, sideways pressure on, 135–136
Lateral sulcus, 19, **19**, 358
Lead pipe resistance, 212
Lee Silverman Voice Treatment (LSVT), 134, 223, 358
Lee Silverman Voice Treatment-LOUD (LSVT LOUD), 234–236
Limb apraxia, 65–66, 300, 354
Limbic system, 27, 358
Lingual apraxia, 300–301
Lip-stretching tasks, 162, 230
Listening, 127
Literal paraphasias, 315–316
Lobe(s), 358
The LOUD Crowd, 235–236
Loudness. *See also* Monoloudness
   average, 234
   decreased, 222–223
   increasing, 167
Loudness displays, 234
Low-grade astrocytoma, 195–196, 358
Low pitch
   in hypokinetic dysarthria, 223
   in spastic dysarthria, 154–155
Lower motor neurons, 48, **49, 52**, 101, 358
LSVT (Lee Silverman Voice Treatment), 134, 223, 358
LSVT LOUD (Lee Silverman Voice Treatment-LOUD), 234–236

M

Mandible, 359
Mandibular musculature evaluation, **88–89**
Manganese poisoning, 218
Masked facies, 211
Massa, Niccolo, 7
Mayo Clinic, 146
Medical history, 71–72, **87**
Medical records, 71, 181

Medulla, 20, **21, 189**, 359
Medulla oblongata, **18**
Meige syndrome, 260
Melodic intonation therapy (MIT), 323, 330–332
Meninges, 8–9, 359
Metastatic tumors, 195, 359
Metronomes, 203, 229
Microglia, 24, 359
Midbrain, **18**, 20, **21**, 359
Middle Ages, 6–7
Middle peduncle, **188, 189**, 189–190, **190**, 359
Minimal contrast drills
   for ataxic dysarthria, 207
   for flaccid dysarthria, 140
   for hypokinetic dysarthria, 232
   for spastic dysarthria, 163–164
   for unilateral upper motor neuron dysarthria, 183
MIT (melodic intonation therapy), 323, 330–332
Mixed dysarthria, 11, 273–293
   of amyotrophic lateral sclerosis, 283–286, **285**, 292
   causes, **60**, 277–288, 292
   definition, 274
   of Friedreich's ataxia, 288
   of multiple sclerosis, 277–281, **280**, 292
   neurologic basis, 274–277
   of olivopontocerebellar atrophy, 283
   of progressive supranuclear palsy, 282
   in Shy-Drager syndrome, 281
   speech characteristics, **60**, 275
   treatment of, 288–292
   of Wilson's disease, 286–288, **287**
Monoloudness, 359
   in ataxic dysarthria, 199
   in dystonia, 263
   in flaccid dysarthria, 123
   in hypokinetic dysarthria, 223
   in spastic dysarthria, 155, 159
Monopitch, 359
   in ataxic dysarthria, 199
   in dystonia, 263

Monopitch *(continued)*
   in flaccid dysarthria, 123
   in hypokinetic dysarthria, 223
   in spastic dysarthria, 155, 159
Motor neurons, 24, 359
Motor speech disorders. *See also specific disorders*
   with intelligible speech, 291
   recommended textbooks, 128
   treatment of, 124–127
Motor speech evaluation, 68–70
   auditory-perceptual, 78–85
   examination form, **87–97**
   goals, 57–58
   instructions for, 70–78
   questions to ask during, 58
   standardized tests for apraxia, 65–68
   standardized tests for dysarthria, 63–65
   stress testing, 82
Motor speech programmer, 302–304, 333, 359
Motor steadiness, 70
Motor strip, **19**, 20, 359
Motor system, 2, 15–54, 359
   components of, 16–27
   structure and function of, 27–53, **28**
Motor system disorders, 2
   evaluation of, 55–97
   historical review, 1–13
Multiple sclerosis (MS), 11, 151–152, 277–281, **278**, 292
   course, 279
   speech characteristics, **280**, 280–281
Multisystems atrophy, 281–283, 359
Muscle atrophy, 124
Muscle strength, 68–69
Muscle tone, 70
Muscles, face and jaw, 72–74
Muscular dystrophy, 119, 359
Myasthenia gravis, 116–117, 359
   causes, 116, **116**
   screening for, 82, **93**, 124
Myelin, 22–23, 359

Myoclonus
   hyperkinetic dysarthria of, 254–255, 264
   palatopharyngolaryngeal, 254–255, 360

N

Nasal emissions, 120, 359
Neologistic jargon, 7
Nerves, 24–25, 359
Nervous system cells, 22–26
Neural tracts, 24–25, 359
Neuroleptic-induced parkinsonism, 216–217
Neurology, 359
Neuromuscular dysarthria. *See* Flaccid dysarthria
Neuromuscular junction(s), 50–53, **52**, 359–360
Neurons, 22, **23**, 27, 360
   lower motor. *See* Lower motor neurons
   types of, 23–24
   upper motor. *See* Upper motor neurons
Neurotransmitters, 25, **26**, 360
19th century, 9–13
Nonverbal oral apraxia, 12–13, 300–301
   definition, 354
   testing for, 82–83, **94**

O

Occipital association area, 30, **30**
Occipital lobe, 18, **19**, 360
Oculomotor nerve (cranial nerve III), **21**
Oligodendroglia, 24, 360
Olivopontocerebellar atrophy, 282–283
Olivopontocerebellar degeneration, 360
Optic nerve (cranial nerve II), **21**, 25, 360
Optimal breath group, 202, 238

Oral apraxia
  nonverbal. *See* Nonverbal oral apraxia
  standardized tests for, 65–66
Oral reflexes, diminished or absent, 124
Organic (essential) tremor, 256–257
Orofacial apraxia, 300–301
Oromandibular dystonia, 259, 268
Overarticulation, 360
  for ataxic dysarthria, 206–207
  for flaccid dysarthria, 139–140
  for spastic dysarthria, 163

P

Pacing boards, **227**, 227–228, 360
Palatal augmentation prosthesis, 131–132
Palatal lift, 131, 166, 360
Palatopharyngolaryngeal myoclonus, 254–255, 360
Palilalia, 221, 360
Palsy
  bulbar, 13, 157
  definition, 360
  progressive bulbar, 119, 361
  pseudobulbar, 157
Parietal association area, **30**, 30–31, 360
Parietal lobe, 18, **19**, 360
Parkinson, James, **10**, 10–11
Parkinsonism, 210, 215
  arteriosclerotic, 218
  causes of, 213–215, **214**, 245
  characteristics of, 211–213
  definition, 360
  neuroleptic-induced, 216–217
  pharmacologic treatments for, 224–225
  postencephalitic, 217
  surgical treatments for, 225–226
  symptoms of, 239
  vascular, 218
Parkinson's disease, 11, 33, 277
  causes of, 213, **214**
  characteristics of, 213, 221–223

  idiopathic, 215–216, 239
  LSVT LOUD for, 234
  progression, 117
Parkinson's syndrome, 215
Paulus Aegineta, 6–7
Perceptual analysis, 360
Peripheral nervous system (PNS), 17, **17**, 27, 360
Perisylvian area, **303**, 303–304, 360
Pharmacologic treatments
  for hyperkinetic dysarthria, 265–266
  for hypokinetic dysarthria, 223
  for parkinsonism, 224–225
Pharyngeal flap procedure, 130, 166, 360
Pharyngeal wall augmentation, posterior, 130, 361
Pharynx, 76–77
Phonation, 61, 360
  in apraxia of speech, 308–309
  in ataxic dysarthria, 199
  in chorea, 252–253
  in dystonia, 263
  early stop, 202, 237–238
  easy-onset, 160, 268
  evaluation of, 81–82
  in flaccid dysarthria, 121–122
  in hypokinetic dysarthria, 221–222
  in spastic dysarthria, 154–155, 159
  in unilateral upper motor neuron dysarthria, 179–180
Phonation treatments, 134–136, 159–160, 232–236
Phonatory incompetence, 121–122, 360
Phonatory-respiratory system
  assessment of, 79–80
  examination form, **91**, **92–93**
Phonemes
  prolonged, 198–199, 251–252, 262–263
  prolonged intervals between, 198–199
  repeated, 221, 223
  substitutions, 306

Phonemic drills, 329–330
Phonetic placement
  for ataxic dysarthria, 206
  for flaccid dysarthria, 139
  for hypokinetic dysarthria, 231
  for spastic dysarthria, 162–163
  for unilateral upper motor neuron dysarthria, 182
Physical trauma, 114–115
Physiology, 3, 361
Pitch. *See also* Monopitch
  low, 154–155, 223
Pitch range exercises, 136–137, 164, 204–205
PNS. *See* Peripheral nervous system
Poisoning, toxic metal, 218
Polio, 119, 361
Pons, **18**, 20, **21, 188, 189**, 361
Postcentral gyrus, **19**, 20, 361
Postencephalitic parkinsonism, 217
Posterior pharyngeal wall augmentation, 130, 361
Postural reflexes, 213, 361
Posture, 140–141
Precentral gyrus (primary motor cortex), **19**, 20, **29**, 30, 37–39, **39**, 361
Premotor area, 39, **40**, 361
Primary auditory cortex, 29, **29**, 361
Primary cortex, 29, **29**, 361
Primary dystonia, 361
Primary motor cortex (precentral gyrus), **19**, 20, **29**, 30, 37–39, **39**, 361
Primary sensory cortex, 20, 29, **29**, 361
Primary visual cortex, **19**, 29, **29**, 361
Progressive bulbar palsy, 119, 361
PROMPT program, 323, 332
Prosodic treatments, 136–138, 164–165, 202–205, 238–239
Prosody, 62–63, 361
  in apraxia of speech, 307–308
  in ataxic dysarthria, 198–199
  in chorea, 251
  in dystonia, 263
  in flaccid dysarthria, 123
  in hypokinetic dysarthria, 219–220, 223
  in spastic dysarthria, 155–156, 159
  treatment of problems with, 202–205
  in unilateral upper motor neuron dysarthria, 180–181
Prosthetic treatments
  characteristics of best candidates, 131
  compensatory devices, 141
  for oromandibular dystonia, 268
  palatal augmentation, 131–132
  for velopharyngeal incompetence, 130–132
Pseudobulbar affect, 156–157, 361
Pseudobulbar palsy, 157
Punch drunk encephalopathy, 218, 361
Pushing and pulling procedures, 233
Putamen, 32, **33**, 213, 243, **244**, 362
Pyramidal decussation, 41, 355–356
Pyramidal system, 38, 40–44, **42, 43,** 362

R

Range of movement, 69, 362
Rate and rhythm procedures
  for apraxia of speech, 321–322
  melodic intonation therapy (MIT), 323, 330–332
Reactive speech, 307
Reading material, cued, 203–204
Reason, localization of, 7–9, **9**
Reciting syllables to a metronome, 203, 229
Reflex(es), 362
  diminished or absent, 124
  gag, 77, 124

hyperreflexes, 124
oral, 124
postural, 213, 361
Relaxation, head and neck, 160
Relaxation therapy, 269–270, 322
Renaissance, 6–7
Repeated phonemes, 221
Repeating words, 67, 310
Resonance, 61–62, 362
　in apraxia of speech, 308
　in ataxic dysarthria, 199
　in chorea, 253
　in dystonia, 263–264
　in flaccid dysarthria, 120–121
　in hypokinetic dysarthria, 222–223
　in spastic dysarthria, 155, 159
　treatment for, 130, 165
　in unilateral upper motor neuron dysarthria, 180
Resonation system
　evaluation of, 80–82
　examination form, **92–93**
Respiration, 59–61, 362
　evaluation of, 81–82
　examination form, **92–93**
　optimal breath group, 202, 238
Respiratory problems
　in apraxia of speech, 308
　in ataxic dysarthria, 200
　in chorea, 253
　compensatory prosthetic devices for, 141
　in dystonia, 263
　in flaccid dysarthria, 122
　in hypokinetic dysarthria, 222
　in spastic dysarthria, 156
　tasks for gaining better control during speech, 201–202
　treatment of, 140–142, 236–238
　in unilateral upper motor neuron dysarthria, 180–181
Respiratory system
　assessment of, 79–80
　examination form, **91**
Resting tremor, 211, 362
Reticular formation, 44, 362

Reticulospinal tract, 44–47, **46**, 48, 362
Rigidity, 34, 212, 362
Role playing, 325
Rubrospinal tract, 44, **45**, 48, 362

S

Saint Vitus's dance, 247
Scanning speech, 13, 196, 362
Schwann cells, 24, 362
See-Scape, 131
Self-correction, 127
Sensory neurons, 24, 362
Sensory strip, 20, 362
Sensory tricks, 258–259, 267, 362
Sentence repetition, 67
Sequential motion rate (SMR), 69, 362
　in apraxia of speech, 67, 82, 310
　examination form, **93**
　standardized tests, 67–68
Shaking palsy, 9–11, **10**
Short phrasing, 155–156, 159
Shy-Drager syndrome, 281
Silences, inappropriate, 223, 263, 308
SMR. *See* Sequential motion rate
Sound pressure level meters, 233–234
Sound Production Treatment (SPT), 321, 323, 325–328
Spasm, hemifacial, 254, 357
Spasmodic dysphonia, 260–261, 265–266, 362–363
Spasmodic torticollis, 259–260, 363
Spastic dysarthria, 48, 145–168
　causes, **60**, 146, **147**, 150–152, **172**
　definition, 146, 363
　differential diagnosis, 157–158
　vs flaccid dysarthria, 157–158
　key evaluation tasks, 158–159
　neurologic basis, 146–149, **147**, 171, **172**
　speech characteristics, **60**, 152–157, **153**, 167
　treatment of, 159–168

Spasticity, 149, 212, 363
SPEAK OUT!, 235–236
Speech
  automatic, 307
  cerebellum and, 191–192
  connected, 84–85, **96–97**
  conversational. *See*
    Conversational speech
  immediately on exhalation, 141,
    201–202, 237
  intelligible, 291
  modification of, 133–134
  reactive, 307
  voluntary, 307
Speech Intelligibility Test for
  Windows, 64
Speech production
  components and disorders,
    58–63
  cranial nerves of, 101–113,
    142
  errors in amyotrophic lateral
    sclerosis, **285**, 285–286
  errors in ataxic dysarthria, 197,
    197
  errors in flaccid dysarthria, 120,
    120
  errors in hyperkinetic
    dysarthria, 251, **252**
  errors in hypokinetic dysarthria,
    219, **219**
  errors in multiple sclerosis, **280**,
    280–281
  errors in spastic dysarthria,
    152–153, **153**
  errors in unilateral upper
    motor neuron dysarthria,
    177, **178**
Speech rate
  control procedures, 203–204,
    227–229
  rate and rhythm procedures,
    321–322
  reducing, 167, 227–229
  slow or irregular, 156, 199
  tasks for increasing awareness
    of, 203–204

Speech stress test, 124
Speed of movement, 69
Spinal cord, **18**
Spinal nerves, 17, **17**, 47–48, **50**,
    51–52, 113–114
  definition, 363
  nuclei, 48–50
SPT (Sound Production Treatment),
    321, 323, 325–328
Standardized tests
  for apraxia, 65–68
  for dysarthria, 63–65
Stem-cell implantation, 226
Stop consonants, 220
Strained-strangled vocal quality,
    154, 363
Stress, 62, 363
  equal and excess, 198
  reduced, 159, 223
Stress and intonation exercises,
    204–205
  contrastive stress drills, 137,
    165, 204, 238–239
Stress testing, 69, 82, **93**
Stretching tasks
  for hypokinetic dysarthria,
    230–231
  lip-stretching exercises, 162
  for spastic dysarthria, 161–162
  tongue-stretching tasks, 161–
    162, 230
Striatum, 32, 243, 246, 363
Stridor, inhalatory, 78, 124, 357
Stroke(s)
  in apraxia of speech, 304
  brainstem, 115–116
  in hyperkinetic dysarthria, 249
  in hypokinetic dysarthria, 218
  in spastic dysarthria, 150–151
  in unilateral upper motor
    neuron dysarthria, 174–175,
    176
Substantia nigra, 34, **34**
  definition, 363
  in Parkinson's disease, 213,
    214
Substitutions, 306

Sulcus, 18, 363
Superior peduncle, **188, 189**, 190, **190**, 363
Supplementary motor area, 39, **40**, 363
Surgical treatments
　for parkinsonism, 223, 225–226
　for vagus nerve damage, 130–132
Sydenham's chorea, 247
Syllables
　blurring of, 223
　reciting to metronome, 203, 229
Synaptic clefts, 25, **26**, 363
Syntactic units, chunking utterances into, 137, 165, 205, 239

T

Talking therapeutically, 126–127
Tapping, finger or hand, 203, 228
Tardive dyskinesia, 249–250, 363
Tardive dystonia, 260, 363
TBI (traumatic brain injury), 134, 177
Tectospinal tract, 44, 47–48
Teflon paste, 130, 166
Temporal association area, 30, **30**, 31, 363
Temporal lobe, 18, 363
Tensilon, 117
Terminal boutons, 22, 363–364
Terminal ramifications, 22, 364
Testing
　for apraxia of speech, 83–84, **95–96**
　for nonverbal oral apraxia, 82–83, **94**
　standardized tests for apraxia, 65–68
　standardized tests for dysarthria, 63–65
　stress, 69, 82, **93**
Tetrabenazine, 265
Thalamus, **18, 33**, 37, **38, 188**, 364

Therapeutic talk, 126–127
Tic(s), 255, 364
Tic disorders, 255–256
　behavioral treatment of, 268–270
　characteristics of, 265
Tongue muscles
　evaluation of, 74–76
　examination form, **89–90**
　extrinsic, 111, **113**
　innervation of, 111, **113**
　intrinsic, 111, **113**
Tongue-stretching tasks, 161–162, 230
Torticollis, spasmodic, 259–260, 363
Tourette's syndrome, 255–256, 266, 269–270, 357
Toxic metal poisoning, 218
Tracts, 364
Trauma, 304
Traumatic brain injury (TBI), 134, 177
Traumatic head injury, 151, 195, 217–218
Treatment, 124–128
Tremor(s), 34, 364
　action, 256–257
　essential (or organic), 256–257, 265–266, 356
　familial, 256
　intention, 37, 357
　resting, 211, 362
　voice, 364
Trifluoperazine, 217
Trigeminal nerve (cranial nerve V), 101, 103
　assessment of, 72–74
　branches, 103, **104**
　root, **21**
　treatment for damage to, 129
Trochlear nerve (cranial nerve IV), **21**
Tumor(s), 364
　in apraxia of speech, 304–305
　in ataxic dysarthria, 195–196
　in flaccid dysarthria, 119

Tumor(s) *(continued)*
  metastatic, 195, 359
  in unilateral upper motor neuron dysarthria, 175–177

U

Unilateral upper motor neuron dysarthria, 12, 43, 169–184
  causes, **60**, 174–177, 183
  definition, 170, 364
  key evaluation tasks, 181
  neurologic basis, 171–174, **173, 175**
  speech characteristics, **60**, 170, 177–181, **178**, 183–184
  treatment of, 181–184
Upper motor neurons, 48
  bilateral damage, 171, **172**
  definition, 364
  facial nerve, 105–107, **106**
  in spastic dysarthria, 147–149
  unilateral damage, 171–174, **173**
Utterances, chunking into syntactic units, 137, 165, 205, 239

V

Vagus nerve (cranial nerve X), 101–102, 107–111
  assessment of, 76–77
  external superior laryngeal nerve branch, **109**, 110
  pharyngeal branch, 108–110, **109**
  recurrent nerve branch, **109**, 110–111
  root, **21**
  treatment for damage to, 129–138
Valproic acid, 265
Vascular parkinsonism, 218
Vegetative movements, 83
Velar hypertonicity, 166
Velar strengthening exercises, 132
Velopharyngeal function, 80–81, **90**
Velopharyngeal incompetence, 130–132, 364
Velum, 76–77
Ventricles, cerebral, 8, **9, 188**
Vermis, **188**, 192, 364
Vesalius, 8
Vestibulocochlear nerve (cranial nerve VIII), **21**
Vestibulospinal tract, 44, 47–48
Viral encephalitis, postencephalitic parkinsonism, 217
Viral infections, 196
Visual association area, 31–32, 364
Visual feedback, 166
Vital capacity, 122–123, 364
Vitamin B12 deficiency, 195
Vitamin E deficiency, 195
Vocal quality
  in ataxic dysarthria, 199–200
  breathy, 122, 124, 222, 354
  in flaccid dysarthria, 122, 124
  harsh, 154, 179–181, 199–200, 222, 252–253, 357
  in hyperkinetic dysarthria, 252–253
  in hypokinetic dysarthria, 222–223
  in Parkinson's disease, 221–222
  in spastic dysarthria, 154
  strained-strangled, 154, 363
  in unilateral upper motor neuron dysarthria, 179–181
Vocal tics, 255
Voice amplifiers, 233
Voice stoppage, 253, 364
Voice tremor, 199, 364
Voluntary movement, 27–28
Voluntary speech, 307
Vowels
  distorted, 251–252, 262–263
  prolonged, 67, 124, 159, 181, 223, 264

W

Weak pressure consonants, 120, 364
Wernicke, Carl, **12**, 12–13
Wernicke's area, **19**, 303, 315
Whispering, 222
White matter, 20, **33**, 364
Willingness to change, 126
Wilson's disease, 195, 286–288, **287**, 364
Word repetition, 67

Y

Yawn-sigh exercises, 160